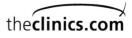

CHILD AND ADOLESCENT PSYCHIATRIC CLINICS OF NORTH AMERICA

Psychopharmacology

GUEST EDITORS
Andrés Martin, MD, MPH, and
Jeff Q. Bostic, MD, EdD

CONSULTING EDITOR
Melvin Lewis, MBBS, FRCPsych, DCH

CONSULTING EDITOR (ACTING)
Andrés Martin, MD, MPH

January 2006 • Volume 15 • Number 1

SAUNDERS

An Imprint of Elsevier, Inc.
PHILADELPHIA   LONDON   TORONTO   MONTREAL   SYDNEY   TOKYO

W.B. SAUNDERS COMPANY
A Division of Elsevier Inc.

Elsevier, Inc. • 1600 John F. Kennedy Boulevard • Suite 1800 • Philadelphia, Pennsylvania 19103-2899

http://www.childpsych.theclinics.com

**CHILD AND ADOLESCENT PSYCHIATRIC CLINICS
OF NORTH AMERICA** Volume 15, Number 1
January 2006 ISSN 1056-4993
Editor: Sarah E. Barth ISBN 1-4160-3382-3

Reprints: For copies of 100 or more, of articles in this publication, please contact the Commercial Reprints Department, Elsevier Inc., 360 Park Avenue South, New York, New York 10010-1710. Tel. (212) 633-3813 Fax: (212) 462-1935 email: reprints@elsevier.com

The ideas and opinions expressed in *Child and Adolescent Psychiatric Clinics of North America* do not necessarily reflect those of the Publisher. The Publisher does not assume any responsibility for any injury and/or damage to persons or property arising out of or related to any use of the material contained in this periodical. The reader is advised to check the appropriate medical literature and the product information currently provided by the manufacturer of each drug to be administered to verify the dosage, the method and duration of administration, or contraindications. It is the responsibility of the treating physician or other health care professional, relying on independent experience and knowledge of the patient, to determine drug dosages and the best treatment for the patient. Mention of any product in this issue should not be construed as endorsement by the contributors, editors, or the Publisher of the product or manufacturers' claims.

Child and Adolescent Psychiatric Clinics of North America (ISSN 1056-4993) is published quarterly by W.B. Saunders Company. Corporate and editorial offices: Elsevier, Inc., 1600 John F. Kennedy Boulevard, Suite 1800, Philadelphia, PA 19103-2899. Accounting and circulation offices: 6277 Sea Harbor Drive, Orlando, FL 32887-4800. Periodicals postage paid at Orlando, FL 32862, and additional mailing offices. Subscription prices are $185.00 per year (US individuals), $95.00 per year (US students), $280.00 per year (US institutions), $210.00 per year (Canadian individuals), $115.00 per year (Canadian and foreign students), $330.00 per year (Canadian and foreign institutions), and $235.00 per year (foreign individuals). Foreign air speed delivery is included in all *Clinics* subscription prices. All prices are subject to change without notice. POSTMASTER: Send address changes to *Child and Adolescent Psychiatric Clinics of North America*, W.B. Saunders Company, Periodicals Fulfillment, Orlando, FL 32887-4800. **Customer Service: 1-800-654-2452 (US). From outside the US, call 1-407-345-4000. E-mail:** hhspcs@harcourt.com.

Child and Adolescent Psychiatric Clinics of North America is covered in *Index Medicus, ISI, SSCI, Research Alert, Social Search, Current Contents,* and *EMBASE/Excerpta Medica.*

Printed in the United States of America.

CONSULTING EDITOR

MELVIN LEWIS, MBBS, FRCPsych, DCH, Professor Emeritus, Senior Research Scientist, Yale Child Study Center, Yale University School of Medicine, New Haven, Connecticut

CONSULTING EDITOR (ACTING)

ANDRÉS MARTIN, MD, MPH, Associate Professor of Child Psychiatry and Psychiatry, Yale Child Study Center, Yale University School of Medicine; and Medical Director, Children's Psychiatric Inpatient Service, Yale-New Haven Children's Hospital, New Haven, Connecticut

GUEST EDITORS

JEFF Q. BOSTIC, MD, EdD, Assistant Clinical Professor of Psychiatry, Harvard Medical School, Massachusetts General Hospital, Boston, Massachusetts

ANDRÉS MARTIN, MD, MPH, Associate Professor of Child Psychiatry and Psychiatry, Yale Child Study Center, Yale University School of Medicine; and Medical Director, Children's Psychiatric Inpatient Service, Yale-New Haven Children's Hospital, New Haven, Connecticut

CONTRIBUTORS

GUY BEAUZILE, MD, Chief Unit Psychiatrist, Sagamore Children's Psychiatric Center, Dix Hills, New York

AMY L. BECKER, MD, Child and Adolescent Psychiatry Fellow, Yale University School of Medicine, Child Study Center, New Haven, Connecticut

JEFF Q. BOSTIC, MD, EdD, Assistant Clinical Professor of Psychiatry, Harvard Medical School, Massachusetts General Hospital, Boston, Massachusetts

MAREN CARBON, MD, North Shore University Hospital, North Shore—Long Island Jewish Health System, Manhasset, New York

CHRISTOPH U. CORRELL, MD, The Zucker Hillside Hospital, North Shore—Long Island Jewish Health System, Glen Oaks, New York

MELISSA P. DELBELLO, MD, Associate Professor of Psychiatry and Pediatrics, Departments of Psychiatry and Pediatrics, University of Cincinnati Medical Center and Cincinnati Children's Hospital Medical Center, Cincinnati, Ohio

KEITH DITKOWSKY, MD, Chief Unit Psychiatrist, Division of Child and Adolescent Psychiatry, Schneider Children's Hospital, North Shore—Long Island Jewish Health System, New Hyde Park, New York

C. NEILL EPPERSON, MD, Director, Yale Behavioral Gynecology Program; and Associate Professor of Psychiatry and Obstetrics and Gynecology, Yale University School of Medicine, New Haven, Connecticut

GINNY GERBINO-ROSEN, MD, Chief, Older Adolescent Inpatient Service, Bronx Children's Psychiatric Center; and Associate Clinical Professor of Psychiatry, Department of Psychiatry, Albert Einstein College of Medicine, Bronx, New York

INIKA N. HENDERSON, PsyD, Associate Psychologist, Bronx Children's Psychiatric Center, Bronx, New York

TARIQ JAVED, MD, The Zucker Hillside Hospital, North Shore—Long Island Jewish Health System, Glen Oaks, New York

SHASHANK V. JOSHI, MD, Director of Training in Child and Adolescent Psychiatry, Stanford University School of Medicine, Stanford, California

HANA M. KESTER, BA, Research Coordinator, Department of Psychiatry Research, Zucker Hillside Hospital, North Shore—Long Island Jewish Health System, Glen Oaks, New York

BRYAN H. KING, MD, Professor; Vice Chair of Psychiatry and Behavioral Sciences; and Director of Child and Adolescent Psychiatry, Children's Hospital and Regional Medical Center, University of Washington, Seattle, Washington

ROBERT A. KOWATCH, MD, Professor of Psychiatry and Pediatrics, Departments of Psychiatry and Pediatrics, University of Cincinnati Medical Center and Cincinnati Children's Hospital Medical Center, Cincinnati, Ohio

HARVEY N. KRANZLER, MD, Clinical Professor of Psychiatry, Department of Psychiatry, Albert Einstein College of Medicine; and Clinical Director, Bronx Children's Psychiatric Center, Bronx, New York

SANJIV KUMRA, MD, Assistant Professor of Psychiatry, Department of Psychiatry, Albert Einstein College of Medicine, Bronx; and Research Psychiatrist, Department of Psychiatry Research, Zucker Hillside Hospital, North Shore—Long Island Jewish Health System, Glen Oaks, New York

ANIL K. MALHOTRA, MD, The Zucker Hillside Hospital, North Shore—Long Island Jewish Health System, Glen Oaks; and Albert Einstein College of Medicine, Bronx, New York

ANDRÉS MARTIN, MD, MPH, Associate Professor of Child Psychiatry and Psychiatry, Yale Child Study Center, Yale University School of Medicine; and Medical Director, Children's Psychiatric Inpatient Service, Yale-New Haven Children's Hospital, New Haven, Connecticut

TAHIR MUGHAL, MD, The Zucker Hillside Hospital, North Shore—Long Island Jewish Health System, Glen Oaks, New York

UMESH H. PARIKH, MD, The Zucker Hillside Hospital, North Shore—Long Island Jewish Health System, Glen Oaks, New York

JULIE B. PENZNER, MD, Weill Cornell Medical College, New York, New York

JEFFERSON B. PRINCE, MD, Department of Child Psychiatry, Massachusetts General Hospital, Harvard Medical School, Boston; and Director, Child and Adolescent Psychiatry, North Shore Medical Center, Salem, Massachusetts

JOSEPH M. REY, MBBS, PhD, FRANZCP, Professor of Child and Adolescent Psychiatry, University of Sydney, Potts Point, New South Wales, Australia

YANNI RHO, MD, MPH, Harvard Medical School, Cambridge Hospital, Cambridge, Massachusetts

VINOD SRIHARI, MD, Postdoctoral Fellow, Department of Psychiatry, Yale University School of Medicine, New Haven; and Special Fellow, Department of Psychiatry, Veterans Administration Medical Center, West Haven, Connecticut

LYNELLE E. THOMAS, MD, Research Psychiatrist, PRIME Research Clinic; and Assistant Professor, Child Study Center, Yale University School of Medicine, New Haven, Connecticut

BENEDETTO VITIELLO, MD, Chief, Child and Adolescent Treatment and Prevention Intervention Research Branch, National Institute of Mental Health, Bethesda, Maryland

BRUCE WASLICK, MD, Associate Professor of Psychiatry, Tufts University School of Medicine, Boston; and Department of Psychiatry, Baystate Medical Center, Springfield, Massachusetts

SCOTT W. WOODS, MD, Director, PRIME Research Clinic; and Professor of Psychiatry, Yale University School of Medicine, New Haven, Connecticut

JOSEPH YOUNGERMAN, MD, Chief, Younger Adolescent Inpatient Service, Bronx Children's Psychiatric Center; and Associate Clinical Professor of Psychiatry, Department of Psychiatry, Albert Einstein College of Medicine, Bronx, New York

Cover art courtesy of Socorro Rivera, Mexico City, Mexico.

CONTENTS

In the last 10 years, the National Institute of Mental Health has funded a number of multisite clinical trials in pediatric psychopharmacology. Trials have been completed or are in progress in attention-deficit hyperactivity disorder, depression, autism, schizophrenia, bipolar disorder, obsessive-compulsive disorder, and other anxiety disorders. Direct comparison between different treatment modalities, such as pharmacotherapy and psychotherapy, alone or in combination, has been the focus of a number of these studies, to inform clinicians and families of the relative therapeutic benefits of alternative interventions. This article presents a brief overview of these studies.

This article reviews data on the safety, tolerability, and efficacy of the extended-delivery stimulant preparations and atomoxetine, including nine methylphenidate formulations, five amphetamine formulations, and one norepinephrine reuptake inhibitor, now indicated for treatment of attention-deficit hyperactivity disorder (ADHD). Six of the nine methylphenidate formulations, three of the five compounds, and the norepinephrine reuptake inhibitor are long-acting, potentially once-daily agents. Data on treatment of common adverse events are described, and data on investigational treatments of ADHD are reviewed.

research is needed before the balance of long-term risks and benefits can be confidently assessed. Other medications or psychotherapies might benefit these patients as well. Some centers are beginning to examine if and how currently used prodromal diagnostic strategies and intervention studies might inform recognition and treatment of younger patients possibly prodromal for childhood-onset schizophrenia.

Treatment-refractory early-onset schizophrenia is a rare but severe form of the disorder associated with poor premorbid function and long-term disability. The currently available evidence suggests that clozapine remains the most efficacious treatment for the amelioration of both positive and negative symptoms of the disorder and problematic aggressive behaviors. Clozapine use in children and adolescents, however, is limited by its association with hematologic adverse events and an increased frequency of seizure activity. Further studies are needed to examine the usefulness of antipsychotic combinations and of augmentation therapies to antipsychotic medications in order to treat persistent residual psychotic symptoms in children and adolescents who have schizophrenia and who have not responded to several sequential trials of antipsychotic monotherapy.

Increasingly recognized over the past 20 years, autism spectrum disorders (ASD) are heterogeneous. Medication treatments remain fundamentally ameliorative, so prioritizing symptoms and matching medications to the patient's constellation of symptoms remains the psychopharmacologic approach to ASD. Atypical antipsychotic medications and glutamatergic agents are receiving increased attention, and antidepressants are being examined for specific symptoms and for younger patients who have autism. Large multisite networks (Research Units on Pediatric Psychopharmacology; Studies to Advance Autism Research and Treatment) have been constructed to expedite studies to elucidate effective treatments for ASD. Findings from these networks are coupled with those from recent independent trials.

II. Side Effects: Developmental Impact

Although second-generation antipsychotics (SGAs) are used increasingly in children and adolescents, data on the effectiveness and safety in pediatric populations are still sparse. Much of the safety information is derived from studies conducted in adults. This derivation is problematic because children and adolescents are exposed to SGAs during a phase of unparalleled physical and psychologic development that can affect pharmacokinetic and pharmacodynamic drug actions, efficacy, and side-effect patterns. This article presents an overview of SGA-related side effects in children and adolescents and strategies to monitor health outcomes effectively in youngsters receiving SGAs.

During puberty, girls may present with psychiatric illness necessitating treatment with psychotropic medications. Pubertal girls are especially vulnerable to medication-associated adverse events. Atypical antipsychotics and antidepressants have the potential to elevate prolactin levels, altering pubertal progression. Selection of prolactin-sparing atypical antipsychotics is recommended, as is treatment with the lowest effective dose of selective serotonin reuptake inhibitors. Monitoring of serum prolactin levels may be necessary.

This article reviews the existing evidence regarding whether selective serotonin reuptake inhibitors increase suicidal behaviors in children and examines the implications of the findings for clinical practice and research. When balanced against the fact that depression in the young is a serious, recurring condition that produces personal suffering and can lead to suicide, the overall weight of the evidence favors pharmacologic treatment over nontreatment in moderate to severe depression. Nevertheless, the need for careful clinical monitoring of suicidality and attention to behavioral activation, manic switching, and medication compliance or withdrawal are clearly warranted.

III. Conceptual Psychopharmacology: Bridging the Generation (Rx) Gap

All child psychiatrists' interactions with patients and families have important potential meanings, and the act of prescribing medication is no exception. As psychopharmacologic practice has increased in child psychiatry, facility with psychotherapeutic skills, such as establishing an alliance, identifying and treating symptoms, and promoting adherence must follow to enhance clinical outcomes. This article addresses the role of the therapeutic alliance in pediatric work, the psychological implications of administering medications, developmental issues altering psychopharmacologic efforts, the role of the dual alliance (allying both patients and parents), and recommendations for clinical practice and further research.

Evidence-based medicine (EBM) represents a powerful model for clinicians to translate everyday clinical tasks of finding and applying scientific literature into explicit and systematic steps. This article uses a question about treating adolescent depression to illustrate this approach in the context of a particular patient and his family. By helping the clinician apply population data to the 'bedside,' EBM can supplement information from individual patient narratives and can facilitate informed decisions.

Psychopharmacology practice seeks to fit specific treatments to specific disease processes. Although categorical diagnoses have improved focus on observable symptom constellations, these approximately 300 categories have limited benefits for illuminating underlying disease pathophysiology. Existing medications do not couple well to the symptom constellations of given disorders. Rather, current medications ameliorate symptoms overlapping among various disorders. Harnessing technology to identify a patient's wider symptom constellation, prioritizing and targeting symptoms across disorders, considering symptoms more dimensionally instead of "present or not," and eliciting factors necessary to improve adherence may allow medication selections to be tailored better to individual patients.

FORTHCOMING ISSUES

RECENT ISSUES

ELSEVIER
SAUNDERS

Child Adolesc Psychiatric Clin N Am
15 (2006) xv–xvii

CHILD AND
ADOLESCENT
PSYCHIATRIC CLINICS
OF NORTH AMERICA

Foreword

The Lewis Lab: An Appreciation

> . . .graves at my command
> Have waked their sleepers, oped, and let 'em forth
> By my so potent art. But this rough magic
> I here abjure.

—William Shakespeare, *The Tempest*

Along any scientific discipline's path of incremental gains, books and periodicals have long held a privileged position: journals reflecting the latest discoveries and keeping the energy and momentum going, books serving as repositories for the regular harvests that the abundance of discovery makes a necessity. The *Clinics of North America* do not fit snugly into the roles of either journals (as relatively little original research is published in them) or—despite deceiving hard covers—of books (the issues are periodical by design, and over the past few years have become formally indexed in Medline). The *Clinics* are hybrids by nature, and it may be this quality, among others, that has contributed to their popularity—and to their diffusion into all branches of medicine.

Fourteen years ago, child and adolescent psychiatry gained entry into the *Clinics of North America* series. Such a milestone reflected the field's coming of age; having developed into something more than psychiatry of the small, and finding a voice unique in its particular approaches and methodologies. Child psychiatry had taken much from its parent disciplines of psychiatry and pediatrics, but was ready for its own seat at the dinner table. A well-deserved seat for sure, but one for which proper guidance was still needed if the guest in question aspired to become a regular. As its first consulting editor, Melvin Lewis secured much more than the regularity of such presence: he made sure that the *Child and Adolescent Psychiatric Clinics of North America* thrived.

Mel Lewis had been an obvious choice as inaugural editor for the newborn series. Editing works in child and adolescent psychiatry came as naturally to him as did breathing—and almost as regularly. Mel had served between 1975 and 1987 as the third editor for the flagship *Journal of the American Academy of Child and Adolescent Psychiatry* and contributed critically to the building of solid foundations we rely on to this day. In 1991 he single-handedly took on the Herculean task of editing one of the first major textbooks in pediatric mental health: *Child and Adolescent Psychiatry—A Comprehensive Textbook* has become a benchmark classic in the three editions published to date (Lippincott Williams and Wilkins, 1991, 1996, 2002). Mel knew his editing well, and was more than superficially acquainted with both sides of the pedigree the new hybrid *Clinics* would be conceived from.

"Children are not little adults" is a refrain well-known to pediatric practitioners of all stripes. In the case of pediatric mental health, the slogan has become a battle cry of sorts: children's needs are unique and not to be confused with or lost under those of their elders; children have rights too. As a relatively young field, child psychiatry has had to make good on such noble and fine-sounding aspirations—and increasingly, it has been able to do just that, to which 56 issues of the *Child and Adolescent Psychiatric Clinics of North America* edited under Mel's watch can patently attest.

Lines of medical inquiry have been traditionally divided into basic and clinical camps. Although Mel was familiar with the tenets of the former and routinely contributed to the latter (most comfortably in the pediatric wards, tending to medically compromised preschoolers), his unique talent and originality lay elsewhere: it was in providing opportunities for growth to young scholars. Over the years, the *Clinics* became a virtual Lewis Lab: its pages his growth cultures (or was it his culture of growth?), a place where new ideas and projects—but mostly rising individuals—could test their wings. Looking back at the whole series today, one sees not only the maturing of a discipline, but that of its "who's who" as well: those child psychiatrists and allied professionals who have gone on to build major research projects and careers, to set innovative clinical programs in motion, to train an entire new generation—indeed to edit and write the field anew.

As chronicled in the preface that follows, my comments are not abstract: I have been one of the many fortunate beneficiaries of the Lewis Lab. As such, I cherish this opportunity to salute my teacher, my mentor, and my friend. Mel dubbed me "Mini-Mel" some years ago, a nod to our shared enthusiasm for the *Austin Powers* character Mini-Me—and to my own appreciation for a role model to emulate: one whose laboratory so thoroughly lived in the written pages of edited works, and who so deeply respected the fresh intelligence of medical students and others starting off on their trajectory.

Prospero's magic of releasing trapped spirits seems apt. Like *The Tempest*'s hero, Mel allowed so many to find their voice, to clear a path, to secure release through expression. And as Shakespeare's stand-in at career's end, Prospero remains a cherished farewell figure. With this issue of the *Child and Adolescent Psychiatric Clinics of North America*, Melvin Lewis's formidable trajectory comes to a close. It is an honor to serve as guest editor (together with my colleague Jeff Bostic) for this issue assigned as the last under Mel's consulting editorship. Jeff and I join Editor Sarah Barth from Elsevier, and her predecessor Catherine Bewick (publishing the series under the Saunders imprint at the time) in showing our respect and gratitude to Professor Lewis. With the next issue of this series, I will take over as consulting editor, and as first order of business welcome Mel back into these pages in his new role of Editor Emeritus. I will become entrusted with the unique privilege (and the tall challenge) of following in this mighty giant's footsteps.

Mighty but gentle. Mel is the ultimate gentleman, the kindest and most generous of individuals. His grace, poise, and beautiful British accent make one think of royalty. His signature modesty may have hidden the fact that for all we know he may in fact be a noble. Whether Her Majesty Queen Elizabeth II has knighted him remains uncertain. But *we* have, his colleagues and disciples all. This issue, and this series henceforth are dedicated to him

–to Sir, with love.

Andrés Martin, MD, MPH
Consulting Editor (Acting)
Yale Child Study Center
Yale University School of Medicine
230 South Frontage Road
New Haven, CT 06520-7900, USA
E-mail address: andres.martin@yale.edu

ELSEVIER
SAUNDERS

Child Adolesc Psychiatric Clin N Am
15 (2006) xix–xxii

CHILD AND
ADOLESCENT
PSYCHIATRIC CLINICS
OF NORTH AMERICA

Preface

Generation Rx

In the spirit of full disclosure, it must be noted that the catchy title *Generation Rx* is not of our own creation, but rather borrowed from the article by Amy Bloom that appeared on March 12, 2000 in the *New York Times Magazine* [1]. Her op ed piece, which was part of the section "The Way We Live Now," was written as a reaction to the publication in the *Journal of the American Medical Association* of Zito and colleague's [2] landmark preschooler paper.

In its original connotation, *Generation Rx* referred to the legions of children, especially kindergartners, who grow up routinely treated with psychotropic medications. As a society suddenly confronted with undeniable trends, the phrase came to embody our communal sigh of wistfulness for the pharmaceutically un-tainted childhoods of yore. Whether we resort to psychiatric drugs for children too often or not often enough remains an unresolved and at times contentious issue. However, there is no arguing with the fact that our profession has changed—profoundly and within a generation at that—because of the expansion of phar-macotherapy in children.

No longer relegated to the occasional cameo appearance, psychotropics are now a routine—if not predominant—presence in our practice. More than our treatment armamentarium has changed as a result: our very identities as child psychopharmacologists now distinguish us from a previous generation of child psychiatrists. It is we, then—more so than our young patients—who represent the true Generation Rx. To consider ourselves from this vantage point may be unflattering and cause unwelcome soul-searching (for surely we are more than glorified prescription-writers?), but it may prove curiously satisfying as well (for often enough our psychotropics prove beneficial to young patients, when not outright liberating). Although the addition of biologic interventions to our toolbox represents a triumph and enormous progress, we also have been led to believe we rely too heavily on psychopharmacology, employing medications to address all kinds of distress and frustrations reported by children, their parents, or teachers. Some history of Generation Rx coming of age, observed through the lens of this series, may help us stay true to our course.

doi:10.1016/j.chc.2005.09.001   *childpsych.theclinics.com*

This issue is the third installment of the *Child and Adolescent Psychiatry Clinics of North America* devoted to psychopharmacology, and so provides a yardstick against which to measure the growth, development, and historical trajectory of our young field. When the first of the three, a two-part issue edited by Mark Riddle, came out in 1995 [3,4], there were few methodologically rigorous studies outside of attention deficit/hyperactivity disorder. The energy was palpable, but the data were scant. The books [5–7] and the journal [8] specifically devoted to pediatric psychopharmacology at the time were largely based on case series or open-label reports. By the time the second installment was published 5 years later [9], federally funded pediatric psychopharmacology study networks had been formed, and large randomized clinical trials had been completed [10] or begun [11,12]. In the epigraph to that issue's preface [13], we spoke of our discipline as though a baby in its cradle:

> If, in Dr. William Osler's famous words "...medicine is a science, the practice of which is an art," it may be said of pediatric psychopharmacology that it too is a science: one in its tender infancy, and whose art has to be practiced with maturity well beyond its years.

As evidenced by the contributions in this most recent installment, while far from fully grown up, the field is well into a later developmental stage from where it was just 6 years ago. At least six more books on the topic published since then [14–19], enough to warrant a recent "meta-review" of sorts [20], further attest to its healthy growth. Failing to thrive, pediatric psychopharmacology definitely is not.

Starting with an overview of the almost too numerous to count (to our great fortune!) federally funded collaborative efforts in pediatric psychopharmacology, the articles in this issue's first part go on to provide six disease-specific updates on attention deficit/hyperactivity disorder, anxiety and bipolar disorders, prodromal and treatment-refractory psychoses, and autism.

The issue's second part provides scientific support for the familiar dictum that children are not little adults: their needs are unique, as can be the side effects they experience when treated with compounds as potent as ours. More than providing definitive answers to problems as varied as obesity, galactorrhea, or treatment-emergent suicidality, the articles in this section may help us approach risk/benefit considerations from an objective stance and better inform the pressing research agenda ahead.

The third and final section explicitly sets out to bridge a generation gap. At first blush, this may be taken to imply the bringing of new tricks (such as evidence-based medicine) to set trades (such as pediatric psychopharmacology). However, a simple thought experiment suggests deeper implications. Were we to imagine ourselves stranded on an island (not the proverbial island of many a *New Yorker* cartoon, but on another one beaming with people, yet entirely devoid of psychotropic medications), we would be hard pressed to envision practicing child psychiatry as we know it today. Without psychopharmacology, what would we do? More to the point perhaps, without medications or prescription pads, who would we be?

The last two articles in this issue remind us that we would still do plenty, that we would still be who we fundamentally are. Our alliance is not contingent on our pills, and our therapeutic agency is only in a limited way predicated on them. Our psychotropics are not ideal or always adequate for patients who come to us for help—but that is a defect now to be cherished, stimulating us to discern what symptoms our medications really do help, which ones beg for better agents, and where medicines are simply less effective than the many other arrows in our therapeutic quiver.

We are grateful and remain indebted to all authors for their contributions and for educating us all on the recent progress in our field. By making use of this collected knowledge—while remaining fully cognizant of how much we can still do with our prescription-writing hands metaphorically tied behind our backs—we will secure a comfortable footing on both sides of the Generation Rx gap.

Andrés Martin, MD, MPH
Yale Child Study Center
Yale University School of Medicine
230 South Frontage Road
New Haven, CT 06520-7900, USA
E-mail address: andres.martin@yale.edu

Jeff Q. Bostic, MD, EdD
Massachusetts General Hospital
15 Parkman Street, WAC 725
Boston, MA 02114, USA
E-mail address: roboz@adelphia.net

References

[1] Martin A. Generation Rx: psychotropic medication utilization and costs among privately insured children and adolescents—1997–2000 patterns and trends [master's thesis]. New Haven (CT): Yale University School of Epidemiology and Public Health; 2002.

[2] Zito JM, Safer DJ, dosReis S, et al. Trends in the prescribing of psychotropic medications to preschoolers. JAMA 2000;283:1025–30.

[3] Riddle M, editor. Psychopharmacology. Child Adolesc Psychiatr Clin N Am 1995;4(1).

[4] Riddle M, editor. Psychopharmacology. Child Adolesc Psychiatr Clin N Am 1995;4(2).

[5] Popper C, editor. Psychiatric pharmacosciences of children and adolescents. Washington (DC): American Psychiatric Press; 1987.

[6] Greene WH. Child and adolescent clinical psychopharmacology. Baltimore (MD): Lippincott Williams and Wilkins; 1991.

[7] Rosenberg DR, Holttum J, Gershon S. Textbook of pharmacotherapy for child and adolescent psychiatric disorders. New York: Brunner/Mazel Publishers; 1994.

[8] Popper CW, Frazier SH, editors. J Child Adolesc Psychopharmacol 1990–1997;1–7.

[9] Martin A, Scahill L, editors. Psychopharmacology. Child Adolesc Psychiatr Clin N Am 2000; 9(1).

[10] MTA. A 14-month randomized clinical trial of treatment strategies for attention-deficit/ hyperactivity disorder. The MTA Cooperative Group. Multimodal Treatment Study of Children with ADHD. Arch Gen Psychiatry 1999;56:1073–86.

[11] RUPP. Fluvoxamine for the treatment of anxiety disorders in children and adolescents. The Research Unit on Pediatric Psychopharmacology Anxiety Study Group. N Engl J Med 2001;344:1279–85.

[12] Research Unit on Pediatric Psychopharmacology Autism Network. Risperidone in children with autism and serious behavioral problems. N Engl J Med 2002;347:314–21.

[13] Martin A. Child and adolescent psychopharmacology, by S. Kutcher [book review]. Am J Psychiatry 1999;156:1465–6.

[14] Kutcher SP. Child and adolescent psychopharmacology. Philadelphia: W.B. Saunders; 1997.

[15] Greene WH. Child and adolescent clinical psychopharmacology. 3rd edition. Baltimore: Lippincott Williams and Wilkins; 2001.

[16] Kutcher SP, editor. Practical child and adolescent psychopharmacology. Cambridge (UK): Cambridge University Press; 2002.

[17] Rosenberg DR, Davanzo PA, Gershon S. Textbook of pharmacotherapy for child and adolescent psychiatric disorders. 2nd edition. New York: Marcel Dekker; 2002.

[18] Martin A, Scahill L, Charney DS, et al, editors. Pediatric psychopharmacology: principles and practice. New York: Oxford University Press; 2003.

[19] Bezchlibnyk-Butler KZ, Virani AS, editors. Clinical handbook of psychotropic drugs for children and adolescents. Cambridge (MA): Hogrefe and Huber Publishers; 2004.

[20] Kowalik SC. A comparison of recently published child and adolescent psychopharmacology books. J Child Adolesc Psychopharmacol 2005;15:127–45.

ELSEVIER
SAUNDERS

Child Adolesc Psychiatric Clin N Am
15 (2006) 1–12

CHILD AND
ADOLESCENT
PSYCHIATRIC CLINICS
OF NORTH AMERICA

An Update on Publicly Funded Multisite Trials in Pediatric Psychopharmacology

Benedetto Vitiello, MD

National Institute of Mental Health, Room 7147, 6001 Executive Boulevard, MSC 9633, Bethesda, MD 20892-9633, USA

The field of pediatric psychopharmacology has undergone major changes during the last 10 years. As the clinical use of psychotropic medications to treat children and adolescents has grown, so has research to evaluate the efficacy and safety of this practice. This article provides an update of multisite clinical trials in pediatric psychopharmacology that recently have been funded by the National Institute of Mental Health (NIMH). Included are controlled trials of psychotropic medications conducted in subjects under age 19 years and involving three or more separate clinical sites. This article includes (1) a summary of the changing clinical and regulatory context relevant to pediatric psychopharmacology; (2) a commentary on how publicly funded and industry-funded research can best collaborate and complement each other while avoiding duplication; (3) an update on the status of selected NIMH-funded multisite trials (Table 1), and (4) a discussion of the limitations of current multisite trials as a step toward developing novel approaches.

The clinical and regulatory context

A substantial increase in the use of psychotropic medications by children and adolescents occurred during the 1990s [1–3]. Likely contributors to this increased use have been an increased awareness among families and clinicians that mental illness can and often does affect children, a more accepted medical model to conceptualize behavioral and emotional disturbances of childhood, the availability of novel medications with improved safety and tolerability profiles,

E-mail address: bvitiell@mail.nih.gov

Table 1
Recent National Institute of Mental Health–sponsored multisite clinical trials in child and adolescent psychopharmacology

Study	Main aim	Psychopathology	Subjects (N)	Subjects' age (y)	Design and duration	Status [reference]
Multimodal Treatment of Attention-Deficit Hyperactivity Disorder (MTA)	To compare the effectiveness of intensive pharmacotherapy versus behavior therapy versus their combination versus community control group	ADHD (hyperactive or combined type)	579	7–9	Randomized, parallel groups 14 mo	Completed [13] Naturalistic follow-up in progress [15,16]
Preschoolers with ADHD Treatment Study (PATS)	To test efficacy and tolerability of methylphenidate in decreasing ADHD symptoms	ADHD (hyperactive or combined)	165 (randomized)	3–5	Sequential phases (cross-over, parallel groups, and open-label)	Completed [24]
Risperidone in Children with Autism and Serious Behavioral Problems	To test the acute efficacy and tolerability of risperidone in decreasing aggression, self-injury and severe tantrums	Autism	101	5–17	Randomized placebo-controlled parallel groups 8 wk	Completed [21]
Longer-Term Risperidone Treatment of Autistic Disorder	To examine extended tolerability and efficacy of risperidone in controlling aggression, self-injury, and severe tantrums	Autism	63 (open-label maintenance) 32 (controlled blinded discontinuation)	5–17	Open-label risperidone for 4 mo, then placebo-controlled discontinuation Total duration 6 mo	Completed [23]
Methylphenidate in the Treatment of Hyperactivity and Impulsiveness in Children with PDD	To test the efficacy and tolerability of methylphenidate in decreasing ADHD	Autism and other PDD	72	5–14	Randomized, placebo-controlled within subjects 5 wk plus open-label maintenance	Completed [22]

Study	Purpose	Condition	N	Age	Design	Status
Citalopram for Children with Autism and Repetitive Behavior	To test the efficacy and tolerability of citalopram in decreasing repetitive behavior and improving functioning	Autism and other PDD	144 (projected)	5–17	Randomized, parallel groups, placebo-controlled	In progress (http://www.clinicaltrials.gov/ct/show/NCT00086645?order=2)
Risperidone and Behavior Therapy in Children with PDD	To compare the relative efficacy of combined pharmacologic and behavioral therapy versus pharmacologic treatment alone in improving functioning	Autism and other PDD	120 (projected)	4–13	Randomized, parallel groups 24 wk	In progress (http://www.clinicaltrials.gov/ct/show/NCT00080145?order=13)
Treatment for Adolescents with Depression Study (TADS)	To compare the effectiveness of fluoxetine or CBT, alone and in combination	Major depressive disorder	439	12–17	Randomized, parallel groups, placebo-controlled 12 wk plus 24-wk continuation	Completed [19] Follow-up in progress
Treatment of Resistant Depression in Adolescents (TORDIA)	To compare the effectiveness of alternative antidepressant medications alone and in combination with CBT	Major depressive disorder nonresponsive to adequate trial of antidepressant medication	400 (projected)	12–18	Randomized factorial 12 wk	In progress (http://clinicaltrials.gov/show/NCT00018902)
Treatment of Adolescent Suicide Attempters (TASA)	To test the feasibility of a trial comparing pharmacologic and CBT modalities, alone or in combination, for decreasing recurrence of suicidal behavior	Depression and recent history of suicidal attempt	120 (projected)	12–18	Randomized or patient choice 6 mo	In progress (http://clinicaltrials.gov/ct/show/NCT00080158?order=1)
Pediatric Bipolar Mood Stabilizer Trial	To test efficacy and tolerability of lithium and valproate as monotherapy	Bipolar disorder, manic or mixed phase	150 (projected)	8–17	Randomized, parallel groups, placebo controlled 8 wk	In progress

(continued on next page)

Table 1 (*continued*)

Study	Main aim	Psychopathology	Subjects (N)	Subjects' age (y)	Design and duration	Status [reference]
Treatment of Early Age Mania (TEAM)	To test the effectiveness of lithium, valproate, and risperidone, alone or in combination	Bipolar disorder, manic or mixed phase	550 (projected)	6–14	Stratified randomization, parallel groups 8–16 wk	In progress (http://www.clinicaltrials. gov/ct/gui/show/ NCT00057681;jsessionid= 604FB8D0FB74B4249CC 2F11E812F188E?order=3)
Treatment of Early Onset Schizophrenia Spectrum	To compare the effectiveness of risperidone, olanzapine, and molindone	Schizophrenia or schizoaffective disorder	168 (projected)	8–19	Randomized, parallel groups 8 wk followed by 44-wk maintenance	In progress (http://www.clinicaltrials. gov/ct/gui/show/ NCT00053703?order=1)
Pediatric Obsessive-CompulsiveTreatment Study (POTS)	To test the efficacy of sertraline and CBT, alone or in combination in decreasing obsessions and compulsions	Obsessive-compulsive disorder	112	7–17	Randomized, parallel groups, placebo-controlled 12 wk	Completed [25]
Fluvoxamine for the Treatment of Anxiety Disorders in Children and Adolescents	To test efficacy and tolerability of fluvoxamine in anxiety	Generalized anxiety disorder, separation disorder, or social phobia	128	6–17	Randomized, placebo-controlled, parallel groups 8 wk	Completed [20]
Children and Adolescents Anxiety Multimodal Treatment (CAMS)	To compare the effectiveness of sertraline and CBT, alone or in combination in decreasing anxiety	Generalized anxiety disorder, and/or separation disorder and/or social phobia	318 (projected)	7–17	Randomized, parallel groups, placebo-controlled 12 wk	In progress (http://www.clinicaltrials. gov/ct/show/ NCT00052078?order=4)

Abbreviations: ADHD, attention-deficit hyperactivity disorder; CBT, cognitive behavioral therapy; PDD, pervasive developmental disorder.

and the spread of managed care with its emphasis on rapid symptom control for achieving clinical stabilization.

The growing off-label use of medications in children across all areas of medicine brought to the attention of researchers, policy makers, and the lay public the unacceptable imbalance between the extent of community medication use and the paucity of empiric evidence supporting such a practice [4]. The ensuing debate and controversy spawned a number of initiatives that have profoundly affected pediatric psychopharmacology research. In 1997, the US Congress passed legislation giving the Food and Drug Administration (FDA) the authority to grant manufacturers an additional 6 months of drug exclusivity in return for conducting specific studies in children [5]. This program, which was later reconfirmed and extended in time by the US Congress [6], has given industry a powerful financial incentive to conduct pediatric research. In parallel, more recently introduced legislation has given FDA the authority to require industry to conduct specific pediatric investigations as a condition for approving new drugs for adults when off-label use in children can be anticipated [7].

As a consequence, the number and size of pediatric clinical trials funded by industry has increased substantially during recent years. As of January 31, 2005, pediatric studies had been requested by the FDA for 298 drugs, of which 40 (13%) were neuropharmacologic medications [8]. Although pharmacokinetics studies often accounted for these requests, many were also for clinical trials. Thus, under this initiative, pediatric multicenter trials have been conducted testing the efficacy of medications such as fluoxetine [9], sertraline [10], paroxetine, citalopram [11], escitalopram, nefazodone, mirtazapine, and venlafaxine in depression. Only a few of these trials have been published thus far.

Together with the strengths of the pediatric exclusivity program, however, one should also acknowledge its limitations. Typically, marketing exclusivity is granted for conducting agreed-upon studies but not necessarily for providing definitive conclusions about efficacy or safety of the drug in children. The financial incentive is to complete the studies in a timely manner rather than to determine if the balance between potential benefits and risks justifies the medication's clinical use. Moreover, the pediatric studies conducted under the additional-exclusivity program involve drugs that have already been marketed for adults and often extensively used off-label in children. The exclusivity program seems to be an effective way to address the existing off-label use but not to prevent off-label use of future drugs. For this purpose, the Pediatric Equity Research Act [7] has been enacted, but it is still too early to determine its impact.

Another limitation of industry-sponsored trials, which is relevant although not specific to pediatric psychopharmacology, is that the data collected in these studies are proprietary and belong to the sponsor. Consequently, the results of some studies have not been published, particularly results of "negative" trials that could not distinguish active medication from placebo. For instance, as of today, studies of mirtazapine and citalopram that did not find any statistically significant treatment differences remain unpublished. This problem may be corrected, at least in part, by the implementation of the Best Pharmaceuticals for

Children Act, which mandates the final study reports of industry-sponsored trials be posted on the FDA web site [6]. In addition, the decision by certain pharmaceutical companies, such as Eli Lilly and GlaxoSmithKline, to make public the results of the antidepressant studies they had sponsored must be acknowledged as a positive development.

These limitations notwithstanding, there is little doubt that the legislative initiatives of the late 1990s and early 2000s have substantially changed the overall scenario of pediatric clinical trials by encouraging major involvement by industry in pediatric research. This development has occurred at a time when public funding of pediatric psychopharmacology has also increased dramatically. In fact, public, private, or joint funding for treatment research relevant to child psychopharmacology more than tripled between 1997 and 2003.

Publicly versus privately funded research in pediatric psychopharmacology

The NIMH had been the source of almost all funding of child psychopharmacology research until the late 1990s. In fact, most of the pediatric research on tricyclic or typical neuroleptic medications was publicly funded. There had been notable and important exceptions, such as the testing of clomipramine in children with obsessive-compulsive disorder (OCD) [12], but, in general, industry had played a minor role in the development and testing of medications in child psychiatry. Also, until the early 1990s, multisite trials were uncommon in child psychopharmacology. Single-site trials, however, are often limited in scope by low sample size and lack of generalizability. The launching of the Multimodal Treatment of attention-deficit hyperactivity disorder (ADHD) study (MTA) constituted a major paradigm shift for psychiatric treatment research in children because of its large sample and the inclusion of multiple active comparisons which necessitated multiple sites to recruit more than 500 children within a 2-year period and include a variety of different settings and investigator expertise [13].

With the recently kindled interest of industry in pediatric psychopharmacology, the interface between privately and publicly funded research has changed [14]. In the interest of complementarity and to avoid duplication, industry has funded primarily placebo-controlled trials aimed at testing acute efficacy. The NIMH has broadened its scope by launching multisite trials to compare the therapeutic benefits of alternative treatments for particular conditions, such as comparisons between active medications or between medications and psychosocial interventions, either alone or in combinations. In fact, although the traditional placebo-controlled trial remains the most efficient way of detecting a signal of medication efficacy, this design lacks full ecologic validity because placebo, on one hand, does not equal lack of treatment and, on the other hand, is not a viable alternative in usual practice. For clinicians, patients, and families to make evidence-based choices among credible treatment alternatives, it is important to have access to information concerning the relative effectiveness of different interventions. The direct testing of alternative interventions within the same clinical trial is the most valid way of comparing their relative efficacy because comparisons across separate trials, each testing one intervention at a time against placebo, are likely to be biased by differences in patient selection, methods, and experimental error.

In addition to efficacy research, another important area in which publicly funded multisite trials seem to be needed is the testing of novel interventions that build on neuroscience advances, especially in the case of conditions such as autism, Tourette's disorder, and OCD, which are not likely to be priorities for industry. Indeed, translational research offers potential opportunities for collaborations between private and public research in pediatric psychopharmacology [14].

Update on ongoing publicly funded multisite trials

The MTA, launched in the early 1990s as a cooperative agreement between six academic sites and the NIMH, signified a paradigm shift in child mental health research because it incorporated both traditional efficacy (eg, placebo-controlled titration) and novel effectiveness features (eg, comparisons between treatment strategies rather than single medications, long-term perspective, multiple outcomes) [13]. The study documented that carefully adjusted pharmacotherapy is the most effective approach for decreasing symptoms of ADHD and improving functioning among school-aged children. The MTA sample is currently being followed after the completion of the 14-month study treatment to ascertain the possible impact of the interventions on distal outcomes. A differential treatment effect was still detectable, although much attenuated, about 1 year after exiting the trial [15]. The data thus far analyzed also have better documented and quantified the effect of stimulant medications on physical growth. During the 2-year period of observation, children who were continuously medicated with stimulants grew in height about 1 cm per year less than never-medicated children [16]. The currently ongoing extended follow-up of the MTA sample, which is funded under NIMH contracts with additional funding from the US Department of Education and the Department of Justice, is unique for randomized clinical trials in pediatric psychopharmacology and possibly in adult psychopharmacology as well. The collection of follow-up data is expected to be completed in the next 2 years.

The Treatment for Adolescents with Depression Study (TADS) is a 13-site randomized clinical trial comparing different treatment interventions for youths with major depressive disorder: antidepressant treatment with fluoxetine, cognitive behavioral therapy (CBT), their combination, and clinical management with a pill placebo [17]. TADS is funded under an NIMH contract. Like the MTA, TADS incorporated both classic elements of efficacy methodology, such as the placebo control, and effectiveness features, such as broad protocol entry criteria that enhanced patient representativeness [18]. Consistent with the need for extended consolidation and maintenance treatment of depression to achieve remission and recovery beyond symptom improvement, the TADS design includes an acute phase of 12 weeks, followed by additional 6 months of treatment and an extended follow-up 1 year after the completion of the entire 9 months. The primary analyses have shown that combined treatment with fluoxetine and CBT is the most effective intervention with respect to both therapeutic response and safety [19]. The rate of improvement was 71% for the combined treatment group, 61% for medication alone, 43% for CBT alone, and 34% for placebo, although the CBT and placebo groups were not statistically different from each other. Additional analyses are in progress to examine possible moderators and mediators of treatment, elucidate safety outcomes better, and examine possible treatment effects on level of functioning. Also in progress are the data analyses of the 9-month treatment phase, which should become available in 2005.

The Treatment of Resistant Depression in Adolescents is a six-site randomized trial of pharmacologic and combined interventions for adolescents who have major depression and have not improved during an adequate antidepressant trial. This trial addresses the clinically important and timely question of how to deal with treatment nonresponse. Given that many depressed youths are treated with a selective serotonin reuptake inhibitor (SSRI) antidepressant and that, based on previous controlled trials, about one third do not improve adequately, it is important to determine the most effective second-step treatment be for SSRI nonresponders. Using a factorial design with four treatment arms, the trial randomly assigns adolescents suffering from depressive disorder who have not responded to an SSRI medication to receive another SSRI or venlafaxine, either alone or in combination with CBT. This study, coordinated by D. Brent of the University of Pittsburgh, is in progress and is actively recruiting subjects (http://clinicaltrials.gov/show/NCT00018902).

The Research Units on Pediatric Psychopharmacology (RUPPs) were originally launched in 1996 under research contracts with the primary aim of testing the acute efficacy and safety of medications used off label in the community [20,21]. The research scope was later broadened as a cooperative agreement to include the testing of psychosocial interventions as well. The RUPPs currently form two groups, one focused on autism and other pervasive developmental disorders (PDD), and the other on depressed adolescents at high risk for suicidal behavior. The former group, after completing two multisite placebo-controlled trials, one of risperidone in children who have autism and severe behavioral disturbances [21] and the other of methylphenidate among children who have PDD and ADHD symptoms [22], is now engaged in a three-site trial of the combined use of risperidone and behavior therapy versus risperidone alone in children who have PDD and severe behavioral problems. In fact, risperidone is quite effective for the management of aggression, self-injury, and tantrums in autism, but it is associated with substantial weight gain, and its discontinuation usually results in relapse of symptoms [23]. A currently ongoing trial intends to test whether combining behavioral therapy with risperidone would result in better level of functioning and increased likelihood of sustaining behavioral improvement after drug discontinuation (http://www.clinicaltrials.gov/ct/show/NCT00080145?order=13).

The other RUPP group is conducting a pilot five-site trial in youths who have recently attempted suicide and currently suffer from depression. This trial, the Treatment of Adolescent Suicidal Attempters, tests three alternative approaches: a special type of CBT for suicidal youths, antidepressant medication algorithmic treatment, and a combination of the two modalities (http://clinicaltrials.gov/ct/show/NCT00080158?order=1). The trial is a five-site pilot study to test the feasibility of conducting a clinical trial in an important clinical area, that of suicide attempt, which has been previously avoided systematically by investigators because of the high-risk patient population involved. Recruitment is now in progress.

The Studies to Advance Autism Research and Treatment Network was established in 2002–2003 under a cooperative agreement funded by NIMH, the National Institute of Child Health and Human Development, the National Institute of Neurological Disorders and Stroke, and the National Institute of Deafness and Communicative Disorders (http://www.nimh.nih.gov/autismiacc/staart.cfm). As part of this network, a multisite trial to test the efficacy of citalopram in autism was recently started (http://www.clinicaltrials.gov/ct/show/NCT00086645?order=2).

The Preschoolers with ADHD Treatment Study is a six-site clinical trial funded under an NIMH cooperative agreement with the aim of testing the efficacy and tolerability of methylphenidate in children 3 to 5 years of age who have ADHD. The protocol was articulated with different phases, which include an initial course of parental training in behavior therapy, in an effort to prevent unnecessary exposure of these young children to medication, followed, for nonresponders to behavior therapy, by a pharmacologic, placebo-controlled, within-subject trial, a parallel-group phase, and an extended open-label maintenance for several months. The trial has been completed and the report is forthcoming [24]. The aim of the within-subject trial was to test the effects of different fixed oral doses of methylphenidate, ranging from 1.25 mg to 7.5 mg three times per day, in the same subject as the most efficient way of describing the dose–response effects of the drug. The parallel-group phase was meant to confirm the efficacy of the best dose of methylphenidate for each subject (identified with the within-subject design) as compared with placebo over several weeks of treatment. Finally, the extended effectiveness and tolerability of methylphenidate was examined in the open-label maintenance.

The Treatment of Early Onset Schizophrenia Spectrum Disorders (TEOSS) is a four-site trial comparing the effects of risperidone, olanzapine, and molindone in the treatment of children and adolescents (8–19 years of age) who have schizophrenia or schizoaffective disorder (http://www.clinicaltrials.gov/ct/gui/show/NCT00053703?order=1). TEOSS is the first publicly funded, multisite, controlled clinical trial focused specifically on the effects of typical and atypical antipsychotic medications in pediatric outpatients who have schizophrenia.

The Pediatric Bipolar Collaborative Mood Stabilizer Trial is a randomized clinical trial of the efficacy of lithium and valproate, used as monotherapy, for children and adolescents with manic bipolar disorder. This trial, which uses a double-blind design with a placebo control group, is funded by NIMH grants to the University of Cincinnati (R. Kowatch), Case Western Reserve University (R. Findling), and the University of Wisconsin at Milwaukee (R. Scheffer).

The Treatment of Early Age Mania is a large, multisite, controlled clinical trial of lithium, valproate, and risperidone, used alone or in combination, for children and adolescents (aged 6–14 years) who have bipolar disorder. The trial is now in progress at five academic sites under the coordination of B. Geller of Washington University (http://www.clinicaltrials.gov/ct/gui/show/NCT00057681;jsessio nid=604FB8D0FB74B4249CC2F11E812F188E?order=3). Unlike TEOSS, this trial does not include a placebo; instead, it compares ecologically valid treatment alternatives that are often used in the community but that have inadequate evidence of efficacy.

The Pediatric Obsessive-compulsive Treatment Study is a recently reported three-site clinical trial of sertraline, CBT, and their combination versus pill placebo control in children and adolescents who have OCD. Although there was evidence for the efficacy of both pharmacologic and CBT intervention for pediatric OCD, it was only when these treatment modalities, and their combination, were directly compared in this study that it was possible to appreciate the critical role of CBT as the most effective treatment of OCD [25]. This study, which was funded by NIMH grants, is now being followed by a new trial, conducted by the same research team, which tries to determine if CBT can be efficiently and effectively exported to general mental health clinicians or requires more specialized providers instead.

The Child and Adolescent Anxiety Multimodal Study (CAMS) is a currently ongoing six-site randomized, clinical trial that compares sertraline with CBT, either alone or in combination, for the treatment of children and adolescents (7–17 years old) with generalized anxiety, separation anxiety, or social phobia disorders (http://www.clinicaltrials.gov/ct/show/NCT00052078?order=4). The design is similar to that of TADS, with one placebo control condition, two monotherapy conditions (medication or psychotherapy), and a combination of the two. Like TADS, this trial, which is in progress, aims to assess the relative therapeutic benefit of already-proven efficacious interventions by directly comparing them in the same randomized design.

Other pediatric psychopharmacology multisite trials in Tourette's disorder, ADHD, and autism have been funded by other institutes of the National Institutes of Health and are not included in this brief overview.

Limitations of traditional clinical trials and possible future developments

Although much progress has been made in the area of pediatric psychopharmacology during the last few years, several limitations of the traditional clinical trials have become apparent. Recruitment is often difficult and slow. Trials require several years for completion. Direct advertisement in the community is often necessary to enroll subjects into a trial. Of the patients originally screened, only a relatively small fraction eventually participates in the study. The ability of the study sample to represent usual patients likely to receive the treatment in the community is at times doubtful. In addition, the treatment provided in clinical trials is provided mainly by specialized clinicians in academic settings and may not represent available community treatment standards. Thus, traditional clinical trials tend to have considerable internal experimental validity but limited external validity. These limitations have led some researchers to consider other approaches, such as the large simple trial or practical clinical trial, which has been successfully applied to other areas of medicine such as pediatric oncology [26]. The NIMH has recently funded a research center to develop an infrastructure for practical clinical trials in child psychiatry [27]. Such studies would rely on participation by nonacademic clinicians, in more traditional clinical settings, with broader inclusion criteria to embrace more "real-world" patients. Although conducting treatment research in practice settings poses formidable challenges from a scientific, logistic, organizational, ethical, and legal perspective, the potential benefit of producing highly informative and clinically relevant data makes it a promising approach worthy of further exploration.

References

[1] Olfson M, Marcus SC, Weissman MM, et al. National trends in the use of psychotropic medications by children. J Am Acad Child Adolesc Psychiatry 2002;41:514–21.

[2] Zito JM, Safer DJ, dos Reis S, Gardner JF, et al. Rising prevalence of antidepressants among US youth. Pediatrics 2002;109:721–7.

[3] Olfson M, Gameroff MJ, Marcus SC, et al. Outpatient treatment of child and adolescent depression in the United States. Arch Gen Psychiatry 2003;60:1236–42.

[4] Vitiello B, Jensen PS. Medication development and testing in children and adolescents. Arch Gen Psychiatry 1997;54:871–6.

[5] US Congress. Food and Drug Administration Modernization Act (1997). Public Law 105–115.

[6] US Congress. Best Pharmaceuticals for Children Act (2002). Public Law 107–109.

[7] US Congress. Pediatric Research Equity Act of 2003 (2003). Public Law 108–155.

[8] Food and Drug Administration. Approved moieties to which FDA has issued a written request for pediatric studies under section 505A of the Federal Food, Drug, and Cosmetic Act. Available at: http://www.fda.gov/cder/pediatric/wrstats.htm. Accessed February 25, 2005.

[9] Emslie GJ, Heiligenstein JH, Wagner KD, et al. Fluoxetine for acute treatment of depression in children and adolescents: a placebo-controlled, randomized clinical trial. J Am Acad Child Adolesc Psychiatry 2002;41:1205–15.

[10] Wagner KD, Ambrosini P, Rynn M, et al. Efficacy of sertraline in the treatment of children and adolescents with major depressive disorder: two randomized controlled trials. JAMA 2003;290:1033–41.

[11] Wagner KD, Robb AS, Findling RL, et al. A randomized, placebo-controlled trial of citalopram for the treatment of major depression in children and adolescents. Am J Psychiatry 2004;161(6):1079–83.

[12] DeVeaugh-Geiss J, Moroz G, Biederman J, et al. Clomipramine hydrochloride in childhood and

adolescent obsessive-compulsive disorder—a multicenter trial. J Am Acad Child Adolesc Psychiatry 1992;31:45–9.

[13] MTA Cooperative Group. A 14-month randomized clinical trial of treatment strategies for attention-deficit/hyperactivity disorder (ADHD). Arch Gen Psychiatry 1999;56:1073–86.

[14] Vitiello B, Heiligenstein JH, Riddle MA, et al. The interface between publicly funded and industry-funded research in pediatric psychopharmacology: opportunities for integration and collaboration. Biol Psychiatry 2004;56:3–9.

[15] MTA Cooperative Group. National Institute of Mental Health Multimodal Treatment Study of ADHD follow-up: 24-month outcomes of treatment strategies for attention-deficit/hyperactivity disorder. Pediatrics 2004;113:754–61.

[16] MTA Cooperative Group. National Institute of Mental Health Multimodal Treatment Study of ADHD follow-up: changes in effectiveness and growth after the end of treatment. Pediatrics 2004;113:762–9.

[17] Treatment for Adolescents with Depression Study Team. Treatment for Adolescents with Depression Study (TADS): rationale, design, and methods. J Am Acad Child Adolesc Psychiatry 2003;42(5):531–42.

[18] Treatment for Adolescents with Depression Study Team. The Treatment for Adolescents with Depression Study (TADS): demographics and clinical characteristics. J Am Acad Child Adolesc Psychiatry 2005;44:28–40.

[19] Treatment for Adolescents with Depression Study Team. Fluoxetine, cognitive-behavioral therapy, and their combination for adolescents with depression: Treatment for Adolescents with Depression Study (TADS) randomized controlled trial. JAMA 2004;292(7):807–20.

[20] Research Units on Pediatric Psychopharmacology Anxiety Study Group. Fluvoxamine for the treatment of anxiety disorders in children and adolescents. N Engl J Med 2001;344:1279–85.

[21] Research Units on Pediatric Psychopharmacology Autism Network. Risperidone in children with autism and serious behavioral problems. N Engl J Med 2002;347:314–21.

[22] Research Units on Pediatric Psychopharmacology Autism Network. A randomized controlled crossover trial of methylphenidate in pervasive developmental disorders and hyperactivity. Arch Gen Psychiatry, in press.

[23] Research Units on Pediatric Psychopharmacology Autism Network. Risperidone treatment of autistic disorder: longer-term benefits and blinded discontinuation after six months. Am J Psychiatry 2005;162(7):1361–9.

[24] Greenhill LL, Vitiello B, Abikoff H, Kollins S, et al. Outcome results from the NIMH multisite preschool ADHD treatment study (PATS). Presented at the 51th Annual Meeting of the American Academy of Child and Adolescents Psychiatry. Washington (DC), October 19–24, 2004.

[25] Pediatric Obsessive-Compulsive Treatment Study. Cognitive-behavior therapy, sertraline, and their combination for children and adolescents with obsessive-compulsive disorder: the Pediatric OCD Treatment Study (POTS) randomized controlled trial. JAMA 2004;292(16):1969–76.

[26] March J, Silva S, Compton S, et al. The case for practical clinical trials in psychiatry. Am J Psychiatry 2005;162(5):836–46.

[27] March JS, Silva SG, Compton S, et al. The Child and Adolescent Psychiatry Trials Network (CAPTN). J Am Acad Child Adolesc Psychiatry 2004;43(5):515–8.

ELSEVIER
SAUNDERS

Child Adolesc Psychiatric Clin N Am
15 (2006) 13–50

CHILD AND
ADOLESCENT
PSYCHIATRIC CLINICS
OF NORTH AMERICA

Pharmacotherapy of Attention-Deficit Hyperactivity Disorder in Children and Adolescents: Update on New Stimulant Preparations, Atomoxetine, and Novel Treatments

Jefferson B. Prince, MD[a,b,*]

[a]*Department of Child Psychiatry, Massachusetts General Hospital, Harvard Medical School, 6900 Yawkey Building, 15 Parkman Street, Boston, MA 02114, USA*
[b]*Child and Adolescent Psychiatry, North Shore Medical Center, 57 Highland Avenue, Salem, MA 01970, USA*

Attention-deficit hyperactivity disorder (ADHD) is a common psychiatric condition shown to occur in 3% to 10% of school-aged children worldwide [1–3]. The classic triad of impaired attention, impulsivity, and excessive motor activity characterizes ADHD, although up to one third of children may manifest only the inattentive aspects of ADHD [4]. In most patients ADHD persists to some degree from childhood through adolescence and into adulthood [5,6]. Pharmacotherapy remains the cornerstone of ADHD treatment [7–10]. As the number of children and adolescents diagnosed with and treated for ADHD tripled during the 1990s [11], research on the pharmacotherapy of ADHD has grown, enhancing the understanding of youth who have ADHD.

Recent developments have improved the care of youth who have ADHD. First, the development and availability of novel delivery systems for methylphenidate (MPH) and mixed amphetamine salts (MAS) make it possible to extend coverage by a single dose. Second, the noradrenergic medication atomo-

Dr. Prince has received research funding, honoraria, consulting fees, and speaker bureau funding from McNeil, Lilly, Forest, Novartis, Shire, GlaxoSmithKline, Astra-Zeneca, and Pfizer Pharmaceuticals.

* Department of Child Psychiatry, Massachusetts General Hospital, Harvard Medical School, 6900 Yawkey Building, 15 Parkman Street, Boston, MA 02114.

E-mail address: jprince@partners.org

doi:10.1016/j.chc.2005.08.002
childpsych.theclinics.com

Table 1
Available treatments approved by the Food and Drug Administration for attention-deficit hyperactivity disorder

Generic name (brand name)	Formulation and mechanism	Duration of activity (hours)	How supplied	Usual absolute and (weight based) dosing range (mg/kg/d)	FDA-approved maximum dose for ADHD
MPH (Ritalin)[a]	Tablet of 50:50 racemic mixture D,l-threo-MPH	3–4	5, 10, and 20 mg tablets	(0.3–2.0)	60 mg/d
Dex-MPH (Focalin)[a]	Tablet of D-threo-MPH	3–5	2.5-, 5-, 10 mg tablets (2.5 mg Focalin equivalent to 5 mg Ritalin)	(0.15–1.0)	20 mg/d
MPH (Methylin)[a]	Tablet of 50:50 racemic mixture D,l-threo-MPH	3–4	5, 10 & 20 mg tablets	(0.3–2.0)	60 mg/d
MPH-SR (Ritalin-SR)[a]	Wax based matrix tablet of 50:50 racemic mixture D,l-threo-MPH	3–8, variable	20 mg tablets (amount absorbed appears to vary)	(0.3–2.0)	60 mg/d
MPH (Metadate ER)[a]	Wax based matrix tablet of 50:50 racemic mixture D,l-threo-MPH	3–8, variable	10 & 20 mg tablets (amount absorbed appears to vary)	(0.3–2.0)	60 mg/d
MPH (Methylin ER)[a]	Hydroxypropyl methylcellulose base tablet of 50:50 racemic mixture D,l-threo-MPH; No preservatives	8	10- and 20-mg tablets; 2.5-, 5-, and 10-mg chewable tablets; 5 mg/5 mL and 10 mg/5 mL oral solution	(0.3–2.0)	60 mg/d
MPH (Ritalin LA)[a]	Two types of beads give bimodal delivery (50% immediate release and 50% delayed release) of 50:50 racemic mixture D,l-threo-MPH	8	20-, 3-0, and 40-mg capsules; can be sprinkled	(0.3–2.0)	60 mg/d
MPH (Metadate CD)[a]	Two types of beads give bimodal delivery (30% immediate release and 70% delayed release) of 50:50 racemic mixture D,l-threo-MPH	8	10-, 20-, and 30-mg capsules; can be sprinkled	(0.3–2.0)	60 mg/d
MPH (Concerta)[a]	Osmotic pressure system delivers 50:50 racemic mixture D,l-threo-MPH	12	18-, 27-, 36-, and 54-mg caplets	(0.3–2.0)	72 mg/d

Drug	Description	Half-life (h)	Dosage forms	Dose (mg/kg/d)	Maximum dose
Dex-MPH XR (Focalin XR)[a,b]	Two types of beads give bimodal delivery (50% immediate release and 50% delayed release) of D,threo-MPH	12	5-, 10-, and 20-mg capsules	0.15–1.0	20 mg/d
AMPH[c] (Dexedrine tablets)	D-AMPH tablet	4–5	5-mg tablets	(0.15–1.0)	40 mg/d
AMPH[c] (Dextrostat)	D-AMPH tablet	4–5	5 & 10 mg tablets	(0.15–1.0)	40 mg/d
AMPH[c] (Dexedrine spansules)	Two types of beads in a 50:50 mixture short and delayed absorption of D-AMPH	8	5-, 10-, and 15-mg capsules	(0.15–1.0)	40 mg/d
Mixed salts of AMPH[c] (Adderall)	Tablet of D,l-AMPH isomers (75% D-AMPH and 25% L-AMPH)	4–6	5-, 7.5-, 10-, 12.5-, 15-, 20-, and 30-mg tablets	(0.15–1.0)	40 mg/d
Mixed salts of AMPH[a,b] (Adderall-XR)	Two types of beads give bimodal delivery (50% immediate release and 50% delayed release) of 75:25 racemic mixture D,l-AMPH	At least 8, but seems to last much longer in certain patients	5-, 10-, 15-, 20-, 25-, and 30-mg capsules; can be sprinkled	(0.15–1.0)	30 mg/d in children; recommended dose is 20 mg/d in adults
Magnesium pemoline (Cylert)[a,d]	Tablets of magnesium pemoline	12	18.75-, 37.5-, and 75-mg tablets	Up to 3; FDA recommends checking liver panel every 2 wk	112.5 mg/d
Atomoxetine (Strattera)[a,b]	Capsule of atomoxetine	5-h plasma half-life, but central nervous system effects seem to last much longer	10-, 18-, 25-, 40-, 60-, and 80-mg capsules	1.2	1.4 mg/kg/d or 100 mg

[a] Approved to treat ADHD age 6 years and older.
[b] Specifically approved for treatment of ADHD in adults.
[c] Approved to treat ADHD age 3 years and older.
[d] Because of its association with life-threatening hepatic failure, FDA recommends monitoring liver function tests every 2 weeks during treatment.

xetine (ATMX) has been approved for the treatment of ADHD. Third, laboratory schools provide innovative and unique methods to study the efficacy and pharmacokinetics and pharmacodynamic profiles of ADHD medications.

This article reviews data on the safety, tolerability, and efficacy of the extended-delivery stimulant preparations and ATMX. Table 1 lists the nine MPH formulations, five amphetamine formulations, and one norepinephrine reuptake inhibitor now indicated for treatment of ADHD. Six of the nine MPH formulations, three of the five compounds, and the norepinephrine reuptake inhibitor are long-acting, potentially once-daily agents. In addition, data on treatment of common adverse events are described. Finally, data on investigational treatments of ADHD are reviewed.

Stimulants

For more than 60 years, stimulants have been used safely and effectively in the treatment of ADHD [12]. The stimulants most commonly used are MPH, MAS, and dextroamphetamine. In recent years novel drug delivery systems have been developed for stimulants, and these formulations have become routine in clinical practice. Recent controlled trials of these medications in pediatric ADHD are described in Table 2.

Recent clinical trials of second-generation stimulant preparations

OROS-MPH

OROS-MPH, available since August 2000, uses an osmotic pump process to deliver a 50:50 racemic mixture of D,l-threo-MPH. Swanson and colleagues [13] demonstrated that a single morning dose of OROS-MPH could provide effective coverage for up to 12 hours and reduce tachyphylaxis (eg, acute tolerance) in the afternoon. The 18-mg caplet of OROS-MPH provides an initial 4-mg bolus, then delivers additional MPH in an ascending profile equivalent to 5 mg of immediate-release MPH (IR-MPH) administered three times/day.

The efficacy of OROS-MPH has been examined in three randomized, controlled trials [14–16]. Wolraich and colleagues [15] examined three dosages of MPH, comparing 18 mg OROS-MPH versus 5 mg IR-MPH, 36 mg OROS-MPH versus 10 mg IR-MPH, and 54 mg OROS-MPH versus 15 mg IR-MPH. All MPH preparations were superior to placebo and equivalent to each other in reducing ADHD symptoms [15]. The effect sizes of OROS-MPH and IR-MPH were 1.05 and 1.02, respectively, and were similar to the effect size of IR-MPH administered three times/day (0.8–1.0) in the National Institute of Mental Health's Multimodal Treatment of ADHD (MTA) study [17]. Generally, both MPH preparations were well tolerated with mild side effects of headache, appetite, and abdominal symptoms. Irritability, depression, and tic (twitching) led to discontinuation of the study in one subject each from the OROS-MPH, IR-MPH administered three times/day, and placebo arms.

The other two controlled trials of OROS-MPH occurred in laboratory school settings. Pelham and colleagues [14] compared the efficacy of OROS-MPH, IR-MPH, and placebo with each child receiving each condition in random order for 7-day intervals. Both MPH treatments equally and significantly reduced ADHD symptoms, with an effect size of 2.0. Significant improvement in peer relations and reductions in oppositional behaviors were noted in the MPH groups. Headache and abdominal pain were the most common side effects in the MPH groups, although both tics and reduced appetite were also reported. Swanson and colleagues [16], using the same dosing levels, observed similar positive effects of OROS-MPH administered once daily and IR-MPH administered three times/day, compared with placebo. Patients receiving MPH, in either condition, displayed significant improvements in academic productivity, classroom behaviors, and peer relations according to parents and laboratory school teachers [16].

Additional controlled studies with OROS-MPH clarify its effect on ADHD symptom clusters. Stein and colleagues [18] found that subjects who have ADHD-inattentive type showed larger decreases in symptoms as the dose of OROS-MPH increased from 0 to 18 mg than with increases from 18 to 36 mg or from 36 to 54 mg. Subjects who have ADHD-combined type showed greater reductions in symptoms of inattention and hyperactivity/impulsivity as the dose of OROS-MPH increased from 36 to 54 mg than with increases from 0 to 18 mg or from 18 to 36 mg. Greenhill and colleagues [19] studied adolescents and found that OROS-MPH, in doses up to 72 mg/day, was well tolerated and effective in controlling ADHD symptoms in adolescents.

Trials of long-term, open-label use of OROS-MPH have been described. Steele and colleagues [19a] reported an OROS-MPH trial with 48 of 54 youth completing 8 months of open-label of treatment. At a median dose of 36 mg/day, these patients demonstrated sustained reductions in ADHD symptoms over the 8 months. In a larger sample drawn from previous trials, Wilens and colleagues [20,21] reported on the 12- and 24-month results from long-term treatment with OROS-MPH. Of the 407 subjects entering this open-label extension, 289 completed 12 months and 240 completed 24 months of follow-up treatment. Over the course of the 12 months' follow-up, the average daily dose increased from 35 mg/day (1.09 mg/kg/day) to 41 mg/day (1.26 mg/kg/day). During this interval, 40% of these patients required no dose changes, 20% required dose increases, and 38% required both increases and decreases to sustain improvement. This extension study adds evidence of the long-term efficacy and tolerability of stimulants.

Methylphenidate MR

MPH MR contains two types of coated beads, IR-MPH and extended-release MPH (ER-MPH), in a 30:70 ratio. The 20-mg MPH MR capsule consists of 6 mg of IR-MPH and 14 mg of ER-MPH, with initial peak serum concentration

Table 2

Recent trials with stimulants to treat attention-deficit hyperactivity disorder in children and adolescents

Generic name (brand name)	Author/ year	N/age range	Design	Primary outcome measure	Dose	Comments
Efficacy trials						
OROS-MPH (Concerta)	Wolraich et al, 2001	N = 282	Randomized to placebo, MPH tid, or OROS-MPH	Teacher and parents IOWA Conners' Rating Scale	Mean daily dose of OROS-MPH 1.1 ± 0.5 mg/kg/d and IR-MPH 0.9 ± 0.4 mg/kg/d 18, 36, 54 mg OROS-MPH compared with 5, 10, 15 mg IR-MPH tid, respectively	Significant reductions in ADHD symptoms in both IR-MPH and OROS-MPH groups compared with placebo ($P < .001$) but no differences between IR-MPH and OROS-MPH
OROS-MPH	Pelham et al, 2001	N = 68; 6–12 y	Within-subject double-blind comparison of placebo, IR-MPH, OROS-MPH	Teacher IOWA Conners' Rating Scale	18, 36, 54 mg OROS-MPH compared with 5, 10, 15 mg IR-MPH tid, respectively	Both OROS-MPH and IR-MPH given tid showed significant improvements in all measures ($P < .001$)
OROS-MPH	Swanson et al, 2002	N = 32 (28 boys); 7–12 y receiving 5–15 mg MPH bid or tid	Analogue classroom study blinded crossover comparison of placebo, MPH tid, and OROS-MPH: low (n = 7), intermediate (n = 17), high (n = 8)	Activity level SKAMP	MPH mean dose 28.9 mg/d (0.9 mg/kg/d)	Both MPH and OROS-MPH improved classroom and social behavior and hyperactivity; experimental design of bolus plus ascending profile successful
OROS-MPH	Greenhill et al, 2002	N = 177 adolescents with ADHD	DBPC; 13- to 18- y-olds	ADHD-RS	Open titration to dose optimization then randomization to placebo or continue current dose of OROS-MPH:	OROS-MPH seems to be well tolerated and effective in doses up to 72 mg in adolescents; approximately two-thirds of adolescents were dosed with either 54 or 72 mg/d

Drug	Study	Subjects	Design	Measures	Dose	Results
OROS-MPH	Stein et al, 2003	N=47 subjects with ADHD-CT or ADHD-PI	Dose response study	Placebo-controlled crossover study of three doses of OROS-MPH	72 mg OROS-MPH (N=65; 36.7%) 54 mg OROS-MPH (N=50; 28.2%) 36 mg OROS-MPH (N=13; 7.3%) 18 mg OROS-MPH (N=13; 7.3%) Placebo or OROS-MPH 18, 36, or 54 mg/d	Subjects with ADHD-CT benefited form higher doses of OROS-MPH relative to those with ADHD-PI; active OROS-MPH and placebo differed in appearance; parent ratings slightly more sensitive than teacher ratings; insomnia primary AE
Modified release-MPH (Metadate-CD)	Greenhill et al, 2002	N=321 (158 MPH-MR; 163 placebo); 6-16 y	DBPC; randomization for 3 wk	Parent and teacher completed Conners' Global Index	Mean dose = 40.7 mg/d (1.28 mg/kg/d)	Significant reductions in both A.M. and afternoon Conners' Global Index Scores; investigators rated 64% of patients treated with MR-MPH as moderately or markedly improved, compared with 27% receiving placebo
MPH (Ritalin-LA)	Biederman et al, 2002	N=161 (136 available for analysis); 6-12 y	2- to 4-wk single-blind dose titration followed by a 1-wk single-blind placebo washout, followed by 2 wk of DB treatment with either placebo or study medication	CADS-T CADS-P Clinical Global Impression-Severity CGI-I	Dose optimized to 20, 30, 40, 50, or 60 mg/d	All primary and secondary efficacy variables significantly improved relative to placebo; effect size of 0.90; anorexia, insomnia and HA most common AEs

(continued on next page)

Table 2 (*continued*)

Generic name (brand name)	Author/ year	N/age range	Design	Primary outcome measure	Dose	Comments
D-MPH (Focalin)	Wigal et al, 2004	N = 132	1-wk single-blind run-in followed by 4-wk DBPC to D-MPH (n = 46) or D,l-MPH (n = 44) or placebo (n = 42)	Teacher SNAP	D,l-threo-MPH 5–20 mg bid D-threo-MPH 2.5–10 mg bid	66% with D-threo-MPH; 47% with D,l-threo-MPH; 20% with placebo
D-MPH	Arnold et al, 2004	N = 75 (35 D-MPH; 40 placebo)	Three-phase multisite (7) trial with 6-wk open-dose titration followed by 2-wk DBPC discontinuation followed by 18- to 44-wk open-label (data not reported on this phase)	SNAP CGI-I after medication randomization	D-MPH 2.5–10 mg bid	83% response to D-MPH; 39% response to placebo; subjects randomized to placebo three times more likely to have relapse compared with placebo; D-MPH demonstrated efficacy 6 h after dosing based on objective measures and behavioral effects
D-MPH XR (Focalin XR)	Greenhill et al, 2005	N = 103 (66 boys); 6–17 y	Multicenter DBPC randomized	CADS-T CADS-P	D-MPH XR 5–30 mg/d; titrated for 5 wk then maintained for 2 wk	D-MPH XR once daily seems to be effective in significantly reducing symptoms of ADHD and well tolerated without significant AEs
Transdermal MPH	Pelham et al, 2005	N = 36 (33 boys); 6–13 y	8-wk DBPC dose-ranging within-subject	Point system Daily report cards Classroom measures	6.25 cm^2 (0.45 mg/h) 12.5 cm^2 (0.9 mg/h) 25 cm^2 (1.8 mg/h)	Part of summer treatment program; 29 completers; 8% of patches either came off or required taping; mild erythema; transdermal MPH significantly improved all measures of behavior as rated by counselors and teachers

Drug	Study	N/Age	Study design	Dose/Measures	Results
Mixed salts of amphetamine (MAS; Adderall)	Ahmann et al, 2001	N = 154	DBPC crossover trial, 2 wk each condition	Placebo 0.15 mg/kg/d 0.3 mg/kg/d Dosed bid	59% response rate if concurrence between teachers and parents; 82% response rate based on parent rating alone and overall 89% (137/154) response rate with either parent or teacher
Mixed salts of amphetamine extended release (MAS-XR; Adderall-XR)	Biederman et al, 2002	N = 563 (119 girls); 6–12 y	Multicenter (47 sites) DBPC parallel study of three doses of Adderall-XR	Average of A.M. and afternoon Conners' Global Index Scale (Teacher Version) Placebo (n = 210) 10 mg (n = 124) 20 mg (n = 121) 30 mg (n = 129)	All active treatment groups showed significant improvements from baseline to endpoint with a fivefold improvement in active treatment compared with placebo; dose–response relationship observed with greatest improvements noted in the 30 mg XR/d relative to the 10 mg XR/d
Mixed salts of amphetamine extended release (Adderall-XR) versus Addeall tablets versus placebo	McCracken et al, 2003	N = 51 (44 boys); 6–12 y	Analogue classroom study	SKAMP rating scale attention and deportment variables Math problems attempted and correct Placebo 10 mg IR 10 mg IR 20 mg XR 30 mg XR	All active treatment arms with efficacy versus placebo; Adderall XR 20 and 30 mg showed continued activity at 12 h; anorexia a dose-dependent side effect; otherwise well tolerated

(continued on next page)

Table 2 (*continued*)

Generic name (brand name)	Author/ year	N/age range	Design	Primary outcome measure	Dose	Comments
Long-term follow-up studies						
MTA 24-mo follow-up; MPH	MTA Coopera- tive Group, 2004	N = 579; 7–9.9 y	24-mo follow-up on all four groups: MedMgt, Comb, Beh, and CC	Parent and teacher SNAP	Comb: 30.4 mg/d MedMgt: 37.5 mg/d Beh: 25.7 mg/d CC: 24.0 mg/d	MTA medication strategy showed continued benefit over behavioral treatment and routine community care at 24-mo follow-up for symptoms of ADHD and opposi- tional defiant disorder; some children may lose initial benefit of medication; groups using MTA medication strat- egy given higher doses of MPH
OROS-MPH	Wilens et al, 2003	N = 407 enrolled (289 [71%] continued through 1 y; 240 [59%] continued through 2 y)	Open-label treatment for up to 2 y	ADHD-RS	Long-term response rates comparable with those seen in short-term studies	8.8% withdrew because of lack of efficacy; 7.1% were lost to follow-up; high degree of parent satisfaction; side effects included headache, abdominal pain, insomnia; rate of tics were 8% over the 2-y period, similar to naturalistic observations; only mild cardiovascular effects noted and thought not to be clinically signifi- cant; no changes in laboratory values were observed; mild decrease initially in growth but subjects seemed to catch up over time
OROS-MPH	Steele et al, 2005	N = 54 (45 boys); 6–13 y	6-mo open-label extension after 8 wk of treatment	SNAP-IV IOWA Conners' CGI-I	Mean dose 40.7 ± 1.6 mg Median dose 36 mg	48/54 subjects retained for 8 mo; OROS-MPH generally well tolerated and sustained reduction of ADHD symptoms observed

	Study	Sample	Design	Measures	Doses	Results
Mixed salts of amphetamine extended release (Adderall-XR)	McGough et al, 2005	N = 568 enrolled from prior two trials (442 boys); 6–12 y	24-mo open-label extension at 45 sites	10-item Conners' Global Index Scale (Parent Version)	10 mg XR, 20 mg XR, 30 mg XR	273 (48%) completed 24-mo trial; 20 mg XR most common dose; 84 (15%) withdrew because of AEs (18 severe AEs)
PK/PD trials MAS-XR	McGough et al, 2003	N = 51 (44 boys); 6–12 y; ethnicity: white (25), African American (8), Hispanic (12), Asian (3), Other (3); mean duration of prior stimulant treatment 1.7 ± 1.7 y (MPH 30; AMPH 17; not listed 4)	Analogue classroom initial, 1-wk washout followed by single dose of 20 mg followed by 5-wk double-blind crossover	Venous sampling to determine C_{max}, T_{max}, AUC_{0-24}	MAS 10-mg tablet, MAS-XR 10, 20, and 30 mg	Considerable between-subject variability of plasma concentrations of both MAS tablet and XR; longer T_{max} in MAS-XR; increased AUC and C_{max} in African American and Hispanic subjects; increased T_{max} for D-isomer in girls, but one outlier; higher doses led to elevated levels of MAS 14 h after dosing; no clear relationship between MAS concentration and behavioral response
D-MPH	Quinn et al, 2004	N = 31 (males); 9–12 y; ADHD stabilized on at least 20 mg D,l-MPH for at least 1 mo	Multisite (3) DBPC crossover comparing equal doses of D-MPH and D,l-MPH with each other and placebo	Plasma levels Conners' 10-item index CLAM Math test	D-MPH 2.5, 5, and 10 mg; D,l-MPH 5, 10, and 20 mg	Dose-related improvements with both D-MPH and D,l-MPH; PD effects of both D-MPH and D,l-MPH parallel plasma levels; PD effects dose related, higher dose led to longer effects; effects of single dose of 5 or 10 mg D-MPH seemed to last 6 h

(continued on next page)

Table 2 (*continued*)

Generic name (brand name)	Author/ year	N/age range	Design	Primary outcome measure	Dose	Comments
OROS-MPH Proof-of-concept	Swanson et al, 2003	Proof-of-concept: N = 32 (28 boys); 7–12 y	Proof-of-concept: placebo versus MPH tid versus OROS-MPH	Proof-of-concept: SKAMP	Proof-of-concept: 5, 10, 15 mg MPH	Proof-of-concept demonstrated large effect sizes (> 1.5) for both tid and ascending conditions from SKAMP attention; small clinically insignificant increases in heart rate and blood pressure noted
PK/PD properties of MPH		PK/PD: N = 64 (82% boys); mean age 9.2 y	PK/PD: randomized three-way crossover double-dummy procedure	PK/PD: IOWA Conners', SNAP, and CLAM		PK/PD studies demonstrated large effect sizes based on teacher and parent ratings for both OROS-MPH (1.69/1.53) and MPH tid (1.57/1.31); similar onset of effect with OROS-MPH and MPH tid

Abbreviations: ADHD-CT, attention-deficit hyperactivity disorder–combined type; ADHD-PI, attention-deficit hyperactivity disorder–primarily inattentive type; AE, adverse events; AMPH, amphetamine; CADS-P, Conners' ADHD DSM-IV Scale-Parent; CADS-T, Conners' ADHD DSM-IV Scale-Teacher; CGI-I, Clinical Global Impression-Improvement; CLAM, Conners', Looney, and Milich Rating Scale for ADHD; DBPC, double-blind, placebo-controlled; IOWA Conners', Inattention/ Overactivity Subscale; OROS-MPH, Concerta; PD, pharmacodynamics; PK, pharmacokinetics; SKAMP, Swanson, Kotkin, Agler, MyInn, and Pelham teacher rating scale designed to evaluate behaviors over a classroom period that are necessary for success in the classroom; SNAP, Swanson, Nolan, and Pelham Rating Scale for ADHD.

at 1.5 hours after dosing. A second peak occurs with the ER-MPH approximately 4.5 hours after dosing (data on file Celltech [http://www.pharma.ucb-group.com/UCBPharmaImages/Metadate%20CD%20-%20R312F%202-2005_tem62-4443.pdf]). These capsules can be broken and the beads sprinkled on food for patients unable to swallow pills.

Greenhill and colleagues [22] found significant improvements (effect size 0.8) during the morning and afternoon hours in patients treated with MPH MR. Designed to simulate IR-MPH twice-daily dosing, MPH MR may exert greater effects during a shorter "school-day" interval. The mean dose of MPH MR was 41 mg/day (1.28 mg/kg/day). By clinical global impression (CGI) efficacy scores, 64% of MPH MR–treated subjects responded, compared with 27% receiving placebo [8]. MPH MR was generally well tolerated, with anorexia and insomnia reported significantly more often than in placebo-treated patients.

Methylphenidate-ERC

MPH-ERC is available in capsules of 10, 20, 30, and 40 mg, which may be sprinkled on food. MPH-ERC uses the spheroidal oral drug absorption system (SODAS) beaded technology to achieve a bimodal release profile that delivers 50% of its D,l-threo-MPH initially and another bolus approximately 3 to 4 hours later, thus providing approximately 8 hours of coverage.

In a multicenter controlled study, Biederman and colleagues [22a] evaluated the efficacy of MPH-ERC. Dosages most often were titrated to 30 or 40 mg of MPH-ERC daily. MPH-ERC–treated subjects experienced significantly greater reductions in impulsivity/hyperactivity and inattention as compared with placebo ($P < .0001$). The overall effect size for active treatment was 0.9. MPH-ERC generally was well tolerated; anorexia, insomnia, and headache were the most frequently reported adverse side effects in the MPH-ERC group. One subject assigned to MPH-ERC experienced a depression during the double-blind phase, requiring hospitalization and discontinuation from the study.

D-threo-methylphenidate, D-methylphenidate

As originally formulated, MPH was produced as an equal mixture of D, l-threo-MPH and D, l-erythro-MPH. It was quickly recognized that the erythro form of MPH produced cardiovascular side effects, and thus MPH is manufactured as an equal mixture of D- and l-threo-MPH. Studies revealed that the primary active form of MPH is the D-threo isomer [23–25]. Recently, D-threo-MPH has become available for clinical use in tablets of 2.5, 5, and 10 mg. In terms of potency, 5 mg of D-MPH is biologically equivalent to 10 mg of MPH.

Quinn and colleagues [26] compared MPH and D,l-MPH in boys who had ADHD. Significant dose-related improvements were observed in which clinical performance improved up to the peak plasma concentration of D-MPH and then declined as the plasma concentration of D-MPH fell. After administration of D,l-MPH, levels of l-MPH were negligible and not correlated with clinical benefit. The duration of effect from MPH seemed to be dose related, with the medium dose conditions (5 mg D-MPH or 10 mg D,l-MPH) and high dose conditions (10 mg D-MPH or 20 mg D,l-MPH) showing improvement for longer periods of time. No clinically significant adverse events related to D-MPH and D,l-MPH were observed.

Clinical experiences with D-MPH have been described in open trials [27] and controlled studies. Wigal and colleagues [28] compared the effects of placebo, D-MPH, and IR-MPH (D,l-MPH) in children who had ADHD (64% had combined-type ADHD). Subjects randomly assigned to D-MPH received an average of 18.25 mg/day, with 85% titrated to the maximal dose of 10 mg twice daily. The average dose of D,l-MPH was 32.14 mg/day, with 69% of patients titrated to maximal dose of 20 mg twice daily. Large effect sizes of 1.0 for both D-MPH and D,l-MPH emerged. Although the second dose of MPH was administered between 11:30 AM and 12:30 PM, subjects treated with D-MPH showed significant improvement on parent ratings and math test scores at 6:00 PM compared with subjects receiving placebo; subjects treated with D,l-MPH did not show these later-day benefits. The time course of D-MPH may be different from that of D,l-MPH. Treatment with both D-MPH and D,l-MPH seemed to be well tolerated, and no serious adverse events occurred. Three D-MPH–treated subjects required dose reductions, one each because of "over focusing," facial flushing, and mildly increased heart rate with sedation. Similarly, Arnold and colleagues [29] found significant reductions in ADHD symptoms, as assessed by both parent and teacher ratings, at both 3 and 6 hours after dosing of D-MPH. After D-MPH response, subjects randomly assigned to placebo experienced treatment failure compared with subjects continuing treatment with D-MPH (61.5% versus 17.1%; $P = .001$). D-MPH was well tolerated, and no serious medication-related adverse events were observed.

With the use of SODAS beaded technology, D-MPH has been formulated into the extended-delivery preparation D-MPH-XR. The Food and Drug Administration (FDA) approved D-MPH-XR for treatment of ADHD in children, adolescents, and adults in May 2005, and it is available in 5-, 10-, and 20-mg capsules. In a controlled study, Greenhill and colleagues [30] titrated subjects to a mean final dose of 0.67 mg/kg/day D-MPH-XR. Subjects treated with D-MPH-XR had significant reductions in ADHD symptoms, with an effect size of 0.79. D-MPH-XR generally was well tolerated, with decreased appetite the most frequent adverse side effect. Six D-MPH-XR subjects (11%) and none of the placebo subjects lost more than 7% of their baseline body weight.

Methylphenidate transdermal patch

Innovative but still investigational MPH preparations have been studied in the treatment of ADHD. For instance, Pelham and colleagues [31] report on a dose-ranging study of a MPH transdermal system (MTS) [31]. Children (aged 6–12 years; 33 boys) who had ADHD participated in this 8-day, double-blind, within-subject crossover study comparing MTS, in doses of 6.25 cm^2

(0.45 mg/hour), 12.5 cm^2 (0.9 mg/hour), and 25 cm^2 (1.8 mg/hour) with placebo. MTS-treated subjects displayed improvements in measures of inattention, overactivity, oppositionality, and certain measures of academic productivity. Erythema occurred in 5% to 21% of the subjects, and the side-effects profile was similar to that of oral MPH, namely dose-related appetite suppression and insomnia.

Mixed amphetamine salts

In recent years both the immediate-release and extended-delivery formulations of MAS have been studied in clinical trials. MAS tablets contain equal portions of D-amphetaine saccharate, D,l-amphetamine asparate, D-amphetamine sulfate, and D,l-amphetamine sulfate. The two isomers have different properties, and some children who have ADHD may respond better to one isomer than to the other. Recent data in children who have ADHD suggest that, when compared with IR-MPH, peak behavioral effects of MAS occur later and are more sustained [32]. Greenhill and colleagues [33] found that 10 mg MAS administered twice daily remained superior to a single 10-mg morning dose, and the twice-daily condition resulted in higher C_{max} (maximal concentration) and AUC_{0-24} (area under curve 0–24 hours) than the single morning dose, although the terminal half-life remained similar, approximately 7.5 hours for D-amphetamine.

Ahmann and colleagues [34] compared two dosages of MAS (0.15 and 0.3 mg/kg/day) with placebo. The investigators enrolled 154 newly diagnosed and stimulant-naive children who had ADHD in this controlled trial. Response rates were 54% based on parent and teacher concurrence of benefit, 81% based on parental reports, and 77% based on teacher reports. There was no effect of gender or ADHD subtype on response to MAS. Children aged 8 and 9 years responded best; efficacy rates were lower in older and younger subjects. Although MAS was generally well tolerated, reduced appetite, insomnia, and stomachaches occurred during treatment.

Mixed amphetamine salts–extended release

The extended-delivery preparation of MAS (MAS XR) contains a 50:50 ratio of immediate-release beads designed to release MAS in a fashion similar to MAS tablets and delayed-release beads designed to release MAS 4 to 6 hours after dosing. Pharmacokinetics and clinical profiles of MAS XR have recently been studied in a group of 51 prepubertal children (6–12 years old; 7 girls; 25 white, 12 Latino, 8 African American, 3 Asian, and 3 other ethnicities) who had ADHD (98% combined subtype) [35,36]. Results of the pharmacokinetics profile demonstrate the time of maximal concentration (T_{max}) of MAS XR is increased relative to MAS tablets, suggesting the MAS XR is effective when dosed once daily. Additional variables seemed to influence the pharmacokinetic profile of MAS XR in these children. For instance, the C_{max} was increased in both African American and Latino subjects, whereas the T_{max} was significantly longer in the female subjects (9.29 ± 1.07 hours for girls versus 6.72 ± 0.43 hours for boys; $t = -2.223$; $P = .03$; $df = 48$). These variations underscore the need for individual titration of MAS XR in clinical practice. Compared with placebo, all active forms of treatment (10-mg MAS tablet and 10, 20, and 30 mg MAS XR) resulted in significant improvements in ADHD symptoms. Increasing doses of MAS XR resulted in greater improvements, with the 30-mg MAS XR dose showing an effect size of 1.0 at 6 hours and significant improvements in all measures out to 12 hours. MAS XR seemed to be well tolerated, with dose-dependent anorexia the primary adverse effect.

MAS XR has also been studied in large groups of children and adolescents in naturalistic settings. Biederman and colleagues [37] studied MAS XR at 10-, 20-, and 30-mg doses in 584 children. Although all three MAS XR dosages resulted in significant ADHD improvement, a dose–response relationship was observed. Subjects treated with 30-mg MAS XR had the most robust gains, and these gains were maintained for up to 12 hours. Subanalyses showed that stimulant-naive subjects responded equally as well as those previously treated with stimulants. Furthermore, boys and girls responded equally well to MAS XR. MAS XR–treated subjects experienced significantly more anorexia, insomnia, abdominal pain, and emotional lability, and anorexia increased in a dose-dependent manner. ECGs repeated at different dose levels revealed no significant findings.

Subjects from these two trials of MAS XR were able to enroll in a 24-month extension trial of open-label treatment with MAS XR [38]. Of the 568 initial subjects, 238 (42%) completed less than 12 months, 330 (58%) completed at least 12 months, 284 (50%) completed more than 18 months, and 273 (48%) completed 24 months. The majority of the subjects were treated with 20 mg daily. Long-term treatment with MAS XR resulted in significant improvements in subjects whose treatment was interrupted between studies, and improvement was maintained in patients whose treatment had not been interrupted. Most subjects (92%) experienced some adverse event, usually mild and diminishing over time. The incidence of adverse events increased with increasing MAS XR dosage. The most frequent adverse events associated with discontinuation were weight loss (n = 27), anorexia/decreased appetite (n = 22), insomnia (n = 11), depression (n = 7), and emotional lability (n = 4). Two subjects had convulsions and were withdrawn from the study. Both subjects were found to have an unrecognized preexisting condition, although neither required an anticonvulsant. In general, treatment with MAS XR over 24 months was well tolerated and resulted in significant and sustained clinical benefits.

Pemoline

Pemoline is a central nervous system stimulant, structurally different from both MPH and amphetamine, which seems to enhance central dopaminergic transmission [39,40]. Since pemoline became available in 1975, 15 cases of acute hepatic failure during pemoline treatment have been reported to the FDA, 12 of which resulted in liver transplantation or death (http://www.fda.gov/medwatch/

safety/1999/cylert.htm) [41]. Although generic pemoline remains available, Abbott Laboratories discontinued production of their proprietary product in May 2005 (http://www.fda.gov/cder/drug/shortages/Cylert_Disc.pdf). FDA recommendations for liver function tests to be obtained every 2 weeks have further relegated pemoline to use only in rare circumstances [42].

Adverse effects of stimulants

Cardiovascular safety

A concern about long-term pharmacotherapy of ADHD with stimulants is the impact of the stimulants on the cardiovascular system. Stimulants seem to have a variable effect on heart rate, systolic blood pressure (SBP), and diastolic blood pressure (DBP). Rapport and Moffitt [43] recently reviewed studies of IR-MPH–associated cardiovascular side effects in studies from 1972 to 1999. These studies indicate clinically minor increases in heart rate (3–10 beats per minute), SBP (3.3–8 mm Hg) and DBP (1.5–14 mm Hg) that seem to be linearly related to dose. Findling and colleagues [44] studied the cardiovascular effects of short-term treatment with three different doses of MPS and MPH compared with placebo. During treatment with either MAS or MPH, subjects experienced statistically significant but clinically insignificant dose-related increases in heart rate (<5 beats per minute) and DBP (<5 mm Hg), but not in SBP. Stowe and colleagues [45] used 24-hour ambulatory blood pressure monitoring in boys (aged 7 to 11 years) who had ADHD and who were stabilized on either MAS (n = 9) or MPH (n = 8) [45]. These investigators found significant dose-related increases in heart rate, SBP, and DBP during both MAS and MPH treatment. During treatment two subjects (one treated with MAS and one with MPH) met criteria for hypertension, and, while off treatment, one subject receiving MAS met criteria for hypertension. These results underscore the need to screen vital signs before initiating pharmacotherapy and for monitoring during ongoing treatment. Wilens and colleagues [46,47] have recently reported cardiovascular effects of long-term treatment with OROS-MPH and MAS XR. Statistically significant but clinically minor increases in heart rate, SBP, and DBP occurred at months 3, 6, 9, and 12 of follow-up. These cardiovascular changes appeared in the first month of treatment, persisted, and seemed to be unrelated to dose or gender. Age-related decreases in heart rate and increases in BP emerged, and subjects with higher baseline vital signs experienced the least change with treatment. Wilens and colleagues [47] reported on the cardiovascular effects of MAS XR in 287 adolescents (aged 13–17 years) who had ADHD treated over 4 weeks. Once again, statistically significant but clinically insignificant increases in heart rate were observed in the 20- and 50-mg/day groups, and no other differences were observed in heart rate, SBP, DBP, or ECG parameters in any of the treatment groups relative to placebo.

Cardiac effects and the MAS XR ban in Canada

On February 9, 2005, Health Canada banned the sale of MAS XR in Canada (http://www.hc-sc.gc.ca/english/protection/warnings/2005/2005_01.html).[1] This ban was based on concerns from postmarketing reports in the United States of 12 sudden, unexplained deaths in pediatric patients prescribed MAS or MAS XR (MAS tablets were never approved in Canada). Five of the 12 cases occurred in patients who had underlying structural heart defects (eg, abnormal arteries or valves, abnormally thickened walls) that increase risks of sudden death. The remaining case histories were complicated by family history of ventricular tachycardia, association of death with heat exhaustion, dehydration, near-drowning, very rigorous exercise, fatty liver, heart attack, above-toxic blood levels of amphetamine, and type 1 diabetes mellitus. The duration of MAS treatment varied from 1 day to 8 years. The number of cases of sudden deaths reported for MAS/MAS XR is only slightly greater, per million prescriptions, than the number reported for MPH products, which are also commonly used to treat pediatric patients who have ADHD (http://www.fda.gov/cder/drug/advisory/adderall.htm). The FDA is continuing to evaluate these and other postmarketing reports of serious adverse events in children, adolescents, and adults treated with MAS-related products. The rate of sudden death in pediatric patients treated with MAS products does not seem to be greater than the number of sudden deaths that would be expected to occur in this population without treatment. For this reason, the FDA has not decided to take any further regulatory action at this time. Because it seemed that patients who have underlying heart defects might be at increased risk for sudden death, however, the labeling for MAS XR was changed in August 2004 to include a warning that these patients might be at particular risk and that these patients ordinarily should not be treated with Adderall products. Information sheets and updates on this issue are available at http://www.fda.gov.

Sleep disturbance

Parents often report sleep disturbances in children who have ADHD [48–50]. A recent comprehensive review of sleep disturbances in ADHD identified 47 research studies (34 naturalistic; 13 during stimulant treatment) of sleep in youth (aged 3–19 years; 60% male) who had ADHD [51]. Sleep in ADHD youth was assessed using various methods including subjective reports by parents and children (n = 25), polysomnography (n = 16), and actigraphy (n = 6). Objective measures of sleep in ADHD youth generally demonstrate increased nighttime activity, reduced

---

[1] After suspending sale of MAS XR, Health Canada assigned a new drug committee (NDC) to review its safety data. In August 2005, the NDC made several recommendations including labeling changes to MAS XR to emphasize that MAS XR should not be used in patients with structural cardiac defects and to advise about the dangers of misusing amphetamines. The NDC also recommended that the manufacturer support independent-enhanced education for professionals about sudden unexplained death and enhance postmarketing surveillance by providing safety information to Health Canada on a regular basis. Health Canada accepted these recommendations and agreed to make MAS XR available again in Canada.

rapid eye movement sleep, notable daytime sleepiness in unmedicated children, little sleep-disordered breathing, and possibly increased occurrence of periodic limb movements. A recent observational study by O'Brien and colleagues [52] evaluated the effect of stimulant medication by using subjective (parental surveys) and objective (polysomnographic) assessments. These investigators report an increased prevalence of sleep disturbance in children who have ADHD but found the use of stimulant medication had little detrimental effect on the sleep characteristics (as subjectively and objectively assessed) of the ADHD child. Solutions to sleep problems might include a decrease in late-day dosing, adjusted timing of dosing, behavior modification, or a small dose of clonidine [8,53].

Melatonin, a circadian rhythm–regulating hormone secreted by the pineal gland, has been studied in children who have ADHD and sleep problems [54,55]. Tjon Pian Gi and colleagues [56] described short-term (1–4 weeks; n=24) and long-term (3 months; n=13) effects of melatonin in 27 MPH-treated children who had ADHD and sleep disturbances [56]. Significant reductions in time needed to fall asleep were observed during short-term treatment with melatonin and seemed to be maintained over 3 months. Two subjects dropped out of the study, one because nightmares, and one because of increased aggression.

Appetite suppression

Patients treated with stimulants often experience dose-related reductions in appetite and, in some cases, weight loss [43]. In many, but not all, patients, appetite suppression wanes over time [20]. Clinicians should give guidance on improving the patient's nutritional options with higher caloric intake to balance the consequences of decreased food intake [8]. Cyproheptadine, a medication with both antihistaminergic and antiserotoninergic effects, is FDA approved to treat allergy symptoms in patients as young as 2 years [57] and has been used to stimulate appetite in a variety of pediatric conditions. Daviss and colleagues [58] reviewed charts of 28 ADHD youth treated with cyproheptadine for stimulant-associated appetite suppression or insomnia. These patients were treated with various stimulants including MAS (n=11), OROS-MPH (n=5), MAS XR (n=2), dextroamphetamine (n=2), and MPH (n=1) for a mean duration of 145 ± 144 days. Cyproheptadine was initiated at 2 mg at bedtime and titrated up to 4 to 8 mg depending on clinical response, for a mean dose of 4.9 ± 1.5 mg. During cyproheptadine treatment (mean duration, 104.7 ± 95.7 days) all patients gained weight (mean gain, 2.2 ± 1.4 kg), and 19 of 21 patients had significant increased weight velocity. During cyproheptadine treatment, insomnia symptoms were "much" (n=8) or "very much" (n=3) improved in 11 of 17 patients, although one patient had new-onset insomnia.

Growth

The impact of stimulant treatment on the rate and extent of growth remains a concern, and the data are conflicting. For instance, at 24-month follow-up in the

MTA study, growth deceleration about 1 cm/year was noted in children who had ADHD and who were treated with continuous stimulant medication [59]. The group treated intermittently with medications experienced less deceleration in growth. Overall, growth remained within the normal curves for all children except those in the lowest percentile for height. Current clinical use of these data to predict growth parameters for patients or to support temporary periods of discontinuation of medication to minimize growth effect is not quite supported [59]. As noted by the MTA investigators, long-term stimulant treatment may slow the rate but extend the duration of growth.

In contrast to these results, Biederman and colleagues [60] recently reported on growth deficit in girls who had ADHD. Although statistically significant differences were observed between ADHD girls and controls, these deficits were modest, were evident only in early adolescence, were unrelated to weight deficits or stimulant treatment, and were not significant after correcting for age and parental height. Current consensus is that stimulants may infrequently produce a small, negative (deficit) impact on growth velocity; however, this delay may be related more to ADHD than to its treatment [61].

Stimulant alternatives in attention-deficit hyperactivity disorder

Atomoxetine

ATMX, a highly selective norepinephrine reuptake inhibitor, recently has been approved for the treatment of ADHD in children, adolescents, and adults. Unlike the stimulants, ATMX is not a controlled substance; therefore, clinicians can provide samples and prescribe refills. ATMX acts by blocking the norepinephrine reuptake pump on the presynaptic membrane, thus increasing the availability of intrasynaptic norepinephrine.

After initial encouraging results in open trials [62], the efficacy of ATMX has been reported in five controlled studies [63–66] and in an open-label extension study over 9 months [67]. Controlled studies of ATMX for ADHD are summarized in Table 3. Spencer and colleagues [63] reported results of two multicenter trials that assessed ATMX's safety, tolerability, and efficacy in children who have ADHD. A total of 291 youth aged 7 to 13 years (mean age, 9.8 years; 147 stimulant-naive; 81% males) who had ADHD (81% who had combined-type ADHD) were randomly assigned to ATMX or placebo administered twice daily for 9 weeks. Treatment with ATMX led to significant reductions on the ADHD rating scale (Study 1: ATMX baseline, 41.2 ± 8.9; change, −15.6 ± 13.7; placebo baseline, 41.4 ± 7.9; change, −5.5 ± 11.6; Study 2: ATMX baseline, 37.8 ± 7.9; change, −14.4 ± 13.0; placebo baseline, 37.6 ± 8.0; change, −5.9 ± 13.0; all *P* values <.001). The mean dose of ATMX in the combined studies was 1.5 mg/kg/day. Although significant improvements were noted in symptoms of inattention and hyperactivity/impulsivity, the mean end scores left ATMX subjects still in the clinically significant range of ADHD.

The effect sizes for the total ADHD rating scale (ADHD-RS) scores, inattentive, and hyperactive/impulsive scores were 0.72, 0.66, and 0.69 respectively. No significant adverse events were observed during the 1-week discontinuation phase. ATMX was generally well tolerated, and the only side effect that occurred significantly more often in ATMX-treated subjects was decreased appetite (21.7% versus 7.3%; $P < .05$). Information from the classroom teachers was intentionally excluded, which may have influenced these results.

Michelson and colleagues [64] compared the effect of placebo (n = 84) with that of ATMX dosed twice daily to a total dose of 0.5 (n = 44), 1.2 (n = 84), or 1.8 (n = 85) mg/kg/day. Compared with youth randomly assigned to placebo, subjects assigned to ATMX dosed to 1.2 or 1.8 mg/kg/day experienced significant reductions in ADHD-RS scores (-13.6 ± 14.0 and -13.5 ± 14.5, respectively; both P values $< .05$ versus placebo), whereas those dosed to 0.5 mg/kg/day did not (-9.9 ± 14.6; P = not significant). ATMX generally was well tolerated with trends of increasing appetite suppression, somnolence, and minor elevations in pulse and DBP with increasing dose. Although there was a small number of "poor metabolizers" (n = 17) of cytochrome 2D6, they seemed to tolerate ATMX well without any unusual or unexpected adverse events.

Two multisite trials compared the effect of ATMX dosed once daily with placebo. In subjects treated with ATMX (mean final dose of ATMX, 1.3 ± 0.2 mg/kg/day dosed once in the morning), Michelson and colleagues [65] described significant reductions on the ADHD-RS (baseline, 37.6 ± 9.4; endpoint, 24.8 ± 12.4; $P < 0.001$) as early as week one, and endpoint ADHD-RS scores remained approximately 1.5 SD above age/gender norms. Mean treatment effect size was 0.71. Rates of response ($> 25\%$ reduction in ADHD-RS scores: 59.5% for ATMX versus 31.3% for placebo; odds ratio = 3.22; 95% CI = 1.63–6.41; $P \leq .001$) and remission (CGI score of 1 or 2: 50% for ATMX versus 25.3% for placebo; odds ratio = 2.95; CI = 1.46–6.01; P = .001)) were greater in subjects treated with ATMX. Decreased appetite, nausea, and dyspepsia were observed significantly more often in ATMX-treated subjects.

Kelsey and colleagues [66] compared once-daily ATMX with placebo in a group of 197 youth (aged 6–12 years; 71% male) who had ADHD (69% had combined-type ADHD; 35% were comorbid with oppositional defiance disorder). ATMX was administered in the morning and titrated from 0.8 mg/kg/day to a maximum of 1.8 mg/kg/day or 120 mg. The final mean dose was 1.3 ± 0.3 mg/kg/day (44.5 mg/day; range, 10–80 mg/day). ATMX-treated subjects had significant reductions in ADHD-RS scores evident by week one follow-up in the symptom domains of inattention and hyperactivity/impulsivity and continued to improve across the 8 weeks of the study (baseline, 42.1 ± 9.2; endpoint, 25.3 ± 14.3; $P < .05$) compared with placebo (baseline, 42.3 ± 7.1; endpoint, 35.2 ± 12.3; P = not significant). ATMX-treated subjects also showed greater improvements in categorical measures of ADHD ($> 25\%$ reduction in ADHD-RS scores: 62.7% for ATMX versus 33.3% for placebo; 95% CI, 15.2%–43.6%; $P < .001$; CGI-ADHD severity score of 1 or 2: 27.0% for ATMX versus 5.0% for placebo 5.0%; 95% CI, 12.8%–31.2%; $P < .001$).

Table 3
Recent studies of atomoxetine in treatment of attention-deficit hyperactivity disorder in children and adolescents

Generic name (brand name)	Author/year	N/age range	Design	Primary outcome measure	Total dose	Response rate
Efficacy						
Atomoxetine (Strattera)	Kelsey et al, 2004	N = 197; 6–12 y	Multisite (12) randomized 8-wk DBPC; randomization unbalanced (ATMX:placebo, 2:1)	ADHD-RS	Initiated at 0.8 mg/kg/d in A.M. for 3 d then increased to 1.2 mg/kg/d; if after 4 wk significant residual ADHD symptoms, then increase to 1.8 mg/kg/d allowed	ATMX effect size 0.71 on ADHD symptoms; 53% previously treated with stimulant; 26 withdrew, 6 because of AEs (reduced appetite, somnolence, fatigue); documented benefit into evening hours from once-daily A.M. dosing
ATMX	Spencer et al, 2002	N = 291; study 1: n = 147 (seven sites), study 2: n = 144 (10 sites), boys (n = 201) and girls (n = 52); 7–12 y	Stimulant-naive subjects randomized to ATMX or MPH or placebo; subjects previously exposed to stimulant randomized to ATMX or placebo	ADHD-RS	25% reduction in ADHD-RS; study 1: 64.1% ATMX versus 24.6% placebo, $P < .001$; study 2: 58.7% ATMX versus 40.0% placebo, $P < .048$; mean dose: 1.5 mg/kg/d at last visit	Intentionally unbalanced randomization ATMX:placebo:MPH 3:3:2; significant reductions in ADHD-RS in ATMX-treated subjects; decreased appetite only statistically significant adverse events
ATMX	Michelson et al, 2002	N = 170; 85 ATMX and 85 placebo; 6–16 y; primarily combined and inattentive subtypes	DBPC double-dummy for 6 wk	Total score on ADHD-RS	Dosed once daily; 0.5 mg/kg/d for 3 d; 0.75 mg/kg/d for 4 d; 1 mg/kg/d thereafter	59.5% ATMX; 31.3% placebo; odds ratio = 3.22; 95% CI 1.63–6.41; $P \leq .001$; effect size 0.71

		N	Design	Measures	Dose	Outcomes
Atomoxetine (Strattera)	Michelson et al, 2001	N=297 (212 boys and 85 girls); 8–18 y	Randomized DBPC dose–response for 8 wk	ADHD-RS	0.5 mg/kg/d (9.9 decrease on ADHD-RS pNS, [95% CI, 8.9, 0.9]); 1.2 mg/kg/d (13.6 decrease on ADHD-RS $P<.001$, [95% CI, 12.1, −4.0]); 1.8 mg/kg/d (13.5 decrease on ADHD-RS $P<.001$, [95% CI, 11.9, −3.7])	ATMX superior to placebo in 1.2 mg/kg/d and 1.8 mg/kg/d groups; evidence of a graded dose–response
ATMX	Spencer et al, 2001	N=30; 7–14 y	Open dose-ranging 11 wk	ADHD-RS	1.9 mg/kg/d 10–90 mg	75% of subjects showed $>25\%$ reduction on ADHD-RS scores
Long-term follow-up ATMX	Michelson et al, 2004	N=416	12-wk initial treatment followed by 9-mo open treatment	ADHD-RS Clinical Global Impression-Severity Child Health Questionnaire	1.57mg/kg/d, dosed bid	ATMX longer time to relapse than placebo (218 d versus 146 d)
Safety ATMX	Wernicke et al, 2001	N=142 (112 children ages 7–11 y and 30 adolescents ages 12–17 y)	10-wk open label to establish efficacy followed by an extension for 1 y of open treatment	Laboratory values	Not specified	Only slight increases in DBP and pulse observed; no medication-related QT_c prolongation observed; height and weight increased in both groups

Abbreviations: DBPC, double-blind, placebo-controlled; QT_c, corrected QT interval.

Somnolence, fatigue, weight loss, and decreased appetite occurred significantly more often in ATMX-treated subjects. ATMX's effect size for reducing ADHD-RS scores was 0.7, similar to effect sizes observed in studies using twice-daily dosing. Kelsey and colleagues [68] recently reported that ATMX dosed in either the morning or evening resulted in significant improvements in ADHD symptoms across the day, although ATMX dosed in the evening was better tolerated.

Michelson and colleagues [67] studied the effects of 9 months of treatment with ATMX or placebo on ADHD symptoms. Of 603 subjects completing 12 weeks of open-label treatment, 416 subjects were randomly assigned to continue treatment either with ATMX (n = 292) or with placebo (n = 124). The mean dose at randomization was 1.57 mg/kg/day dosed evenly twice daily. The primary outcome measure was time to relapse, defined as an increase in ADHD-RS total score to 90% of baseline. Subjects randomly assigned to ATMX had a substantially longer time to relapse than those receiving placebo (217.7 ± 5.5 days for ATMX versus 146.1 ± 7.2 days for placebo; $P < .001$). These results add to the literature on long-term pharmacotherapy of ADHD and support the clinical practice of maintaining ongoing pharmacotherapy for ADHD in patients whose symptoms respond to initial treatment.

Although benefit may be seen early in treatment, the full benefit of ATMX may take several weeks. Although plasma levels generally are not used to direct ATMX dosing, a recent presentation correlated ATMX plasma levels and response [69]. ATMX-treated patients with plasma levels above 800 ng/mL showed trends toward greater improvements in ADHD symptomatology, although some patients required dosing up to 2.4 mg/kg/day to achieve this level. Increased rates of adverse events were observed in patients treated with higher doses of ATMX. Because long-term pharmacotherapy of ADHD is often necessary, missed doses of medication can be expected and may be problematic. Wernicke and colleagues [70] studied the effects of sudden discontinuation of ATMX in children and adults. When ATMX was suddenly discontinued in children aged 7 to 12 years who had ADHD and who had been treated with ATMX in divided twice-daily doses up to 2 mg/kg/day, symptoms of ADHD worsened, but few if any discontinuation-emergent adverse events were seen. Tapering ATMX rapidly seems to be safe.

Using atomoxetine with stimulants

Combining ATMX with stimulants has been described in case reports [71], although investigations studying the combination of these medications are underway. Brown [71] recently reported on a case series of four pediatric patients successfully treated with this combination. In two of the cases an extended-delivery stimulant was added to ATMX (27 mg/day OROS-MPH or 20 mg MAS-XR), and in two cases ATMX was added to an extended-delivery stimulant (ATMX dosed at 18 mg/day or 40 mg twice daily). Brown reports tolerability of the combination and positive benefit in all four cases. Reports of significant hepatotoxicity in two patients taking ATMX (of two million patients exposed to

ATMX) have recently been described. Both patients recovered upon discontinuation of ATMX. The manufacturer recently added a bold-face warning to the labeling about hepatotoxicity (http://www.fda.gov/bbs/topics/ANSWERS/2004/ANS01335.html). The warning indicates that ATMX should be discontinued in patients who have jaundice and that patients should contact their doctors if they develop pruritus, jaundice, dark urine, right upper quadrant tenderness, or unexplained flulike symptoms. At this time, laboratory monitoring outside of routine medical care usually is not necessary [72].

Similarly, the impact of ATMX on the cardiovascular system seems to be minimal [73]. ATMX was associated with mean increases in heart rate of 6 beats per minute and increases in SDP and DBP of 1.5 mm Hg. Extensive ECG monitoring indicates that ATMX has no apparent effect on QTc intervals, and ECG monitoring outside of routine medical care does not seem to be necessary.[2]

Bupropion

Bupropion hydrochloride, FDA-approved for treatment of depression and as an aid for smoking cessation in adults, is now available in three forms: immediate release, sustained release, and extended release. Several controlled reports have shown that children and adolescents with ADHD may respond favorably to the immediate-release form of bupropion [74,75]. In addition, bupropion has been studied in small groups of adolescents who have ADHD and nicotine dependence [76] as well as ADHD and depression [77]. In the adult population both the sustained-release and extended-release forms of bupropion have been shown in short-term controlled trials to help reduce symptoms of ADHD [78,79]. Although helpful, the magnitude of effect of bupropion is less than that seen with either stimulants or ATMX.

Neuroimaging indicates bupropion occupies only 22% of dopamine transporter proteins, bringing into question the current understanding of its pharmacodynamic properties [80]. Daviss and colleagues [81] reported on steady-state pharmacokinetics of bupropion in 19 youth aged 13 to 18 years who were prescribed bupropion for ADHD or depressive disorders. In all subjects the mean terminal half-life was 12.1 hours, suggesting the need to dose sustained-release bupropion SR twice daily in the adolescent population.

---

[2] On September 29, 2005, the FDA issued an advisory about a small but statistically significant increase in suicidal thinking in patients treated with atomoxetine. In pooled data from 12 clinical trials, approximately 0.37% of ATMX-treated subjects (5/1357) experienced suicidal thinking compared to none out of 851, and one subject made a nonfatal suicide attempt. Based on this information, the FDA has advised adding a black box warning to ATMX's label. In particular, patients who are started on therapy should be observed closely for clinical worsening, suicidal thinking or behaviors, or unusual changes in behavior. Families and caregivers should be advised to closely observe the patient and to communicate changes or concerning behaviors with the prescriber. This information is contained in the Heath Professional's Advisory issued on September 29, 2005. Updated information can be obtained at http://www.fda.gov.

Bupropion may cause irritability and agitation and has been reported to exacerbate tics [82]. As in adults, the medication should be given in divided doses; no single dose of should exceed 150 mg for the immediate-release formulation, 200 mg for the sustained-release formulation, or 300 mg for the extended-release formulation.

Alpha-adrenergic agonists

Clonidine is an imidazoline derivative with alpha-adrenergic agonist properties; it has been used primarily in the treatment of hypertension [83]. At low doses, it seems to stimulate inhibitory presynaptic autoreceptors in the central nervous system [84]. Although clonidine reduces symptoms of ADHD [85], its overall effect is less than those of the stimulants [86] and probably is smaller than those of atomoxetine, tricyclic antidepressants, and bupropion. Clonidine may be particularly helpful in patients who have ADHD and comorbid conduct or oppositional defiant disorder [87,88], tic disorders [89,90], and ADHD-associated sleep disturbances [53,91]. Current guidelines are to monitor blood pressure when initiating and tapering clonidine treatment, but ECG monitoring usually is not necessary [92].

A clonidine-like but more selective alpha-2 adrenergic agonist compound, guanfacine, has been used as an alternative to clonidine for the same indications [93,94]. Possible advantages of guanfacine over clonidine include less sedation and a longer duration of action. In open-label trials, school-aged children with ADHD and comorbid tic disorder were treated with guanfacine in doses ranging from 0.5 mg twice daily to 1.0 mg three times/day. These patients showed reduction in both tics and ADHD [95]. Recent data from a controlled trial demonstrated the benefit of guanfacine in reducing tic severity and ADHD symptomology [96]. Guanfacine treatment was associated with minor, clinically insignificant, decreases in blood pressure and pulse rate. Adverse effects of guanfacine most commonly include sedation, irritability, and depression. Recently, several cases of apparent guanfacine-induced mania have been described [97].

Novel medications for the treatment of attention-deficit hyperactivity disorder

Multiple novel medications are being investigated for treatment of ADHD. Many of these agents reflect different mechanisms of action to treat ADHD symptoms. Some of the agents currently being investigated are described in Table 4.

Modafinil

A novel stimulant distinct from amphetamine, modafinil is FDA approved for the treatment of narcolepsy [98]. Modafinil seems to activate specific hypothalamic regions [99,100]. Modafinil at 4 mg/kg/day has been shown to improve cognitive and meta-cognitive functioning in healthy, non–sleep-deprived adults [101]. In a controlled study of 20 adults who had ADHD, modafinil treatment improved short-term and visual memory, spatial planning, vigilance, and accuracy while reducing response latency [102]. Published trials of modafinil in the treatment of pediatric ADHD include one 6-week controlled study in 24 youth who had ADHD (5- to 15-year-olds, 15 males, 67% had combined-type ADHD). A mean dose of modafinil (264 ± 50 mg/day) administered as a single morning dose significantly improved ADHD symptoms. Biederman and colleagues [103] presented results of two multisite, double-blind, placebo-controlled trials of modafinil in children who had ADHD. With doses up to 300 mg/day, children who had ADHD experienced significant reductions in ADHD-RS scores. The overall effect size for modafinil was 0.52 when dosed at 200 mg/100 mg and 0.58 when dosed at 300 mg/0. Based on these significant positive results, in December 2004 the makers of modafinil submitted a supplemental new drug indication for treatment of children and adolescents with ADHD (http://www.cephalon.com/research/clinical_research.html). Modafinil has the potential to exacerbate mania [104].

GW320659

Because the neurochemical dysfunction in ADHD seems to be mediated primarily by dopaminergic and adrenergic systems [105], DeVeaugh-Geiss and colleagues [106] studied GW320659, a chemically novel norepinephrine and dopamine reuptake inhibitor. Of 51 subjects entering this study, 46 completed the study and were treated with a mean dose of 14.2 mg/day of GW320659. By the end of the titration and treatment phases, respectively, 65% and 76% of subjects were considered responders. The most common drug-related treatment-emergent adverse events observed included headaches (31%), gastrointestinal discomfort/pain (25%), emotional lability (20%), anorexia (18%), insomnia (14%), and nausea/vomiting (12%). Increases in standing and supine heart rate (10 beats per minute) and supine SBP (5–6 mm Hg) occurred during treatment.

Reboxetine

A selective norepinephrine reuptake inhibitor approved for the treatment of depression in Europe, reboxetine has recently been studied in pediatric ADHD. Ratner and colleagues [106a] studied the effects of reboxetine in 31 youth (25 boys; mean age, 11.7 ± 2.9 years) who had combined-type ADHD. All subjects either did not respond to or could not tolerate treatment with MPH. Reboxetine was started and maintained at 4 mg/day given once daily in the morning. The 24 subjects completing 6 weeks of treatment had significant reductions in ADHD-RS scores beginning by week two and continuing over the ensuing weeks. Ratings of both hyperactivity/impulsivity and inattention improved, and by week two of treatment 70% of the completers were responders. The most common adverse events included drowsiness/sedation (29%), decreased appetite (23%), and gastrointestinal complaints.

Table 4
Recent developments in investigational medications used in pharmacotherapy of pediatric attention-deficit hyperactivity disorder

Generic name (brand name)	Author/ year	N/age range	Design	Primary outcome measure	Total dose	Response rate
Modafinil	Rugino and Samsock, 2003	N = 22 (seven boys and four girls in each group)	6-wk DBPC using flexible dosing to effect	Test of Variable Attention and CPRS CTRS ADHD-RS	N = 4 at 200 mg/d N = 7 at 300 mg/d Dosed once daily in A.M.	10/11 reported significant improvement with modafinil; one subject withdrew because of emesis otherwise no significant AEs noted
Modafinil	Biederman, 2003	N = 191 (boys and girls); 6–13 y	Multisite DBPC; randomization to placebo or one of three doses of modafinil	Teacher completed ADHD-RS	n = 51 placebo n = 48 100/200 n = 49 200/100 n = 50 300/0	New drug application with FDA (submitted 12/04); modafinil dosed A.M. and noon; eight subjects discontinued because of AEs; no significant effects on white blood cell count or absolute neutrophil count noted; significant positive reductions in 200/100 and 300/0 groups from baseline; effect sizes of 0.52 200/100 and 0.58 for 300/0
GW 320659	DeVeaugh-Geiss, 2002	N = 51	Open-label dose titration over 11 wk	CPRS/CTRS and Clinical Global Impression-Improvement	14.2 mg/d	65% responded by end of titration phase and 76% responded by end of treatment
Reboxetine	Ratner et al, 2005	N = 31 (25 males); 8–18 y	6-wk open-label study	ADHD-RS	24 completed study; significant reductions in ADHD-RS and other measures noted by 2 wk of treatment	Reboxetine reduced symptoms of both inattention and hyperactivity/impulsivity; most common side effects were drowsiness, sedation, and gastrointestinal complaints;

Drug	Study	Sample	Design	Rating scales	Dose	Results
					and continued improvement with time; 20/30 with >40% reduction in ADHD-RS and 23/30 with >25% reduction in ADHD-RS	five subjects discontinued because of lack of efficacy
Reboxetine	Mozes et al, 2005	N=15 (11 boys); 5–14 y (mean age, 10.32 ± 2.15 y); hyperkinetic disorder	12-wk open-label trial	CTRS-abbreviated Yudofsky Overt Aggression Scale Plutchick Impulsivity Scale Revised Children's Manifest Anxiety Scale Hamilton Depression Rating Scale	4–8 mg/d Mean dose 4.39 ± 1.76 mg/d	9/15 subjects taking additional psychotropic medications; mean CTRS score reduced from baseline 20.2 ± 6.35 to 9.53 ± 5.15; $P<.0001$; reductions in impulsivity, anxiety, and depression scores noted; no reduction in aggression observed; well tolerated with reduced appetite commonly observed
Selegiline versus MPH	Mohammadi et al, 2004	N=40 (31 boys); 6–15 y	10-wk double-blind randomization to MPH or selegiline	ADHD-RS	MPH initiated at 5 mg bid with max 40 mg/d Selegiline initiated at 2.5 mg bid with maximum of 10 mg/d	MPH and selegiline both significantly improved ADHD symptoms; generally mild AEs with HA and labile mood were seen in two selegiline-treated subjects
Selegiline versus MPH	Akhondzadeh et al, 2003	N=28 (20 boys)	4-wk double-blind trial randomized to either MPH or selegiline	ADHD-RS Teacher and Parent	MPH: 1 mg/kg/d Selegiline: age <5 y (5 mg/d) and age >5 y (10 mg/d)	Both treatments significantly reduced ADHD symptoms per parents and teachers; HA, decreased appetite, and insomnia seen more often in MPH group

(continued on next page)

Table 4 (*continued*)

Generic name (brand name)	Author/ year	N/age range	Design	Primary outcome measure	Total dose	Response rate
Nicotine	Potter and Newhouse, 2004	N=8 nonsmoking adolescents with ADHD	Crossover comparison of transdermal nicotine (7mg patch) versus MPH (mean 0.21 mg/kg/d) versus placebo	Stop-signal reaction time Stroop	Transdermal nicotine patch (7 mg) MPH: 0.21 mg/kg mean Placebo	Three patients experienced severe nausea and vomiting on nicotine which prevented their participation; both nicotine and MPH improved cognitive performance
Theophylline	Mohammadi et al, 2004	N=32	6-wk double-blind randomized to either theophylline or MPH	CTRS CPRS	MPH: 1 mg/kg/d Theophylline: age <12 y (4 mg/kg/d) and age >12 y (3 mg/kg/d)	At 2-, 4-, and 6-wk follow-up both theophylline- and MPH-treated subjects demonstrated improvements in ADHD symptoms per parents and teachers; both treatments well tolerated

Duration of medication trial includes placebo phase.

Abbreviations: AE, adverse events; CPRS, Conners' Parent Rating Scale; CTRS, Conners' Teacher Rating Scale; DBPC, double-blind, placebo-controlled; HA, headache.

Selegiline

An irreversible type B monoamine oxidase inhibitor that is metabolized into amphetamine and methamphetamine, selegiline has recently been compared with MPH in two trials of youth who had ADHD [107,108]. Previous work with selegiline in children who had ADHD and Tourette's syndrome suggested that it may reduce symptoms of ADHD [109,110]. Akhondzadeh and colleagues [108] randomly assigned 28 children (aged 4–9 years; mean age, 7.36 ± 1.46 years; 20 boys) who had combined-type ADHD to 4 weeks of treatment with either MPH (titrated to 1 mg/kg/day) or selegiline (5 mg/day if aged <5 years or 10 mg/day if aged >5 years). Twenty-three subjects completed the study. Both treatments resulted in significant and similar reductions in parent-evaluated and teacher-evaluated ADHD-RS scores. Similar percentages of responders were seen in both groups (57.14% for selegiline versus 42.85% for MPH). Both treatments were well tolerated. Significantly more MPH-treated subjects reported headache, decreased appetite, and difficulty falling asleep. Using a similar design, Mohammadi and colleagues [107] randomly allocated 40 youth (aged 6–15 years; 31 boys) who had ADHD to 10 weeks of double-blind treatment with either MPH (starting dose, 5 mg two times/day titrated to 1 mg/kg/day or 40 mg/day) or selegiline (starting dose, 2.5 mg two times/day titrated to a maximum of 10 mg/day). Both treatments led to significant reductions, of similar magnitude, in parent-evaluated and teacher-evaluated ADHD-RS scores. Anorexia, insomnia, and headache were seen more often in MPH-treated subjects. Potentially life-threatening reactions with tyramine-rich foods, such as cheese, impede the use of selegiline in children unlikely to remember or adhere to these diet restrictions.

Anti-Alzheimer agents

Medications used to slow decline in Alzheimer's disease have also generated interest in enhancing cognition and in the treatment of ADHD. Although cholinergic modulation of temporal memory has been investigated [111], the effects of cholinergic-enhancing agents on ADHD remain unclear [112]. To date, studies involving the short- and long-term safety, tolerability, and efficacy of newer cognitive-enhancing medications (eg, donepezil, galantamine, revastigmine, memantine) in youth are limited to case series [113] or investigational agents [114].

Nicotinic agents

Based on the high rates of cigarette smoking in adolescents who have ADHD [115] and the cognitive-enhancing properties of nicotine [116], Potter and colleagues [117] compared the effects of transdermal nicotine, MPH, and placebo on measures of behavioral inhibition in eight nonsmoking adolescents who had ADHD. Single administrations of either nicotine or MPH, in doses of 7 mg and 10 to 20 mg (0.15–0.21 mg/kg), respectively, resulted in improvements in stop-signal reaction time. Nicotine, but not MPH, decreased the Stroop effect (interference by irrelevant stimuli) compared with placebo. These results support the neurobiologic hypothesis of impaired fronto-strial attentional networks. Although cigarette smoking remains an ongoing challenge in the treatment of adolescents who have ADHD, nicotine is, at this point, not a viable or recommended treatment. The nicotinic system remains a potential target for development of novel treatments, however.

Theophylline

An adenosine receptor antagonist, theophylline is a psychostimulant widely used as a bronchodilator. Antagonism of adenosine receptors seems to have effects on central dopaminergic and noradrenergic neurotransmission and may have benefit in a variety of neuropsychiatric conditions such as ADHD [118,119]. Mohammadi and colleagues [120] studied the efficacy of theophylline in the treatment of 32 newly diagnosed youth (aged 6–14 years; 22 boys) who had combined-type ADHD. Subjects were randomly assigned to 6 weeks of treatment with either theophylline (<12 years old, 4 mg/kg/day; >12 years old, 3 mg/kg/day) or MPH (1 mg/kg/day). Both treatments resulted in significant linear reductions of similar magitude in parent-evaluated and teacher-evaluated ADHD-RS scores. Both treatments seemed to be well tolerated, with decreased appetite, sleep disturbances, and palpitations reported in both groups. These pilot data support role for theophylline as a potential treatment for pediatric ADHD.

Summary

The pharmacology of ADHD is directly related to the pathogenesis of ADHD. The neurochemical dysfunction in ADHD seems to be mediated by dopaminergic and adrenergic systems with little direct influence by the serotonergic systems [105,121–123]. The aggregate literature indicates effective pharmacologic treatments for pediatric ADHD include the use of the psychostimulants and ATMX. Bupropion, modafinil, and tricyclic antidepressants have been studied in the treatment of adult ADHD and have a secondary role in treatment. Although interest remains high, data on the efficacy of cognitive enhancers remain minimal, and their role is limited. Further controlled investigations assessing the efficacy of single and combination agents for adults who have ADHD are necessary, with careful attention to diagnostics, comorbidity, symptom and neuropsychologic outcomes, long-term tolerability and efficacy, and use in specific ADHD subgroups.

References

[1] Pediatrics AAO Committee on Quality Improvement SoA-DHD. Diagnosis and evaluation of the child with attention-deficit/hyperactivity disorder. Pediatrics 2000;105:1158–70.

[2] Faraone SV, Sergeant J, Gillberg C, et al. The worldwide prevalence of ADHD: is it an American condition? World Psychiatry 2003;2(2):104–13.

[3] Biederman J, Faraone SV. Attention deficit hyperactivity disorder: a worldwide concern. J Nerv Ment Dis 2004;192(7):453–4.

[4] Goldman L, Genel M, Bezman R, et al. Diagnosis and treatment of attention-deficit/ hyperactivity disorder in children and adolescents. JAMA 1998;279(14):1100–7.

[5] Wilens T, Biederman J, Spencer T. Attention deficit hyperactivity disorder. Annu Rev Med 2002;53:113–31.

[6] Biederman J, Faraone S, Mick E. Age dependent decline of ADHD symptoms revisited: impact of remission definition and symptom subtype. Am J Psychiatry 2000;157:816–7.

[7] National Institute of Mental Health Multimodal Treatment Study of ADHD follow-up: 24-month outcomes of treatment strategies for attention-deficit/hyperactivity disorder. Pediatrics 2004;113(4):754–61.

[8] Greenhill LL, Pliszka S, Dulcan MK, et al. Practice parameter for the use of stimulant medications in the treatment of children, adolescents, and adults. J Am Acad Child Adolesc Psychiatry 2002;41(2 Suppl):26S–49S.

[9] Clinical practice guideline: treatment of the school-aged child with attention-deficit/hyper-activity disorder. Pediatrics 2001;108(4):1033–44.

[10] Dulcan M. Practice parameters for the assessment and treatment of children, adolescents, and adults with attention-deficit/hyperactivity disorder. J Am Acad Child Adolesc Psychiatry 1997;36(10):85S–121S.

[11] Olfson M, Gameroff MJ, Marcus SC, et al. National trends in the treatment of attention deficit hyperactivity disorder. Am J Psychiatry 2003;160(6):1071–7.

[12] Bradley C. The behavior of children receiving benzedrine. Am J Psychiatry 1937;94:577–85.

[13] Swanson J, Gupta S, Lam A, et al. Development of a new once-a-day formulation of methyl-phenidate for the treatment of attention-deficit/hyperactivity disorder: proof-of-concept and proof-of-product studies. Arch Gen Psychiatry 2003;60(2):204–11.

[14] Pelham WE, Gnagy EM, Burrows-Maclean L, et al. Once-a-day Concerta methylphenidate versus three-times-daily methylphenidate in laboratory and natural settings. Pediatrics 2001; 107(6):E105.

[15] Wolraich ML, Greenhill LL, Pelham W, et al. Randomized, controlled trial of OROS methyl-phenidate once a day in children with attention-deficit/hyperactivity disorder. Pediatrics 2001; 108(4):883–92.

[16] Swanson JM, Gupta S, Williams L, et al. Efficacy of a new pattern of delivery of methyl-phenidate for the treatment of ADHD: effects on activity level in the classroom and on the playground. J Am Acad Child Adolesc Psychiatry 2002;41(11):1306–14.

[17] Multimodal Treatment Study of Children with ADHD Group. A 14-month randomized clinical trial of treatment strategies for attention-deficit/hyperactivity disorder. The MTA Cooperative Group. Multimodal Treatment Study of Children with ADHD. Arch Gen Psychiatry 1999; 56(12):1073–86.

[18] Stein MA, Sarampote CS, Waldman ID, et al. A dose-response study of OROS methylphe-nidate in children with attention-deficit/hyperactivity disorder. Pediatrics 2003;112(5):e404.

[19] Greenhill L. Efficacy and safety of OROS methylphenidate in adolescents with ADHD. Presented at the 49th Annual Meeting of the American Academy of Child and Adolescent Psychiatry. San Francisco (CA), October 22–27, 2002.

[19a] Steele M, Riccardelli R, Binder C. Effectiveness of OROS®-methylphenidate vs. usual care with immediate-release methylphenidate in ADHD children. Presented at the American Psy-chiatric Association Annual Meeting. New York (NY), May 1–6, 2004.

[20] Wilens T, Pelham W, Stein M, et al. ADHD treatment with once-daily OROS methylphe-nidate: interim 12-month results from a long-term open-label study. J Am Acad Child Adolesc Psychiatry 2003;42(4):424–33.

[21] Wilens T, Pelham W, Stein M, et al. ADHD treatment with a once-daily formulation of methylphenidate hydrochloride: a two-year study. Presented at the 155th Annual Meeting of the American Psychiatric Association. Philadelphia (PA), May 18–23, 2002.

[22] Greenhill LL, Findling RL, Swanson JM, for the ADHD Study Group. A double-blind, placebo-controlled study of modified-release methylphenidate in children with attention-deficit/hyperactivity disorder. Pediatrics 2002;109(3):E39.

[22a] Biederman J, Quinn D, Weiss M, et al. Efficacy and safety of Ritalin LA, a new, once daily, extended-release dosage form of methylphenidate, in children with attention deficit hyperactivity disorder. Paediatr Drugs 2003;5:833–41.

[23] Patrick KS, Caldwell RW, Ferris RM, et al. Pharmacology of the enantiomers of threo-methylphenidate. J Pharmacol Exper Ther 1987;241(1):152–8.

[24] Ding YS, Fowler JS, Volkow ND, et al. Chiral drugs: comparison of the pharmacokinetics of [11C]D-threo and L-threo-methylphenidate in the human and baboon brain. Psychopharmacology (Berl) 1997;131(1):71–8.

[25] Ding YS, Gatley SJ, Thanos PK, et al. Brain kinetics of methylphenidate (Ritalin) enantiomers after oral administration. Synapse 2004;53(3):168–75.

[26] Quinn D, Wigal S, Swanson J, et al. Comparative pharmacodynamics and plasma concentrations of D-threo-methylphenidate hydrochloride after single doses of D-threo-methylphenidate hydrochloride and D,l-threo-methylphenidate hydrochloride in a double-blind, placebo-controlled, crossover laboratory school study in children with attention-deficit/hyperactivity disorder. J Am Acad Child Adolesc Psychiatry 2004;43(11):1422–9.

[27] Silva R, Tilker HA, Cecil JT, et al. Open-label study of dexmethylphenidate hydrochloride in children and adolescents with attention deficit hyperactivity disorder. J Child Adolesc Psychopharmacol 2004;14(4):555–63.

[28] Wigal S, Swanson JM, Feifel D, et al. A double-blind, placebo-controlled trial of dexmethylphenidate hydrochloride and D,l-threo-methylphenidate hydrochloride in children with attention-deficit/hyperactivity disorder. J Am Acad Child Adolesc Psychiatry 2004;43(11):1406–14.

[29] Arnold LE, Lindsay RL, Conners CK, et al. A double-blind, placebo-controlled withdrawal trial of dexmethylphenidate hydrochloride in children with attention deficit hyperactivity disorder. J Child Adolesc Psychopharmacol 2004;14(4):542–54.

[30] Greenhill L, Ball R, Levine AJ, et al. Extended-release dexmethylphenidate in children and adolescents with ADHD. Presented at the 158th Annual Meeting of the American Psychiatric Association. Atlanta (GA), 2005.

[31] Pelham WE, Manos MJ, Ezzell CE, et al. A dose-ranging study of a methylphenidate transdermal system in children with ADHD. J Am Acad Child Adolesc Psychiatry 2005;44(6):522–9.

[32] Pliszka SR, Browne RG, Olvera RL, et al. A double-blind, placebo-controlled study of Adderall and methylphenidate in the treatment of attention-deficit/hyperactivity disorder. J Am Acad Child Adolesc Psychiatry 2000;39(5):619–26.

[33] Greenhill LL, Swanson JM, Steinhoff K, et al. A pharmacokinetic/pharmacodynamic study comparing a single morning dose of adderall to twice-daily dosing in children with ADHD. J Am Acad Child Adolesc Psychiatry 2003;42(10):1234–41.

[34] Ahmann PA, Theye FW, Berg R, et al. Placebo-controlled evaluation of amphetamine mixture-dextroamphetamine salts and amphetamine salts (Adderall): efficacy rate and side effects. Pediatrics 2001;107(1):E10.

[35] McGough JJ, Biederman J, Greenhill LL, et al. Pharmacokinetics of SLI381 (ADDERALL XR), an extended-release formulation of Adderall. J Am Acad Child Adolesc Psychiatry 2003;42(6):684–91.

[36] McCracken JT, Biederman J, Greenhill LL, et al. Analog classroom assessment of a once-daily mixed amphetamine formulation, SLI381 (Adderall XR), in children with ADHD. J Am Acad Child Adolesc Psychiatry 2003;42(6):673–83.

[37] Biederman J, Lopez FA, Boellner SW, et al. A randomized, double-blind, placebo-controlled, parallel-group study of SLI381 (Adderal XR) in children with attention-deficit/hyperactivity disorder. Pediatrics 2002;110(2 Pt 1):258–66.

[38] McGough JJ, Biederman J, Wigal SB, et al. Long-term tolerability and effectiveness of once-daily mixed amphetamine salts (Adderall XR) in children with ADHD. J Am Acad Child Adolesc Psychiatry 2005;44(6):530–8.

[39] Sallee FR, Stiller RL, Perel JM. Pharmacodynamics of pemoline in attention deficit disorder with hyperactivity. J Am Acad Child Adolesc Psychiatry 1992;31:244–51.

[40] Patrick KS, Markowitz JS. Pharmacology of methylphenidate, amphetamine enantiomers and pemoline in attention-deficit hyperactivity disorder. Hum Psychopharmacol 1997;12:527–46.

[41] Safer DJ, Zito JM, Gardner JE. Pemoline hepatotoxicity and postmarketing surveillance. J Am Acad Child Adolesc Psychiatry 2001;40(6):622–9.

[42] Willy ME, Manda B, Shatin D, et al. A study of compliance with FDA recommendations for pemoline (Cylert) [comment]. J Am Acad Child Adolesc Psychiatry 2002;41(7):785–90.

[43] Rapport MD, Moffitt C. Attention deficit/hyperactivity disorder and methylphenidate. A review of height/weight, cardiovascular, and somatic complaint side effects. Clin Psychol Rev 2002; 22(8):1107–31.

[44] Findling RL, Short EJ, Manos MJ. Short-term cardiovascular effects of methylphenidate and Adderall. J Am Acad Child Adolesc Psychiatry 2001;40(5):525–9.

[45] Stowe CD, Gardner SF, Gist CC, et al. 24-hour ambulatory blood pressure monitoring in male children receiving stimulant therapy. Ann Pharmacother 2002;36(7–8):1142–9.

[46] Wilens TE, Biederman J, Lerner M. Effects of once-daily osmotic-release methylphenidate on blood pressure and heart rate in children with attention-deficit/hyperactivity disorder: results from a one-year follow-up study. J Clin Psychopharmacol 2004;24(1):36–41.

[47] Wilens T, Spencer TJ, Biederman J, et al. Mixed amphetamine salts XR: cardiovascular safety in adolescents with ADHD. Presented at the 158th Annual Meeting of the American Psychiatric Association. Atlanta (GA), 2005.

[48] Corkum P, Tannock R, Moldofsky H, et al. Actigraphy and parental ratings of sleep in children with attention-deficit/hyperactivity disorder (ADHD). Sleep 2001;24(3):303–12.

[49] Mick E, Biederman J, Jetton J, et al. Sleep disturbances associated with attention deficit hyperactivity disorder: the impact of psychiatric comorbidity and pharmacotherapy. J Child Adolesc Psychopharmacol 2000;10(3):223–31.

[50] Stein MA. Unravelling sleep problems in treated and untreated children with ADHD [comment]. J Child Adolesc Psychopharmacol 1999;9(3):157–68.

[51] Cohen-Zion M, Ancoli-Israel S. Sleep in children with attention-deficit hyperactivity disorder (ADHD): a review of naturalistic and stimulant intervention studies. Sleep Med Rev 2004;8(5): 379–402.

[52] O'Brien LM, Ivanenko A, Crabtree VM, et al. Sleep disturbances in children with attention deficit hyperactivity disorder. Pediatr Res 2003;54(2):237–43.

[53] Prince J, Wilens T, Biederman J, et al. Clonidine for sleep disturbances associated with attention-deficit hyperactivity disorder: a systematic chart review of 62 cases. J Am Acad Child Adolesc Psychiatry 1996;35(5):599–605.

[54] Smits MG, van Stel HF, van der Heijden K, et al. Melatonin improves health status and sleep in children with idiopathic chronic sleep-onset insomnia: a randomized placebo-controlled trial. J Am Acad Child Adolesc Psychiatry 2003;42(11):1286–93.

[55] Macchi MM, Bruce JN. Human pineal physiology and functional significance of melatonin. Front Neuroendocrinol 2004;25(3–4):177–95.

[56] Tjon Pian Gi CV, Broeren JP, Starreveld JS, et al. Melatonin for treatment of sleeping disorders in children with attention deficit/hyperactivity disorder: a preliminary open label study. Eur J Pediatr 2003;162(7–8):554–5.

[57] Physicians Desk Reference. Montvale (NJ): Medical Economics Data Production Company; 2005.

[58] Daviss WB, Scott J. A chart review of cyproheptadine for stimulant-induced weight loss. J Child Adolesc Psychopharmacol 2004;14(1):65–73.

[59] National Institute of Mental Health Multimodal Treatment Study of ADHD follow-up: changes in effectiveness and growth after the end of treatment. Pediatrics 2004;113(4):762–9.

[60] Biederman J, Faraone SV, Monuteaux MC, et al. Growth deficits and attention-deficit/hyperactivity disorder revisited: impact of gender, development, and treatment. Pediatrics 2003; 111(5 Pt 1):1010–6.

[61] Spencer TJ, Biederman J, Harding M, et al. Growth deficits in ADHD children revisited:

evidence for disorder-associated growth delays? J Am Acad Child Adolesc Psychiatry 1996; 35(11):1460–9.

[62] Spencer T, Biederman J, Wilens T, et al. Effectiveness and tolerability of tomoxetine in adults with attention deficit hyperactivity disorder. Am J Psychiatry 1998;155(5):693–5.

[63] Spencer T, Heiligenstein JH, Biederman J, et al. Results from 2 proof-of-concept, placebo-controlled studies of atomoxetine in children with attention-deficit/hyperactivity disorder. J Clin Psychiatry 2002;63(12):1140–7.

[64] Michelson D, Faries D, Wernicke J, et al. Atomoxetine in the treatment of children and adolescents with attention-deficit/hyperactivity disorder: a randomized, placebo-controlled, dose-response study. Pediatrics 2001;108(5):E83.

[65] Michelson D, Allen AJ, Busner J, et al. Once-daily atomoxetine treatment for children and adolescents with attention deficit hyperactivity disorder: a randomized, placebo-controlled study. Am J Psychiatry 2002;159(11):1896–901.

[66] Kelsey DK, Sumner CR, Casat CD, et al. Once-daily atomoxetine treatment for children with attention-deficit/hyperactivity disorder, including an assessment of evening and morning behavior: a double-blind, placebo-controlled trial. Pediatrics 2004;114(1):e1–8.

[67] Michelson D, Buitelaar JK, Danckaerts M, et al. Relapse prevention in pediatric patients with ADHD treated with atomoxetine: a randomized, double-blind, placebo-controlled study. J Am Acad Child Adolesc Psychiatry 2004;43(7):896–904.

[68] Kelsey D, Sutton V, Lewis D, et al. Morning-dosed versus evening-dosed atomoxetine for treating ADHD in children. Presented at the 158th Annual Meeting of the American Psychiatric Association. Atlanta (GA), 2005.

[69] Dunn DW, Turgay A, Weiss M, et al. Use of plasma concentration to guide atomoxetine doses in ADHD patients. Presented at the 158th Annual Meeting of the American Psychiatric Association. Atlanta (GA), 2005.

[70] Wernicke JF, Adler L, Spencer T, et al. Changes in symptoms and adverse events after discontinuation of atomoxetine in children and adults with attention deficit/hyperactivity disorder: a prospective, placebo-controlled assessment. J Clin Psychopharmacol 2004;24(1):30–5.

[71] Brown TE. Atomoxetine and stimulants in combination for treatment of attention deficit hyperactivity disorder: four case reports. J Child Adolesc Psychopharmacol 2004;14(1):129–36.

[72] Wernicke JF, Kratochvil CJ. Safety profile of atomoxetine in the treatment of children and adolescents with ADHD. J Clin Psychiatry 2002;63(Suppl 12):50–5.

[73] Wernicke JF, Faries D, Girod D, et al. Cardiovascular effects of atomoxetine in children, adolescents, and adults. Drug Saf 2003;26(10):729–40.

[74] Conners CK, Casat CD, Gualtieri CT, et al. Bupropion hydrochloride in attention deficit disorder with hyperactivity. J Am Acad Child Adolesc Psychiatry 1996;35(10):1314–21.

[75] Barrickman L, Perry P, Allen A, et al. Bupropion versus methylphenidate in the treatment of attention-deficit hyperactivity disorder. J Am Acad Child Adolesc Psychiatry 1995;34(5):649–57.

[76] Upadhyaya HP, Brady KT, Wang W. Bupropion SR in adolescents with comorbid ADHD and nicotine dependence: a pilot study. J Am Acad Child Adolesc Psychiatry 2004;43(2):199–205.

[77] Daviss WB, Bentivoglio P, Racusin R, et al. Bupropion sustained release in adolescents with comorbid attention-deficit/hyperactivity disorder and depression. J Am Acad Child Adolesc Psychiatry 2001;40(3):307–14.

[78] Wilens TE, Spencer TJ, Biederman J, et al. A controlled clinical trial of bupropion for attention deficit hyperactivity disorder in adults. Am J Psychiatry 2001;158(2):282–8.

[79] Wilens TE, Haight BR, Horrigan JP, et al. Bupropion XL in adults with attention-deficit/hyperactivity disorder: a randomized, placebo-controlled study. Biol Psychiatry 2005;57(7):793–801.

[80] Meyer JH, Goulding VS, Wilson AA, et al. Bupropion occupancy of the dopamine transporter is low during clinical treatment. Psychopharmacology (Berl) 2002;163(1):102–5.

[81] Daviss WB, Perel JM, Rudolph GR, et al. Steady-state pharmacokinetics of bupropion SR in juvenile patients. J Am Acad Child Adolesc Psychiatry 2005;44(4):349–57.

[82] Spencer T, Biederman J, Steingard R, et al. Bupropion exacerbates tics in children with

attention deficit hyperactivity disorder and Tourette's disorder. J Am Acad Child Adolesc Psychiatry 1993;32(1):211–4.

[83] Roden DM, Nadeau JHJ, Primm RK. Electrophysiologic and hemodynamic effects of chronic oral therapy with the alpha₂-agonists clonidine and tiamenidine in hypertensive volunteers. Clin Pharmacol Ther 1988;43:648–54.

[84] Buccafusco JJ. Neuropharmacologic and behavioral actions of clonidine: interactions with central neurotransmitters. Int Rev Neurobiol 1992;33:55–107.

[85] Hunt RD, Inderaa RB, Cohen DJ. The therapeutic effect of clonidine and attention deficit disorder with hyperactivity: a comparison with placebo and methylphenidate. Psychopharmacol Bull 1986;22(1):229–36.

[86] Connor DF, Fletcher KE, Swanson JM. A meta-analysis of clonidine for symptoms of attention-deficit hyperactivity disorder. J Am Acad Child Adolesc Psychiatry 1999;38(12):1551–9.

[87] Connor DF, Barkley RA, Davis HT. A pilot study of methylphenidate, clonidine, or the combination in ADHD comorbid with aggressive oppositional defiant or conduct disorder. Clin Pediatr (Phila) 2000;39(1):15–25.

[88] Schvehla TJ, Mandoki MW, Sumner GS. Clonidine therapy for comorbid attention deficit hyperactivity disorder and conduct disorder: preliminary findings in a children's inpatient unit. South Med J 1994;87(7):692–5.

[89] Singer HV, Brown J, Quaskey S, et al. The treatment of attention-deficit hyperactivity disorder in Tourette's syndrome: a double-blind placebo controlled study with clonidine and desipramine. Pediatrics 1995;95:74–81.

[90] Steingard R, Biederman J, Spencer T, et al. Comparison of clonidine response in the treatment of attention deficit hyperactivity disorder with and without comorbid tic disorders. J Am Acad Child Adolesc Psychiatry 1993;32:350–3.

[91] Wilens TE, Biederman J, Spencer T. Clonidine for sleep disturbances associated with attention deficit hyperactivity disorder. J Am Acad Child Adolesc Psychiatry 1994;33:424–6.

[92] Gutgesell H, Atkins D, Barst R, et al. AHA scientific statement: cardiovascular monitoring of children and adolescents receiving psychotropic drugs. J Am Acad Child Adolesc Psychiatry 1999;38(8):979–82.

[93] Chappell PB, Riddle MA, Scahill L, et al. Guanfacine treatment of comorbid attention-deficit hyperactivity disorder and Tourette's syndrome: preliminary clinical experience. J Am Acad Child Adolesc Psychiatry 1995;34(9):1140–6.

[94] Horrigan JP, Barnhill LJ. Guanfacine for treatment of attention-deficit hyperactivity disorder in boys. J Child Adolesc Psychopharmacol 1995;5(3):215–23.

[95] Scahill L. Controlled clinical trial of guanfacine in ADHD youth with tic disorders. Presented at the 2000 Meeting of the New Clinical Drug Evaluation Unit. Boca Raton (FL), May 30–June 2, 2000.

[96] Scahill L, Chappell PB, Kim YS, et al. A placebo-controlled study of guanfacine in the treatment of children with tic disorders and attention deficit hyperactivity disorder. Am J Psychiatry 2001;158(7):1067–74.

[97] Horrigan JP, Barnhill LJ. Guanfacine and secondary mania in children. J Affect Disord 1999; 54(3):309–14.

[98] US Modafinil in Narcolepsy Multicenter Study Group. Randomized trial of modafinil for the treatment of pathological somnolence in narcolepsy. Ann Neurol 1998;43(1):88–97.

[99] Lin JS, Hou Y, Jouvet M. Potential brain neuronal targets for amphetamine-, methylphenidate-, and modafinil-induced wakefulness, evidenced by c-focs immunocytochemistry in the cat. Proc Natl Acad Sci U S A 1996;93:14128–33.

[100] Lin JS, Gervasoni D, Hou Y, et al. Effects of amphetamine and modafinil on the sleep/wake cycle during experimental hypersomnia induced by sleep deprivation in the cat. J Sleep Res 2000;9(1):89–96.

[101] Baranski JV, Pigeau R, Dinich P, et al. Effects of modafinil on cognitive and meta-cognitive performance. Hum Psychopharmacol 2004;19(5):323–32.

[102] Turner DC, Clark L, Dowson J, et al. Modafinil improves cognition and response inhibition in adult attention-deficit/hyperactivity disorder. Biol Psychiatry 2004;55(10):1031–40.

[103] Biederman J. A double-blind placebo-controlled trial of modafinil in the treatment of attention-deficit/hyperactivity disorder. Presented at the 2003 Annual Meeting of the American Psychiatric Association. San Francisco (CA), 2003.

[104] Vorspan F, Warot D, Consoli A, et al. Mania in a boy treated with modafinil for narcolepsy. Am J Psychiatry 2005;162(4):813–4.

[105] Zametkin A, Liotta W. The neurobiology of attention-deficit/hyperactivity disorder. J Clin Psychiatry 1998;59(7):17–23.

[106] DeVeaugh-Geiss J, Conners CK, Sarkis EH, et al. GW320659 for the treatment of attention-deficit/hyperactivity disorder in children. J Am Acad Child Adolesc Psychiatry 2002;41(8): 914–20.

[106a] Ratner S, Laor N, Bronstein Y, et al. Six-week open-label reboxetine treatment in children and adolescents with attention-deficit/hyperactivity disorder. J Am Acad Child Adolesc Psychiatry 2005;44:428–33.

[107] Mohammadi MR, Ghanizadeh A, Alaghband-Rad J, et al. Selegiline in comparison with methylphenidate in attention deficit hyperactivity disorder children and adolescents in a double-blind, randomized clinical trial. J Child Adolesc Psychopharmacol 2004;14(3):418–25.

[108] Akhondzadeh S, Tavakolian R, Davari-Ashtiani R, et al. Selegiline in the treatment of attention deficit hyperactivity disorder in children: a double blind and randomized trial. Prog Neuropsychopharmacol Biol Psychiatry 2003;27(5):841–5.

[109] Feigin A, Kurlan R, McDermott MP, et al. A controlled trial of deprenyl in children with Tourette's syndrome and attention deficit hyperactivity disorder. Neurology 1996;46(4): 965–8.

[110] Jankovic J. Deprenyl in attention deficit associated with Tourette's syndrome. Arch Neurol 1993;50:286–8.

[111] Meck W, Church R. Cholinergic modulation of the content of temporal memory. Behav Neuroci 1987;101(4):457–64.

[112] Narahashi T, Moriguchi S, Zhao X, et al. Mechanisms of action of cognitive enhancers on neuroreceptors. Biol Pharm Bull 2004;27(11):1701–6.

[113] Wilens TE, Biederman J, Wong J, et al. Adjunctive donepezil in attention deficit hyperactivity disorder youth: case series. J Child Adolesc Psychopharmacol 2000;10(3):217–22.

[114] Wilens T, Biederman J, Spencer T, et al. A pilot controlled clinical trial of ABT-418, a cholinergic agonist, in the treatment of adults with attention deficit hyperactivity disorder. Am J Psychiatry 1999;156:1931–7.

[115] Pomerleau O, Downey K, Stelson F, et al. Cigarette smoking in adult patients diagnosed with attention deficit hyperactivity disorder. J Subst Abuse 1995;7:373–8.

[116] Rezvani AH, Levin ED. Cognitive effects of nicotine. Biol Psychiatry 2001;49(3):258–67.

[117] Potter AS, Newhouse PA. Effects of acute nicotine administration on behavioral inhibition in adolescents with attention-deficit/hyperactivity disorder. Psychopharmacology (Berl) 2004; 176(2):182–94.

[118] Guieu R, Couraud F, Pouget J, et al. Adenosine and the nervous system: clinical implications. Clin Neuropharmacol 1996;19(6):459–74.

[119] Higgins MJ, Hosseinzadeh H, MacGregor DG, et al. Release and actions of adenosine in the central nervous system. Pharm World Sci 1994;16(2):62–8.

[120] Mohammadi MR, Kashani L, Akhondzadeh S, et al. Efficacy of theophylline compared to methylphenidate for the treatment of attention-deficit hyperactivity disorder in children and adolescents: a pilot double-blind randomized trial. J Clin Pharm Ther 2004;29(2):139–44.

[121] Wilens T, Spencer T. Pharmacology of amphetamines. In: Tarter R, Ammerman R, Ott P, editors. Handbook of substance abuse: neurobehavioral pharmacology. New York: Plenum Press; 1998. p. 501–13.

[122] Elia J, Borcherding BG, Potter WZ, et al. Stimulant drug treatment of hyperactivity: biochemical correlates. Clin Pharmacol Ther 1990;48:57–66.

[123] Volkow ND, Wang GJ, Fowler JS, et al. Therapeutic doses of oral methylphenidate significantly increase extracellular dopamine in human brain. J Neurosci 2001;21:1–5.

ELSEVIER
SAUNDERS

Child Adolesc Psychiatric Clin N Am
15 (2006) 51–71

CHILD AND
ADOLESCENT
PSYCHIATRIC CLINICS
OF NORTH AMERICA

Psychopharmacology Interventions for Pediatric Anxiety Disorders: A Research Update

Bruce Waslick, MD[a,b,*]

[a]Department of Psychiatry, Baystate Medical Center, 759 Chestnut Street, Springfield,
MA 01199, USA
[b]Tufts University School of Medicine, Boston, MA, USA

During the past 2 decades, significant progress has been made in a variety of treatment approaches for youth who have anxiety disorders. Simple short-term, randomized clinical trials (RCTs) have been designed and completed demonstrating that pharmacotherapy approaches and psychosocial interventions are potentially safe and effective for youth who have a variety of anxiety disorders. Recently, collaborations between pharmacotherapy researchers and psychotherapy researchers have led to a new generation of comparative RCTs comparing monotherapies (psychotherapy or medication alone) with each other and with combination treatments (psychotherapy plus medication therapy). This article presents the recent progress made in research studies attempting to understand therapeutic approaches to the various pediatric anxiety disorders, with the primary focus on medication modalities. The spectrum of pediatric anxiety disorders, based on the *Diagnostic and Statistical Manual–Fourth Edition, Text Revision (DSM-IV-TR)* [1], are reviewed, with the exception of specific phobia, which generally does not require pharmacologic management in clinical practice. This article relies on recent RCTs to examine the efficacy, risks, and adverse events associated with each medication class. The goal is to provide a solid foundation of information for practitioners to make evidence-based decisions regarding treatment strategies for anxious children and adolescents. The focus here is on published studies, because such reports have generally passed through

Dr. Waslick has received research funding support from the National Institute of Mental Health, Eli Lilly and Company, and Johnson and Johnson, Co. He has served as a paid consultant to Astra-Zeneca.

* Department of Psychiatry, Baystate Medical Center, 759 Chestnut Street, Springfield, MA 01199.

E-mail address: bdw7@columbia.edu

the peer review process that may be absent in posters or preliminary presentations at scientific meetings. Additionally, gaps in current knowledge and suggestions for future research efforts are provided.

Pharmacologic treatment of separation anxiety disorder, generalized anxiety disorder, and social phobia

Overview and initial studies

Separation anxiety disorder (SAD), generalized anxiety disorder (GAD), and social phobia (SPh) are commonly occurring anxiety disorders of childhood, frequent causes of child distress and functional impairment, and regular reasons for referral of children to mental health practitioners. Excellent reviews of the phenomenology, causation, natural history, and diagnostic considerations of these important pediatric anxiety disorders are available [2,3]. These conditions are included together in this section for several reasons:

1. They commonly co-occur in clinical practice.
2. The available medication treatments probably target common underlying neurophysiologic processes.
3. Several important RCTs have been conducted in populations that have any one or combinations of the three disorders.

The landmark National Institute of Mental Health–funded Research Units in Pediatric Psychopharmacology (RUPP) fluvoxamine study is presented in greater detail, including the results of its acute-phase trial, the work on defining moderators and mediators of acute treatment response, and the longer-term follow-on study of treatment responders and nonresponders.

Tricyclic antidepressants

There are few published RCTs examining the use of tricyclic antidepressants (TCAs) for youth who have SAD, GAD, and SPh. The evidence supporting the efficacy of TCAs for these disorders is mixed. One early study suggested that imipramine might be helpful for children who have "school phobia," most of whom seemed to be primarily suffering from SAD [4]. Other early studies examining the role of clomipramine and imipramine for children who have school phobia found no difference between those treated with active medication or placebo [5,6]. Klein and colleagues [7] failed to replicate an earlier finding that imipramine was beneficial for pediatric patients who had SAD and who had failed to respond to a short, intensive, behaviorally oriented psychosocial intervention. Although the study was admittedly underpowered, with only 21 subjects recruited into the RCT phase, little evidence is available from the results of this study to suggest that the risk–benefit ratio of imipramine for this disorder is favorable. Approximately half of the subjects in each group were better at the end of the 6-week medication phase. Bernstein and colleagues [8] found that pediatric patients who had a history of school refusal and who also met criteria for both an anxiety and mood disorder responded better in the short run to symptom-focused CBT combined with imipramine than to CBT plus placebo (described later), but overall there is little empiric support at present for the use of TCAs as a stand-alone treatment for pediatric SAD, GAD, or SPh.

Benzodiazepines

Few published reports are available on well-designed, well-controlled investigations of the use of benzodiazepines for pediatric anxiety disorders. Despite some initial evidence from an open-label trial suggesting that pediatric patients who exhibited school refusal and underlying anxiety problems benefited from treatment with alprazolam, a follow-up RCT found no statistically significant benefit for alprazolam compared with placebo once baseline anxiety scores were factored in as a covariate [5]. Similarly, despite some promising results from an open-label preliminary trial, when Simeon and colleagues [9] enrolled subjects who had *DSM-III* diagnoses of overanxious disorder (similar to *DSM-IV* GAD) and avoidant disorder (similar to *DSM-IV* SPh) in a 4-week RCT of alprazolam and placebo, results obtained suggested that alprazolam had minimal impact on the symptom relief. Graae and colleagues [10] studied the efficacy of clonazepam as a treatment for children who had a variety of anxiety disorders (most were diagnosed with SAD, and most had comorbid concurrent diagnoses) in a double-blind, placebo-controlled crossover study, but clonazepam provided little benefit. Subjects in this study had difficulty tolerating clonazepam, because a nearly every subject experienced drowsiness, irritability, or oppositional behavior during the active treatment period. In summary, a favorable risk–benefit profile for the use of benzodiazepines in the treatment of common pediatric anxiety disorders has yet to be demonstrated.

Selective serotonin reuptake inhibitors

More substantive is the emerging literature on the use of selective serotonin reuptake inhibitors (SSRIs). After a variety of chart reviews [11,12] and open-label trials [13–15] were published suggesting that SSRIs were potentially efficacious and safe in pediatric anxiety disorders, published RCTs have more recently emerged.

Published RCTs that focus on each of these three disorders, as well as RCTs that have combined the three together, are now available. One early study suggested the efficacy of SSRIs in the treatment of selective mutism [16], which, although not formally categorized as a pediatric anxiety disorder, can be seen, at least in some cases, as a variant of SPh in young children. This placebo-controlled RCT provided at least preliminary evidence that fluoxetine may benefit children who have selective mutism. Two other recent studies examined SSRI therapy in patients who had one of the three primary diagnoses examined in this section. In a small (n = 22) RCT examining the efficacy of sertraline for children and adolescents who had primary GAD, Rynn and colleagues [17] found

significant benefit for low doses of sertraline (25–50 mg/day) in global assessments of anxiety severity, improvement in illness, and anxiety symptom
rating scales. Differences between the sertraline and placebo groups were detected
by week four of the 9-week double-blind period. Sertraline was well tolerated in
this study, and the investigators found that several systematically assessed physical
symptoms (dizziness, nausea, and stomach pain) were reported significantly less
often in the sertraline group than in the placebo group, probably reflecting efficacy
of the medication in reducing somatic symptoms of anxiety. In contrast to this
small, single-site study, Wagner and colleagues [18] reported on a large (n = 322),
industry-sponsored, multisite RCT comparing the safety and efficacy of paroxetine in children and adolescents who had SPh. The results of this study robustly
favored the group randomly assigned to paroxetine treatment. Measures of
improvement, illness severity, treatment response, and treatment remission all
suggested that those randomly assigned to paroxetine had much better short-term
outcomes than those randomly assigned to placebo. Adverse events in those taking
paroxetine included increased rates of insomnia, decreased appetite, and vomiting.
In addition, nervousness, hyperkinesia, asthenia, and hostility were more commonly
noted in the younger children randomly assigned to paroxetine.

In a federally funded single-site study, Birmaher and colleagues [19] examined the efficacy of fluoxetine (20-mg fixed dose) for pediatric patients with
primary diagnoses of SAD, GAD, or SPh in a 12-week placebo-controlled RCT.
Seventy-four patients were enrolled in the trial, of whom 80% completed the
trial. Response rates at the end of the trial were 61% for subjects randomly
assigned to the fluoxetine group and 35% for those in the placebo group. Robust
evidence of acute efficacy was demonstrated for fluoxetine in the clinician-rated
and self-reported anxiety rating scales used in the study. Repeated measures
assessments of global function suggested that functional status, in addition to the
observed symptomatic improvement, improved preferentially in the fluoxetine-
treated group. In this study, patients with the diagnosis of SPh fared somewhat
better when taking fluoxetine than did patients with the diagnoses of GAD or
SAD. Patients in the fluoxetine group reported more gastrointestinal distress,
drowsiness, and headaches during initial treatment, but over the course of the entire
study only gastrointestinal side effects were more common in the fluoxetine group.

Other medications

Other medications showing efficacy in adults who have anxiety disorders may
similarly prove useful in children and adolescents, although the safety and efficacy of these agents in juveniles is less clear than for the SSRIs. The published
literature on the use of buspirone in pediatric anxiety disorders is limited to case
reports and case series [20–26]. In contrast to the adult literature, the serotonin-
norepinephrine reuptake inhibitors venlafaxine, mirtazapine, and duloxetine have
not been studied to a significant degree in pediatric anxiety disorders, so published RCTs are lacking. Anticonvulsant medications such as gabapentin, which
may have a role in the management of some types of anxiety in adults, have not
been adequately studied in the pediatric population.

The Research Units in Pediatric Psychopharmacology Anxiety Disorders Study Group fluvoxamine study

In 1996, the National Institute of Mental Health launched the RUPP networks for child psychiatry disorders. These units were set up as infrastructure to facilitate the execution of important investigations in the safety and efficacy of medication treatments for pediatric mental health disorders. One of the major initial efforts of this network was to use a definitive protocol to study the SSRI medication fluvoxamine for common pediatric anxiety disorders, including SAD, GAD, and SPh. The original RUPP Anxiety Disorders Study Group network consisted of five leading child psychiatry academic centers noted for previous experience in the investigation of pediatric anxiety disorders. The pharmaceutical company with patent rights to fluvoxamine in the United States at the time (Solvay, Marietta, Georgia) donated medication and contributed an unrestricted grant to support the trial but was not involved in the design or execution of the trial and had no proprietary rights to the data or any say in the research report writing component of the project.

Acute efficacy study

With recruitment over 2 years, the RUPP Anxiety Disorders Study Group randomly assigned 128 children and adolescents who had a primary diagnosis of SAD, GAD, or SPh to 8 weeks of double-blinded treatment with either fluvoxamine or placebo [27]. Subjects entered the double-blind component of the trial only if they had failed to show evidence of symptomatic improvement during a 3-week lead-in psychoeducational psychosocial intervention. (Only 5 of 153 subjects improved significantly with the lead-in psychosocial intervention.) Dosing of fluvoxamine ranged from a daily minimum of 50 mg to a maximum of 250 mg for children and 300 mg for adolescents. Fluvoxamine was titrated weekly based on clinical response and tolerance. The average dose of fluvoxamine given at the end of the trial for both children and adolescents was 4.0 mg/kg/day. The primary outcome measures were the newly designed Pediatric Anxiety Rating Scale [28] and the clinician-rated Clinical Global Impressions-Improvement (CGI-I) 8-point scale, which was used to dichotomize the subjects into treatment responders (CGI-I scores of 1, 2, or 3) or nonresponders (CGI-I scores of 4 or greater).

The study found a significant advantage in treatment response for subjects randomly assigned to the fluvoxamine group. When compared with those assigned to placebo, subjects in the fluvoxamine group achieved greater reduction in anxiety symptoms as measured by the Pediatric Anxiety Rating Scale (decrease of 9.7 ± 6.9 points, versus placebo group decrease of 3.1 ± 4.8 points, $P < .001$.) and were much more likely to be rated by clinicians as treatment responders (76% acute response in fluvoxamine group versus 29% response in the placebo group). Fluvoxamine was generally well tolerated, although 8% of subjects in the fluvoxamine group discontinued the acute trial because of adverse events, compared with 2% of those in the placebo group. The only adverse events found to occur more commonly in the fluvoxamine group were abdominal discomfort and increased motor activity. Overall, this study demonstrated a striking improvement in clinical status for subjects treated with fluvoxamine compared with placebo.

Predictors, moderators, and mediators

Although group results of an acute clinical trial are important, other important issues can be studied in RCTs with a well-characterized study sample. Understanding baseline characteristics that predict general responsiveness regardless of treatment assignment (predictors) or differential responsiveness to one of the studied treatment interventions (moderators) can enhance clinical care by identifying subgroups of patients who may have lesser or greater likelihood of responding to the treatments under study. Additionally, measuring variables that occur after randomization that may influence clinical response during the course of the trial (mediators) might clarify mechanisms of therapeutic actions of treatments. Although most pediatric psychopharmacology studies have not been designed with sample sizes large enough to make definitive statements about important predictors, moderators, or mediators of treatment response, investigators often engage in at least preliminary exploratory examination of these factors to give further insight as to what subject characteristics or postrandomization events significantly affect outcomes in clinical trials.

The RUPP fluvoxamine study investigators examined several variables that might have had some influence on the results of the acute trial [29]. Baseline characteristics examined included age of the child, gender, race/ethnicity, the presence or absence of the different anxiety disorder diagnoses, anxiety disorder severity, comorbidity, depressive symptoms, intelligence, and family socioeconomic status. Postrandomization variables studied included treatment adherence (days on medication), dosage, treatment-emergent adverse events, and blindness of the rater providing the main outcome measures, typically the child's prescribing clinician.

General predictors of a worse treatment response in the acute trial, regardless of treatment assignment, included the presence of the diagnosis of SPh, higher levels of parent-rated depressive symptoms at baseline, and a greater baseline severity of anxiety illness. The only baseline variable that moderated treatment was parent-reported depressive symptoms in the child: superiority of the fluvoxamine group was more marked in the subgroup of subjects with lower parent-rated depressive scores, as measured by the Children's Depressive Rating Scale. The significance of this finding is not clear, especially because subjects with a current diagnosis of major depression (but not of dysthymic disorder) were excluded from participating in the trial, and that exclusion criterion probably constrained the range of depressive symptoms found at baseline in this sample. Other variables examined had no predictive or moderating influence on the primary outcomes in the trial.

In mediation analyses, two factors seemed to affect treatment response. First, greater adherence to the medication dosing schedule led to a more favorable outcome, so medication compliance was related to treatment results with fluvoxamine, although not with placebo. Second, the child's clinician was asked at the end of the trial, before unblinding, to guess whether the child was taking fluvoxamine or placebo; if the clinician's guess was correct, the child was more likely to have a favorable outcome if he or she was taking fluvoxamine. This finding is probably highly confounded by the primary results, because clinicians seemed to be biased to believe that, if the patient improved, the child was probably taking fluvoxamine. Thus, clinicians tended to use treatment response (and to a lesser extent emergence of adverse events) to guide their guess, and at least in this study, they were more often correct in doing so. Such confounding could have been prevented by using a masked, dual-rater approach (with a primary rater assessing efficacy and a second rater assessing side effects). Such an approach has been used in other pediatric RCTs, notably the RUPP Autism Network risperidone study.

Longer-term follow-up

The RUPP fluvoxamine study included a 6-month open-label extension trial for subjects completing the acute trial [30]. Subjects who responded to fluvoxamine in the original trial were maintained on fluvoxamine for an additional 6 months to assess longer-term safety and maintenance of efficacy. Subjects who were fluvoxamine nonresponders were given a trial of fluoxetine for up to 6 months. Subjects who were placebo nonresponders were treated openly with fluvoxamine for 8 weeks, and then responders were maintained on fluvoxamine for 6 months. Ninety-four percent of subjects with initial good response to fluvoxamine retained their response over the following 6 months, suggesting that, even without dose changes, most subjects with a good acute response will continue to do well over longer periods. Switching to fluoxetine treatment led to good symptomatic response in 10 of 14 fluvoxamine nonresponders (71%). In placebo nonresponders, response to acute, open-label titration was seen in only 59% at 8 weeks, and only 59% were rated as significantly improved at the time of their termination assessment, in contrast with the 76% response rate to double-blinded treatment for 8 weeks in the acute trial. Subjects who tolerated the medication and remained in the trial for the full 8 months achieved a 92% response rate, but only half of the placebo nonresponders were able to do so.

Pharmacologic treatment of obsessive-compulsive disorder

Brief overview of pediatric obsessive-compulsive disorder

Comprehensive reviews of the phenomenology, epidemiology, etiology, and natural history of pediatric obsessive-compulsive disease (OCD) are available for interested readers [31]. OCD is diagnosed in children and adolescents using essentially the same diagnostic criteria as in adults. The *DSM-IV-TR* specifies that an adult is expected to recognize, at some point during the course of the disorder, that the obsessions or compulsions are excessive and unreasonable, but this criterion is waived for children. Prevalence of the disorder in community samples has ranged from 0.05% to 3.0%. Clinical samples of children and adolescents recruited for treatment studies demonstrate significant problems with comorbid internalizing and externalizing psychiatric disorders, which may make treatment more complicated than suggested by single-agent, single-disorder research studies. Significant percentages of adults who have OCD report the onset of their symptoms and impairment from the disorder as beginning in childhood, suggesting that early recognition and early referral for effective intervention may hold promise for decreasing the life-long impact of suffering and disability associated with this disorder.

Acute efficacy studies

There is good support for the use of medication treatment to help alleviate the symptoms of OCD in the short term for pediatric patients. Clomipramine, a serotonergic TCA, and nearly all commonly prescribed SSRIs have been studied in simple, placebo-controlled RCTs, and nearly every study provides substantive evidence for short-term efficacy of medication treatment. Clomipramine, fluvoxamine, sertraline, and fluoxetine all are now approved by the US Food and Drug Administration (FDA) for the treatment of OCD in both children and adolescents. Clomipramine was the first medication adequately studied for use in pediatric OCD, and its efficacy is supported by both federally funded and industry-funded research [32,33]. As described later in the discussion of comparative studies, the more noradrenergic TCAs have seemed to be less effective than this serotonergic agent for OCD. More recently, studies have been published supporting the acute superiority of fluvoxamine, sertraline, fluoxetine, and paroxetine compared with placebo in diminishing symptoms of OCD [34–39]. Studies consistently report that subjects randomly assigned to active medication treatment demonstrate superior improvement in clinician-administered symptom scales (ie, Children's Yale-Brown Obsessive Compulsive Scale: CY-BOCS) as compared with subjects randomly assigned to a placebo group. In general, however, the pool of available studies has been less able to demonstrate short-term advantages of medication when examining alternative outcome measures, such as general improvement measures (CGI), or in functional measures (such as the Children's Global Assessment Scale).

Longer-term studies

Few studies have examined the benefits of medication treatment performed for longer than the typical 8- to 14-week time frame studied in the acute RCTs. OCD tends to require chronic treatment, however, and therefore longer-term studies examining benefits and risks of medication treatment are needed.

No studies examining the long-term benefit of clomipramine for pediatric OCD are currently available, but preliminary studies examining longer-term benefits of SSRI therapy are available. In an open-label, 2-year observational study of the efficacy of citalopram for adolescents who had OCD, approximately 70% of subjects met the study criteria for response status after 1 year of observation [40]. Twenty percent of subjects still had CY-BOCS scores of 20 or greater, making one wonder why the subjects were maintained for that long on an ineffective treatment regimen. In an open-label extension study of sertraline following a placebo-controlled RCT for youth who had OCD, 137 subjects taking sertraline were observed for up to 52 weeks [41,42]. At endpoint, 72% of the children and 61% of the adolescents in the study were considered responders by study criteria. All subjects who were considered responders in the acute trial maintained their response status throughout the 52-week open-label extension period, and no major safety issues with longer-term treatment were uncovered. These initial studies suggest that SSRI therapy may be safe and efficacious in the first 2 years of treatment, but more studies are needed to be definitive.

Predictors, moderators, and mediators

A variety of baseline subject characteristics have been examined as both predictors and moderators of treatment response in the available placebo-controlled RCTs. Variables examined to date include demographics (age, gender), psychopathology (illness severity and duration, comorbidity, symptom patterns), and functional impairment. Age emerged as a significant predictor of acute-treatment response in two studies, both of which found that, regardless of whether they were assigned to active medication or placebo, children had higher response rates than adolescents [36,39]. In one study [39], subjects with higher baseline scores had greater decreases in symptoms, irrespective of treatment group. Other than these findings, no other predictors, moderators, or mediators of treatment response in pediatric OCD have been identified to date. There is no substantive research support at present for using very high doses of medication in pediatric OCD (which is often suggested as clinically necessary), because the studies conducted thus far have mostly been done with fairly standard low-to-moderate range doses. Studies using these dose ranges have reliably separated active treatments from placebo.

Comparative treatment studies

Of substantial interest to researchers, clinicians, parents, youth afflicted with OCD, and policy makers alike are studies that compare and contrast different treatment approaches. Studies aimed at comparing different medication treatment approaches, comparing medication with psychosocial treatment approaches, or comparing combination treatment with monotherapies offer the hope of demonstrating which of the available treatment approaches are the most promising and potentially helping a practitioner select a particular treatment strategy for a patient with a particular clinical profile. In general, few such studies are available in the pediatric therapeutics literature, but there are some important studies examining these issues in youth who have OCD.

There is a dearth of studies comparing medication approaches directly head-to-head. An early 10-week, double-blind, crossover study found that clomipramine was superior in efficacy to the relatively less-serotonergic TCA desipramine [43]. Crossing over to desipramine led to a significant deterioration of therapeutic gains in 64% of acute clomipramine responders. There are no available direct-comparison studies of subjects randomly assigned to clomipramine versus any SSRI.

Indirect comparisons of clomipramine and SSRI therapy by way of meta-analysis may shed some light on the comparative therapeutic efficacy of these two different classes of medication. Geller and colleagues [44] used meta-analytic techniques to examine the available pediatric OCD RCTs to date and concluded that there was some evidence suggesting that treatment with clomipramine may have greater efficacy than SSRI therapy. In addition, there was no substantive evidence in this study that the various available SSRIs could be differentiated from each other in terms of their relative efficacy.

Preliminary attempts to compare psychosocial treatment strategies (ie, cognitive behavior therapy, CBT) with medication treatment and combination treatments have been difficult to interpret because of small sample sizes, lack of suitable control conditions, and lack of appropriate blinding of evaluators providing the primary efficacy outcome data [45–47]. Most of these shortcomings were addressed in the recently published Pediatric OCD Treatment Study (POTS) [48,49], which was the first major RCT in pediatric OCD populations to examine the relative efficacy of acute monotherapies and combination therapy in an adequately characterized and maintained sample.

Findings from the POTS revealed a reduction of symptoms in the main study symptom scale (CY-BOCS). Subjects who received any of the three active treatments (CBT, sertraline, or combination) achieved superior results compared with placebo-treated subjects. Symptom reduction was greater in the combination group than in the groups receiving sertraline and CBT monotherapy, but the sertraline and CBT monotherapy groups did not differentiate from each other. When evaluated with a dichotomous measure of clinical remission (CYBOCS < 10), the combination and CBT groups achieved results that were superior to the placebo group, whereas sertraline monotherapy did not. Additionally, combination treatment was statistically superior to sertraline monotherapy, but not superior to CBT monotherapy. CBT monotherapy and sertraline monotherapy did not statistically separate in the measure of clinical remission of symptoms.

Overall, the POTS provides evidence that combining CBT with medication management may be the most efficacious intervention, when available, for the short-term reduction in symptoms of OCD in pediatric patients. Monotherapy with CBT seems to be somewhat more efficacious than sertraline monotherapy in terms of the observed effect sizes reported in this study, although the sample was too small to for these differences to be statistically significant. One interesting finding is that site differences were observed in the results achieved with monotherapy treatments (but not the combination treatment) in this study. One center had relatively better results with CBT only, whereas the second main center had relatively better results with medication monotherapy. Both centers can be considered expert centers in terms of delivering CBT to children and adolescents who have OCD, but there seemed to be some variability in the results achieved with the different monotherapy treatments, and these differences probably resulted from center-specific variables. In both main centers, however, subjects receiving combination treatment consistently achieved superior results, suggesting that the finding that combination treatment is the most efficacious treatment is robust and potentially important when applying the results of this trial to clinical practice.

Pharmacologic treatment of panic disorder and posttraumatic stress disorder

Panic disorder in children and adolescents

Although panic disorder (PD) in adults has an extensive psychopharmacologic literature suggesting that a variety of medications are helpful in the alleviation of symptoms of the disorder, the pediatric literature lags far behind. This inequity may be caused by differences in the prevalence of the disorder at different developmental time periods; although panic attacks may be relatively prevalent in pediatric populations, it is not clear that *DSM-IV* PD is common in the general population or in treatment-seeking populations of children and adolescents [50–53]. A few preliminary studies examining psychopharmacologic interventions in pediatric PD hve hinted at the efficacy of SSRIs for pediatric PD, but definitive RCTs are not presently available. For example, Masi and colleagues [54] conducted a chart review of 18 pediatric patients who had *DSM-IV* PD in an Italian child psychiatry and neurology clinic. Paroxetine was given at an initial mean dosage of 5 to 10 mg/day and was gradually increased up to 40 mg/day, depending on clinical response and side effects. Clinical status was assessed with the CGI, and adverse effects were assessed retrospectively at each visit. The authors concluded that 15 of the 18 subjects (83.3%) were considered responders and that in general paroxetine was well tolerated in this group. Renaud and colleagues [55] examined a variety of SSRIs in the treatment of PD in 12 children and adolescents in a prospective, open-label study, initially for a period of 6 to 8 weeks and then followed for approximately 6 months. Evaluated with the CGI-I scale, 75% of patients showed much or very much improvement with SSRIs, without experiencing significant side effects. At the end of the 6-month trial, 67% of patients no longer fulfilled criteria for PD, and four patients remained with significant residual symptoms.

Posttraumatic stress disorder in children and adolescents

The pediatric psychopharmacology literature on approaches to children and adolescents with posttraumatic stress disorder (PTSD) or acute stress disorder is sparse. No definitive RCTs are available. Preliminary open-label studies suggest that SSRIs such as citalopram may be beneficial for symptoms of PTSD in children and adolescents [56] and that treatment effects in children and adolescents may be similar to the benefits seen in adult patients with PTSD [57]. The literature is so lacking in this area that little in the way of substantive conclusions can be made, and although pediatric patients who have PTSD and traumatized children and adolescents are routinely encountered in a variety of clinical settings, solid, well-informed, evidenced-based medication recommendations cannot be made at present.

Integrating psychosocial treatments with pharmacologic treatments

Brief overview of psychosocial approaches in pediatric anxiety disorders

Excellent summaries of the psychosocial approaches studied and the RCT data are available, and the interested reader is directed to March and colleagues [58] and Kendall and colleagues [59]. The goal here is to review briefly the most effective psychosocial approaches available and to discuss how these may be used in sequenced or combination strategies that may be of relevance to treatment protocols.

In general, the best studied and most promising psychosocial intervention strategies are subsumed under the heading of CBT. CBT has been studied as an intervention strategy in a variety of pediatric anxiety disorders, especially SAD, GAD, SPh, and OCD [60–76], and to a lesser extent in PD and PTSD [77,78]. There are commonalities to of the treatment approach of CBT that cut across disorders. All CBT protocols include some degree of adequate assessment and diagnostic evaluation, high-quality psychoeducation about the disorder and the approach to treatment, skill-building (helping the child and parent learn new ways to cope with anxiety), and then systematic exposure to and practice in coping with the anxiety-provoking stimuli and situations. CBT-based approaches to the treatment of pediatric anxiety disorders have substantive empiric literature supporting their efficacy. One caveat is the CBT trials in pediatric anxiety have relied on comparing active CBT treatment with wait-list controls rather than with other types of comparative interventions that might better control for the non-specific therapeutic effects of time and attention. Comparing active treatment with wait-list controls probably demonstrates more about the benefits of treatment versus no treatment; the more informative comparison would be the benefits of a specific, theoretically-based, specialized psychosocial intervention versus nonspecialized therapeutic contact. Thus, psychosocial interventions that control for expectancy effects, time, and attention (ie, supportive therapy, treatment-as-usual, pill placebo) may be more valid comparative interventions in RCTs than wait-list controls.

At least theoretically, medication treatment strategies and psychosocial treatment strategies can be integrated in useful research designs. Treatments can be sequenced, so that one treatment is selected and administered and then a second treatment is either substituted or added contingent on a partial response or lack of response to the first intervention. Patients responding to the first treatment are not exposed to the second. First treatment could be either a psychosocial intervention or a medication treatment strategy. Advantages of beginning with a psychosocial treatment strategy are that, from a clinical and consumer perspective, it may be more acceptable to service delivery systems, clinicians, parents, and children to begin with psychotherapy and to reserve pharmacologic strategies to nonresponders. Concerns persist that medication treatment has a higher risk of adverse events or toxicity than do psychosocial interventions, so fewer children might be exposed to this possible risk. Lower numbers of children and adolescents would be exposed to a particular toxicity by reserving medication treatment to those not responding adequately to psychotherapy.

Alternatively, medication treatment could be the first of the sequenced treatments. From a public health perspective, advantages of this sequence are that SSRI therapy may be more readily available in the community (through child psychiatrists, general psychiatrists, pediatricians, family practitioners, and certain medical specialists) and more easily obtainable than the highly specialized CBT demonstrated to be effective in the empiric literature. Therefore there are arguments in favor of reserving the more specialized, less available resource for patients not responsive to the readily available, easily obtainable first intervention.

In contrast, combination treatment strategies might make sense in some situations. Combining treatment interventions, such as medication and psychotherapy, as the initial intervention may make sense if the combination treatment results improve on monotherapy treatment results in general, or even in selected subgroups of patients. For example, in the recently completed Treatments for Adolescents with Depression Study [79,80], examination of the safety and efficacy data suggested that the group receiving combination CBT and fluoxetine from the beginning of treatment in the randomized, controlled trial obtained more benefit after 12 weeks than did subjects in the control condition (pill placebo) or those in the active monotherapy conditions (fluoxetine only or CBT only). Therefore, beginning treatment with both interventions offered the best chance of receiving substantive positive results within the first 3 months of treatment for the subject group as a whole.

Review of research examining integration of psychotherapy with psychopharmacology

To date, there have been few attempts to study medication treatment interventions integrated in either sequenced or combination treatment strategies, but some studies are available. Literature on the sequencing of treatments is sparse. Klein and colleagues [7] and the RUPP fluvoxamine study [27] were designed as quasi-sequential intervention studies. All subjects ultimately randomly assigned to the medication component of both studies had not responded to a very brief behaviorally oriented psychosocial intervention delivered shortly after diagnostic evaluation. To some extent, therefore, these studies are best viewed as medication studies in populations that had not responded to brief psychosocial intervention strategies. In neither of these two studies were subjects exposed to a psychosocial intervention of significant quality and duration such as the leading CBT approaches to pediatric anxiety disorders suggest is necessary for optimal treatment response. Therefore, these studies should not be characterized as studies of psychotherapy-resistant subjects. It seems that the intent of the brief psychosocial exposure in these two medication studies was to eliminate subjects who demonstrated benefit to brief psychosocial interventions for two main reasons:

1. To eliminate exposure to medication risks in children not requiring it
2. To reduce the rate of response to minimal therapeutic attention in the study groups, thereby possibly reducing the placebo response and making the study more powerful to detect medication effects

The RUPP fluvoxamine follow-on study described previously provided preliminary information suggesting that subjects not responding to a first trial of an SSRI (fluvoxamine) may benefit from a trial with a second SSRI (fluoxetine) [30].

Some studies have examined the effects of combining treatment approaches versus monotherapy approaches. The POTS study, detailed previously, found that, overall, beginning treatment with combined sertraline and CBT led to superior short-term treatment results than seen in the comparison control group or in the active monotherapy treatment protocols. Bernstein and colleagues [8] examined combination treatment with imipramine and CBT in a group of adolescents who exhibited significant school refusal and underlying depression and anxiety disorders. In the design of that study, all subjects received CBT focused on school refusal but were randomly assigned to double-blind treatment with imipramine or placebo. Overall, subjects in the imipramine plus CBT group had better short-term outcomes in terms of alleviation of depressive symptoms and improved school attendance than did subjects in the placebo plus CBT group. Beyond the use of imipramine, better school attendance at entry into the study predicted a better outcome in terms of school attendance, and the presence of SAD or avoidant disorder predicted a worse outcome [81]. Girls did worse in terms of school attendance by the end of the trial than boys.

In summary, studies that have addressed integration of psychotherapy with medication approaches for pediatric anxiety suggest that combining empirically supported psychosocial approaches with medication may offer better short-term results than monotherapy approaches with either modality. No published studies are available that examine efficacy of combined treatments over longer periods of time than acute treatment. No adequately designed studies are available to indicate the best approach to sequencing treatments for patients who are partial responders or who do not respond at all to acute treatment.

Risk–benefit considerations in the pharmacologic treatment of pediatric anxiety disorders

Antidepressant medications (tricyclic antidepressants, selective serotonin reuptake inhibitors, serotonin-norepinephrine reuptake inhibitors)

Treatment decisions regarding the use of medication in pediatric anxiety disorders are based not only on the available efficacy data but also must factor in safety data to assess adequately the risk–benefit ratio for use of a particular intervention for a given child. All of the available RCTs provide at least some data on safety considerations and adverse-event profiles for the medications studied to date. In summary, for most antidepressant medications, adverse-event profiles in children and adolescents resemble those seen in studies of adults. Both somatic and psychologic/behavioral adverse reactions have been demonstrated, mostly at low frequencies, in studies of children and adolescents. Although adverse events are commonly reported in children and adolescents taking placebo pills, certain adverse events have been repeatedly demonstrated to occur at higher rates in those taking active medication.

The studies with the largest sample sizes may be more informative here because of increased statistical power. For example, in the RUPP fluvoxamine study [27], higher rates of gastrointestinal distress and hyperkinetic behavior were found in the subjects taking fluvoxamine who had SAD, GAD, and SPh. In Birmaher and colleagues' [19] study of fluoxetine in subjects who had SAD, GAD, or SPh, those taking fluoxetine were found to have higher rates of gastrointestinal problems and neurologic complaints (drowsiness and headaches). In subjects who had SPh, gastrointestinal side effects and insomnia were more commonly reported in those taking paroxetine than in those assigned to placebo in the large industry-sponsored RCT previously described; nonsignificant but elevated rates of nervousness, hyperkinesia, asthenia, and hostility were also reported. Similarly, treatment of pediatric patients with TCAs has been associated with adverse events ranging from somatic events to psychologic/behavioral events. Head-to-head comparisons of SSRIs and TCAs are not currently available, so it is not possible to compare the safety and tolerability profiles of the two classes of medications in youth. The potential for cardiovascular toxicity with intentional or unintentional overdose makes treatment with clomipramine and imipramine inherently more risky and tends to steer clinicians toward SSRIs for treatment of pediatric anxiety disorders.

Recently concern has arisen regarding the association of antidepressant medication therapy in children and adolescents with the development of suicidal thinking and nonfatal suicidal behavior. The FDA has required that, regardless of the disorder being treated, a "black box" warning regarding the association with suicidality in pediatric patients be placed in the labeling of all agents in the various classes of antidepressants. See the article by Rey and Martin elsewhere in this issue for further exploration of this topic. In terms of studies of pediatric anxiety disorders, few have found the suicidality signal in the adverse events data that has been more consistently present in studies of pediatric affective disorders. No individual pediatric anxiety study has found a statistically significant increase in suicidality induction among the studies reviewed here. Because these studies were not intended or powered to measure suicidality, several pediatric anxiety studies excluded subjects who had major depression or who were at elevated risk for suicidal behavior because of a history of previous suicidality or active suicidality at the time of evaluation for the study.

Benzodiazepines

Unfortunately, the paucity of RCTs for pediatric anxiety disorders, as reported in the discussion of efficacy data, precludes any definitive evaluations of the safety of benzodiazepines for youth. Simeon and colleagues [9] suggested that there is no major increased risk of adverse events associated with alprazolam treatment compared with placebo in subjects who had a variety of anxiety disorders, but the statistical power in this study for detecting tolerability differences was very low. Graae and colleagues [10] found suggestions of higher levels of drowsiness, irritability, or oppositional behavior in patients treated with clonazepam for anxiety problems and noted some problems with disinhibition in their patients exposed to relatively low-dose treatment: two of three study dropouts experienced marked disinhibition during the active medication phase.

Future directions

Gaps in current knowledge

This article shows that truly significant research progress has been made identifying safe and effective medication approaches for the treatment of multiple pediatric anxiety disorders. The basic short-term safety and efficacy of agents, such as SSRIs and clomipramine for pediatric OCD and the SSRIs for SAD, GAD, and SPh, are now empirically supported, and this information can contribute meaningfully to evidenced-based pediatric psychiatric practice. Still, many gaps remain in the understanding of the role of medication treatment for pediatric anxiety disorders:

1. There is a dearth of studies examining therapeutic medication approaches to some important anxiety disorders, such as PD, PTSD, and acute stress disorder.

2. Some medication classes with potential for becoming important therapeutic agents for pediatric anxiety disorders, including benzodiazepines and serotonin-norepinephrine reuptake inhibitors, remain significantly understudied.

3. Head-to-head comparisons of the most promising medications for various disorders have not been made as yet (ie, clomipramine versus SSRIs for pediatric OCD, one SSRI versus another in SAD, GAD, or SPh), and therefore definitive risk–benefit comparisons between medication classes or between medications of a given class cannot be made.

4. Few studies have attempted to compare safety and efficacy of medication treatment approaches with psychosocial interventions.

5. Few studies have attempted to compare safety and efficacy of combined medication plus psychotherapy treatment with medication or psychotherapy as monotherapy.

6. No studies have adequately addressed medication treatment options for nonresponders or partial responders to the initial treatment approach, whether the initial treatment is medication or psychotherapy.

7. No studies are available that adequately address the longer-term safety and efficacy of various medication treatment approaches, and no studies are currently informative regarding the optimal duration of medication treatment once adequate acute treatment is achieved.

8. The efficacy of antianxiety medication strategies for common comorbid symptoms and disorders seen in anxious children and adolescents (ie, depressive illness, attention-deficit hyperactivity disorder, other anxiety disorders) and combination medication treatment strategies for complicated anxiety disorder presentations has been understudied at present.

9. Research into subgroups of anxious children more or less likely to respond to various medication treatment approaches (ie, endophenotypes, genotypes) is in its infancy, and the mechanism of action of medication treatment in restoring anxious children to healthy status remains inadequately investigated.

Summary

During the past 20 years, and especially during the last decade, significant progress has been made in understanding the role of medication therapy for a variety of pediatric anxiety disorders. Several recent important RCTs provide evidenced-based risk–benefit decision making about the use of medication to treat pediatric anxiety problems. Major gaps in the current knowledge are being addressed. It is encouraging that the published literature seems to offer a fair representation of all the research to date (unlike the literature in pediatric depression, for which many medication treatment studies remain both negative and unpublished). Significant evidence is accumulating about the important role of medications in the treatment of pediatric anxiety disorders. Further work is needed to define that role more precisely as compared with other interventions or in combination with them.

References

[1] Diagnostic and statistical manual of mental disorders, fourth edition, text revision. Washington (DC): American Psychiatric Association; 2000.

[2] Bernstein GA, Layne AE. Separation anxiety disorder and generalized anxiety disorder. In: Wiener JM, Dulcan MK, editors. Textbook of child and adolescent psychiatry. Washington (DC): American Psychiatric Press, Inc.; 2004. p. 557–74.

[3] Black B, Garcia A, Freeman J, et al. Specific phobia, panic disorder, social phobia and selective mutism. In: Wiener JM, Dulcan MK, editors. Textbook of child and adolescent psychiatry. Washington (DC): American Psychiatric Press, Inc.; 2004. p. 589–608.

[4] Gittelman-Klein R, Klein DF. Controlled imipramine treatment of school phobia. Arch Gen Psychiatry 1971;25:204–7.

[5] Bernstein GA, Garfinkel BD, Borchardt CM. Comparative studies of pharmacotherapy for school refusal. J Am Acad Child Adolesc Psychiatry 1990;29(5):773–81.

[6] Berney T, Kolvin I, Bhate SR, et al. School phobia: a therapeutic trial with clomipramine and short-term outcome. Br J Psychiatry 1981;138:110–8.

[7] Klein RG, Koplewicz HS, Kanner A. Imipramine treatment of children with separation anxiety disorder. J Am Acad Child Adolesc Psychiatry 1992;31(1):21–8.

[8] Bernstein GA, Borchardt CM, Perwien AR, et al. Imipramine plus cognitive-behavioral therapy in the treatment of school refusal [see comment]. J Am Acad Child Adolesc Psychiatry 2000; 39(3):276–83.

[9] Simeon JG, Ferguson HB, Knott V, et al. Clinical, cognitive, and neurophysiological effects of alprazolam in children and adolescents with overanxious and avoidant disorders. J Am Acad Child Adolesc Psychiatry 1992;31(1):29–33.

[10] Graae F, Milner J, Rizzotto L, et al. Clonazepam in childhood anxiety disorders. J Am Acad Child Adolesc Psychiatry 1994;33(3):372–6.

[11] Lepola U, Leinonen E, Koponen H. Citalopram in the treatment of early-onset panic disorder and school phobia. Pharmacopsychiatry 1996;29(1):30–2.

[12] Mancini C, Van Ameringen M, Oakman JM, et al. Serotonergic agents in the treatment of social phobia in children and adolescents: a case series. Depress Anxiety 1999;10(1):33–9.

[13] Birmaher B, Waterman GS, Ryan N, et al. Fluoxetine for childhood anxiety disorders. J Am Acad Child Adolesc Psychiatry 1994;33(7):993–9.

[14] Fairbanks JM, Pine DS, Tancer NK, et al. Open fluoxetine treatment of mixed anxiety disorders in children and adolescents. J Child Adolesc Psychopharmacol 1997;7(1):17–29.

[15] Compton SN, Grant PJ, Chrisman AK, et al. Sertraline in children and adolescents with social anxiety disorder: an open trial. J Am Acad Child Adolesc Psychiatry 2001;40(5):564–71.

[16] Black B, Uhde TW. Treatment of elective mutism with fluoxetine: a double-blind, placebo-controlled study. J Am Acad Child Adolesc Psychiatry 1994;33(7):1000–6.

[17] Rynn MA, Siqueland L, Rickels K. Placebo-controlled trial of sertraline in the treatment of children with generalized anxiety disorder. Am J Psychiatry 2001;158(12):2008–14.

[18] Wagner KD, Berard R, Stein MB, et al. A multicenter, randomized, double-blind, placebo-controlled trial of paroxetine in children and adolescents with social anxiety disorder. Arch Gen Psychiatry 2004;61(11):1153–62.

[19] Birmaher B, Axelson DA, Monk K, et al. Fluoxetine for the treatment of childhood anxiety disorders. J Am Acad Child Adolesc Psychiatry 2003;42(4):415–23.

[20] Salazar DE, Frackiewicz EJ, Dockens R, et al. Pharmacokinetics and tolerability of buspirone during oral administration to children and adolescents with anxiety disorder and normal healthy adults. J Clin Pharmacol 2001;41(12):1351–8.

[21] Thomsen PH, Mikkelsen HU. The addition of buspirone to SSRI in the treatment of adolescent obsessive-compulsive disorder. A study of six cases. Eur Child Adolesc Psychiatry 1999;8(2): 143–8.

[22] Pfeffer CR, Jiang H, Domeshek LJ. Buspirone treatment of psychiatrically hospitalized prepubertal children with symptoms of anxiety and moderately severe aggression. J Child Adolesc Psychopharmacol 1997;7(3):145–55.

[23] Balon R. Buspirone in the treatment of separation anxiety in an adolescent boy. Can J Psychiatry 1994;39(9):581–2.

[24] Zwier KJ, Rao U. Buspirone use in an adolescent with social phobia and mixed personality disorder (cluster A type). J Am Acad Child Adolesc Psychiatry 1994;33(7):1007–11.

[25] Alessi N, Bos T. Buspirone augmentation of fluoxetine in a depressed child with obsessive-compulsive disorder [comment]. Am J Psychiatry 1991;148(11):1605–6.

[26] Kranzler HR. Use of buspirone in an adolescent with overanxious disorder. J Am Acad Child Adolesc Psychiatry 1988;27(6):789–90.

[27] Research Unit on Pediatric Psychopharmacology Anxiety Disorders Study Group. Fluvoxamine for the treatment of anxiety disorders in children and adolescents. The Research Unit on Pediatric Psychopharmacology Anxiety Study Group. N Engl J Med 2001;344(17):1279–85.

[28] Research Unit on Pediatric Psychopharmacology Anxiety Disorders Study Group. The Pediatric Anxiety Rating Scale (PARS): development and psychometric properties. J Am Acad Child Adolesc Psychiatry 2002;41(9):1061–9.

[29] Walkup JT, Labellarte MJ, Riddle MA, et al. Searching for moderators and mediators of pharmacological treatment effects in children and adolescents with anxiety disorders. J Am Acad Child Adolesc Psychiatry 2003;42(1):13–21.

[30] Walkup J, Labellarte M, Riddle MA, et al. Treatment of pediatric anxiety disorders: an open-label extension of the research units on pediatric psychopharmacology anxiety study. J Child Adolesc Psychopharmacol 2002;12(3):175–88.

[31] Freeman J, Garcia A, Swedo SE, et al. Obsessive-compulsive disorder. In: Wiener JM, Dulcan MK, editors. Textbook of child and adolescent psychiatry. Washington (DC): American Psychiatric Press, Inc.; 2004. p. 575–84.

[32] Leonard HL, Swedo SE, Rapoport JL, et al. Treatment of obsessive-compulsive disorder with clomipramine and desipramine in children and adolescents. A double-blind crossover comparison. Arch Gen Psychiatry 1989;46(12):1088–92.

[33] DeVeaugh-Geiss J, Moroz G, Biederman J, et al. Clomipramine hydrochloride in childhood and adolescent obsessive-compulsive disorder—a multicenter trial. J Am Acad Child Adolesc Psychiatry 1992;31(1):45–9.

[34] Riddle MA, Scahill L, King RA, et al. Double-blind, crossover trial of fluoxetine and placebo in children and adolescents with obsessive-compulsive disorder. J Am Acad Child Adolesc Psychiatry 1992;31(6):1062–9.

[35] March JS, Biederman J, Wolkow R, et al. Sertraline in children and adolescents with obsessive-compulsive disorder: a multicenter randomized controlled trial. JAMA 1998;280(20):1752–6.

[36] Riddle MA, Reeve EA, Yaryura-Tobias JA, et al. Fluvoxamine for children and adolescents with obsessive-compulsive disorder: a randomized, controlled, multicenter trial. J Am Acad Child Adolesc Psychiatry 2001;40(2):222–9.

[37] Geller DA, Hoog SL, Heiligenstein JH, et al. Fluoxetine treatment for obsessive-compulsive disorder in children and adolescents: a placebo-controlled clinical trial. J Am Acad Child Adolesc Psychiatry 2001;40(7):773–9.

[38] Liebowitz MR, Turner SM, Piacentini J, et al. Fluoxetine in children and adolescents with OCD: a placebo-controlled trial. J Am Acad Child Adolesc Psychiatry 2002;41(12):1431–8.

[39] Geller DA, Wagner KD, Emslie G, et al. Paroxetine treatment in children and adolescents with obsessive-compulsive disorder: a randomized, multicenter, double-blind, placebo-controlled trial. J Am Acad Child Adolesc Psychiatry 2004;43(11):1387–96.

[40] Thomsen PH, Ebbesen C, Persson C. Long-term experience with citalopram in the treatment of adolescent OCD. J Am Acad Child Adolesc Psychiatry 2001;40(8):895–902.

[41] Cook EH, Wagner KD, March JS, et al. Long-term sertraline treatment of children and

adolescents with obsessive-compulsive disorder. J Am Acad Child Adolesc Psychiatry 2001; 40(10):1175–81.

[42] Wagner KD, Cook EH, Chung H, et al. Remission status after long-term sertraline treatment of pediatric obsessive-compulsive disorder. J Child Adolesc Psychopharmacol 2003;13(Suppl 1): S53–60.

[43] Leonard HL, Swedo SE, Lenane MC, et al. A double-blind desipramine substitution during long-term clomipramine treatment in children and adolescents with obsessive-compulsive disorder. Arch Gen Psychiatry 1991;48(10):922–7.

[44] Geller DA, Biederman J, Stewart SE, et al. Which SSRI? A meta-analysis of pharmacotherapy trials in pediatric obsessive-compulsive disorder [see comment]. Am J Psychiatry 2003;160(11): 1919–28.

[45] Figueroa Y, Rosenberg DR, Birmaher B, et al. Combination treatment with clomipramine and selective serotonin reuptake inhibitors for obsessive-compulsive disorder in children and adolescents. J Child Adolesc Psychopharmacol 1998;8(1):61–7.

[46] de Haan E, Hoogduin KA, Buitelaar JK, et al. Behavior therapy versus clomipramine for the treatment of obsessive-compulsive disorder in children and adolescents. J Am Acad Child Adolesc Psychiatry 1998;37(10):1022–9.

[47] Neziroglu F, Yaryura-Tobias JA, Walz J, et al. The effect of fluvoxamine and behavior therapy on children and adolescents with obsessive-compulsive disorder. J Child Adolesc Psychopharmacol 2000;10(4):295–306.

[48] Franklin M, Foa E, March JS. The pediatric obsessive-compulsive disorder treatment study: rationale, design, and methods. J Child Adolesc Psychopharmacol 2003;13(Suppl 1):S39–51.

[49] Pediatric OCD Treatment Study (POTS) Team. Cognitive-behavior therapy, sertraline, and their combination for children and adolescents with obsessive-compulsive disorder: the Pediatric OCD Treatment Study (POTS) randomized controlled trial. JAMA 2004;292(16):1969–76.

[50] Masi G, Favilla L, Mucci M, et al. Panic disorder in clinically referred children and adolescents. Child Psychiatry Hum Dev 2000;31(2):139–51.

[51] Essau CA, Conradt J, Petermann F. Frequency of panic attacks and panic disorder in adolescents. Depress Anxiety 1999;9(1):19–26.

[52] Reed V, Wittchen HU. DSM-IV panic attacks and panic disorder in a community sample of adolescents and young adults: how specific are panic attacks? J Psychiatr Res 1998;32(6): 335–45.

[53] Bradley S, Wachsmuth R, Swinson R, et al. A pilot study of panic attacks in a child and adolescent psychiatric population. Can J Psychiatry 1990;35(6):526–8.

[54] Masi G, Toni C, Mucci M, et al. Paroxetine in child and adolescent outpatients with panic disorder. J Child Adolesc Psychopharmacol 2001;11(2):151–7.

[55] Renaud J, Birmaher B, Wassick SC, et al. Use of selective serotonin reuptake inhibitors for the treatment of childhood panic disorder: a pilot study. J Child Adolesc Psychopharmacol 1999; 9(2):73–83.

[56] Seedat S, Lockhat R, Kaminer D, et al. An open trial of citalopram in adolescents with post-traumatic stress disorder. Int Clin Psychopharmacol 2001;16(1):21–5.

[57] Seedat S, Stein DJ, Ziervogel C, et al. Comparison of response to a selective serotonin reuptake inhibitor in children, adolescents, and adults with posttraumatic stress disorder. J Child Adolesc Psychopharmacol 2002;12(1):37–46.

[58] March JS, Franklin M, Nelson A, et al. Cognitive-behavioral psychotherapy for pediatric obsessive-compulsive disorder. J Clin Child Psychol 2001;30(1):8–18.

[59] Kendall PC, Hudson JL, Choudhury M, et al. Cognitive-behavioral treatment for childhood anxiety disorders. In: Hibbs ED, Jensen PS, editors. Psychosocial treatments for child and adolescent disorders: empirically based strategies for clinical practice. 2nd edition. Washington (DC): American Psychological Association; 2005. p. 47–73.

[60] Kendall PC, Flannery-Schroeder E, Panichelli-Mindel SM, et al. Therapy for youths with anxiety disorders: a second randomized clinical trial. J Consult Clin Psychol 1997;65(3):366–80.

[61] Kendall PC. Treating anxiety disorders in children: results of a randomized clinical trial. J Consult Clin Psychol 1994;62(1):100–10.

[62] Manassis K, Mendlowitz SL, Scapillato D, et al. Group and individual cognitive-behavioral therapy for childhood anxiety disorders: a randomized trial. J Am Acad Child Adolesc Psychiatry 2002;41(12):1423–30.

[63] Scapillato D, Manassis K. Cognitive-behavioral/interpersonal group treatment for anxious adolescents. J Am Acad Child Adolesc Psychiatry 2002;41(6):739–41.

[64] Muris P, Meesters C, van Melick M. Treatment of childhood anxiety disorders; a preliminary comparison between cognitive-behavioral group therapy and a psychological placebo intervention. J Behav Ther Exp Psychiatry 2002;33(3–4):143–58.

[65] Shortt AL, Barrett PM, Fox TL. Evaluating the FRIENDS program: a cognitive-behavioral group treatment for anxious children and their parents. J Clin Child Psychol 2001;30(4):525–35.

[66] Thienemann M, Martin J, Cregger B, et al. Manual-driven group cognitive-behavioral therapy for adolescents with obsessive-compulsive disorder: a pilot study. J Am Acad Child Adolesc Psychiatry 2001;40(11):1254–60.

[67] Waters TL, Barrett PM, March JS. Cognitive-behavioral family treatment of childhood obsessive-compulsive disorder: preliminary findings. Am J Psychother 2001;55(3):372–87.

[68] Hayward C, Varady S, Albano AM, et al. Cognitive-behavioral group therapy for social phobia in female adolescents: results of a pilot study. J Am Acad Child Adolesc Psychiatry 2000;39(6): 721–6.

[69] Silverman WK, Kurtines WM, Ginsburg GS, et al. Treating anxiety disorders in children with group cognitive-behaviorial therapy: a randomized clinical trial. J Consult Clin Psychol 1999; 67(6):995–1003.

[70] Mendlowitz SL, Manassis K, Bradley S, et al. Cognitive-behavioral group treatments in childhood anxiety disorders: the role of parental involvement. J Am Acad Child Adolesc Psychiatry 1999;38(10):1223–9.

[71] Barrett PM. Evaluation of cognitive-behavioral group treatments for childhood anxiety disorders. J Clin Child Psychol 1998;27(4):459–68.

[72] Franklin ME, Kozak MJ, Cashman LA, et al. Cognitive-behavioral treatment of pediatric obsessive-compulsive disorder: an open clinical trial. J Am Acad Child Adolesc Psychiatry 1998;37(4):412–9.

[73] King NJ, Tonge BJ, Heyne D, et al. Cognitive-behavioral treatment of school-refusing children: a controlled evaluation. J Am Acad Child Adolesc Psychiatry 1998;37(4):395–403.

[74] Last CG, Hansen C, Franco N. Cognitive-behavioral treatment of school phobia. J Am Acad Child Adolesc Psychiatry 1998;37(4):404–11.

[75] Albano AM, Marten PA, Holt CS, et al. Cognitive-behavioral group treatment for social phobia in adolescents. A preliminary study. J Nerv Ment Dis 1995;183(10):649–56.

[76] March JS. Cognitive-behavioral psychotherapy for children and adolescents with OCD: a review and recommendations for treatment. J Am Acad Child Adolesc Psychiatry 1995;34(1):7–18.

[77] March JS, Amaya-Jackson L, Murray MC, et al. Cognitive-behavioral psychotherapy for children and adolescents with posttraumatic stress disorder after a single-incident stressor. J Am Acad Child Adolesc Psychiatry 1998;37(6):585–93.

[78] Deblinger E, Steer RA, Lippmann J. Two-year follow-up study of cognitive behavioral therapy for sexually abused children suffering post-traumatic stress symptoms. Child Abuse Negl 1999; 23(12):1371–8.

[79] Treatment for Adolescents with Depression Study Team. Treatment for Adolescents with Depression Study (TADS): rationale, design, and methods. J Am Acad Child Adolesc Psychiatry 2003;42(5):531–42.

[80] Treatment for Adolescents with Depression Study Team. Fluoxetine, cognitive-behavioral therapy, and their combination for adolescents with depression: Treatment for Adolescents with Depression Study (TADS) randomized controlled trial. JAMA 2004;292(7):807–20.

[81] Layne AE, Bernstein GA, Egan EA, et al. Predictors of treatment response in anxious-depressed adolescents with school refusal. J Am Acad Child Adolesc Psychiatry 2003;42(3):319–26.

ELSEVIER
SAUNDERS

Child Adolesc Psychiatric Clin N Am
15 (2006) 73–108

CHILD AND
ADOLESCENT
PSYCHIATRIC CLINICS
OF NORTH AMERICA

Pediatric Bipolar Disorder: Emerging Diagnostic and Treatment Approaches

Robert A. Kowatch, MD*, Melissa P. DelBello, MD

*Departments of Psychiatry and Pediatrics, University of Cincinnati Medical Center &
Cincinnati Children's Hospital Medical Center, MSB 7261, PO Box 670559,
Cincinnati, OH 45267-0559, USA*

Pediatric bipolar disorders are prevalent psychiatric disorders that seriously disrupt the lives of children, adolescents, and their families [1–3]. Numerous studies have shown that children and adolescents who have bipolar disorder have significantly higher rates of morbidity and mortality, including psychosocial morbidity with impaired family and peer relationships [4], impaired academic performance with increased rates of school failure and school dropouts [5], increased levels of substance abuse, increased rates of suicide attempts and completion, legal difficulties, and multiple hospitalizations [2,6]. It is important that these disorders be recognized early so that the appropriate treatments may be started and these negative outcomes minimized.

Prevalence

The population prevalence of bipolar disorder in adolescents seems to be similar to the adult rate of approximately 1.5% [1,7,8]. In clinical settings, however, the prevalence of bipolar disorder or "base rate" is much higher, approximately 20% to 30%. Youngstrom and Daux [9] recently reported that the rate of bipolar disorder in children and adolescents varied from 0 to 0.6% in

Dr. Kowatch has financial affiliations with Bristol-Myers Squibb, GlaxoSmithKline, Janssen, Astra-Zeneca, and Abbott. Dr. DelBello has financial affiliations with AstraZeneca, Bristol-Myers Squibb, Pfizer, Abbott, Janssen, OrthoMcNeil, Lilly, and GlaxoSmithKline.

* Corresponding author.
E-mail address: robert.kowatch@uc.edu (R.A. Kowatch).

epidemiologic samples to 17% to 30% in clinical samples. The reasons for this wide range of rates include varying diagnostic criteria, who is interviewed, who does the interviewing, the type of diagnostic instrument used, and the type of setting where the patients are seen. For example, in an epidemiologic study of the incidence of mood disorders in adolescents in six Oregon high schools, Lewinsohn and colleagues [1] reported an overall lifetime prevalence of 1% for bipolar disorders which included bipolar I disorder, bipolar II disorder, and cyclothymia. In more specialized psychiatric settings such as a pediatric psychopharmacology clinic, the occurrence of pediatric bipolar disorder is often much greater than that found in the general population. Wozniak and colleagues [10] reported that of 262 children consecutively referred to a specialty pediatric psychopharmacology clinic, 16% met *Diagnostic and Statistic Manual, edition 3 revised* (*DSM-III-R*) criteria for mania. Isaac [11] reported that 8 of 12 students in a special education class met *DSM-III-R* criteria for a bipolar disorder [11]. On child/adolescent inpatient units it is common to find that 30% to 40% of patients have bipolar disorder.

Children with a parent with bipolar disorder are also at an increased risk for developing a mood disorder [12]. In a review of bipolar offspring studies that included studies that evaluated children and adolescents, rates of mood disorders ranged from 8% to 67%, compared with rates in offspring of healthy volunteers of 0 to 38%. A recent meta-analysis found that children with a biologic parent who had bipolar disorder average a fivefold increase in their risk of developing a bipolar disorder [13].

Diagnosis

In a child or adolescent, the diagnosis of bipolar disorder is often difficult because of the developmental differences in symptom expression, the frequent presence of comorbid disorders, and the lack of biologic tests to confirm this disorder. The *DSM-IV* criteria for mania/hypomania were developed for adults, and none of these criteria take into account developmental differences between bipolar adults and bipolar children or adolescents. Clinicians who evaluate such children often attempt to use the *DSM-IV* course modifier rapid cycling but find that this description does not fit children very well: children often do not have clearly delineated episodes of mania but seem to be chronically cycling [14–17].

Barbara Geller at Washington University, one of the leaders in the diagnosis and phenomenology of pediatric bipolar disorder, has developed and validated a structured interview based on the Schedule for Affective Disorders and Schizophrenia for School-Age Children (K-SADS), the Washington University K-SADS (WASH-U K-SADS), with more age-appropriate items for mania (Appendix 1) [17]. The WASH-U K-SADS has been widely used in research involving children and adolescents who have mood disorders. Geller and colleagues [18] recently reported the results of a 4-year longitudinal study of a sample of 93 consecutive outpatients ascertained to have bipolar disorder. During the course of this study, the WASH-U-KSADS was blindly administered by research nurses to the subjects' mothers and to children/adolescents about themselves. In this study, Geller and colleagues elected to require current *DSM-IV* mania or hypomania with elated mood or grandiosity as their inclusion criterion for bipolar disorder. The "caseness" of these subjects was established by consensus conferences that included diagnostic and impairment data, teacher and school reports, agency records, videotapes viewed by Dr. Geller, and medical charts. Geller and colleagues defined a manic episode as the entire length of the illness and cycling as mood changes within an episode. They reported that the persons who had bipolar disorder in this study were aged 10.9 ± 2.6 years, had a current episode length of 3.6 ± 2.5 years, and had an age at onset of 7.3 ± 3.5 years. No significant differences were found by gender, puberty, or comorbid attention-deficit hyperactivity disorder (ADHD) on rates of mania criteria, mixed mania, psychosis, rapid cycling, suicidality, or comorbid oppositional defiant disorder. This is the first longitudinal study of children who have mania, and it demonstrates that children who have bipolar I disorder present differently from adults, with episodes that are longer, mixed in nature and chronic in course.

Assessment of manic symptoms in children and adolescents

When evaluating a child or adolescent for a possible bipolar disorder, two questions become important: does the patient have a bipolar disorder, and, if so, how severe is it? The former is important for prediction and the latter for planning and monitoring treatment. When determining the presence or absence of manic symptoms, clinicians can use a variation of the frequency, intensity, number, and duration strategy to make this determination. The original guidelines for this strategy, developed by Mary Fristad at Ohio State University, are modified here to include

- Frequency of symptoms: how many days in a week is the patient symptomatic?
- Intensity: Are the patient's symptoms severe enough to cause severe dysfunction in one domain or moderate disturbance in two or more domains?
- Number: What is the number of *DSM-IV* manic symptoms?
- Duration: How long is the patient symptomatic on an average day when manic or hypomanic?

In the *DSM-IV* the diagnosis of a bipolar disorder requires a history of one of the following mood episodes:

1. A manic episode
2. A hypomanic episode and a major depressive episode or
3. An episode of mixed mania and depression

A single manic episode will result in a diagnosis of bipolar disorder type I by *DSM-IV* criteria. A child or adolescent who has had one or more episodes of major depression, no episodes of mania, and at least one episode of hypomania is classified in the *DSM-IV* as having bipolar II disorder. A mixed episode by *DSM-IV* criteria is characterized by both manic and depressive symptoms lasting at least 1 week. Typically, prepubertal patients with bipolar disorder I have multiple mood swings each day, have mixed episodes with short periods of euphoria mixed with longer periods of irritability, and have several other comorbid disorders such as ADHD, oppositional defiant disorder, or conduct disorder [10,15,18].

Bipolar II disorder, hypomania with depressive episodes, presents more typically in adolescence, and the major depressive episode is usually noticed first clinically. A hypomanic episode is characterized in the *DSM-IV* as an abnormally and persistently elevated, expansive, or irritable mood that lasts at least 4 days. In contrast to a bipolar I disorder, the illness caused by bipolar II disorder is not severe enough to cause marked impairment in occupational functioning (school functioning in children and adolescents), to interfere with social activities or relationships with others, or to necessitate hospitalization, and there are no psychotic features. Often, past episodes of hypomania may be missed unless a careful history is taken.

Cyclothymia is a bipolar disorder in which there are hypomanic episodes and minor depressive episodes without a history of major depressive episodes. Cyclothymia can be difficult to diagnose, because the hypomania and depressive symptoms are not as severe as in bipolar I or bipolar II disorder. In cyclothymia, the child or adolescent is not without symptoms for more than 2 months at a time. Retrospective studies of adults with cyclothymia have shown that adolescence is the most common age of onset for cyclothymia [20]. A significant proportion of adolescents who have cyclothymia are at risk of progressing to bipolar disorder. In a study by Akiskal and colleagues [21] of the offspring of adults who have bipolar disorder, 7 of 10 adolescents who had cyclothymia progressed to mania or hypomania within 3 years of diagnosis [21]. Prospective mood charting is often helpful to diagnose cyclothymia. Examples of mood charts appropriate for pediatric patients can be found at http://www.bpkids.org/site/PageServer?page name=lrn_mood.

Bipolar disorder–not otherwise specified (BP-NOS) represents a large group of patients with bipolar symptoms [22]. Children without clearly defined episodes, whose episodes do not meet *DSM-IV* duration criteria for bipolar I disorder, bipolar II disorder, or cyclothymia, or who have too few manic symptoms are often diagnosed as having BP-NOS [23]. The diagnosis of BP-NOS can also be given when a bipolar disorder is present but secondary to a general medical condition (eg, fetal alcohol syndrome or an alcohol-related neurodevelopmental disorder) [24]. Little is known about prepubertal BP-NOS, including whether it will evolve into bipolar I or bipolar II disorder. An overview of these four *DSM-IV* bipolar subtypes is presented in Table 1.

Table 1
Pediatric bipolar disorder subtypes using frequency, intensity, number, and duration strategy

DSM-IV bipolar subtype	Frequency of symptoms	Intensity (functioning)	Number of DSM-IV manic symptoms	Duration of symptoms
Bipolar I	3–4 severe mood swings/d for 5/7 d	Manic symptoms cause significant dysfunction; parents cannot manage the patient in public because of severity of symptoms; symptoms occur at home or in school	3 if manic 4 if irritable	Mood swings last min–h with >4 h/d total
Bipolar II	2–3 severe mood swings/d for 4/7 d	Hypomanic symptoms do not cause significant dysfunction but are still noticed by the patient's caretakers	3 if manic 4 if irritable	Mood swings last min–h with >3 h/d total
Cyclothymia	Chronic, not without symptoms for >2 mo at a time	Significant, chronic dysfunction	2–3	>50%/d
Bipolar (not otherwise specified)	2–3 severe mood swings/d for 2/7 d	Some dysfunction but not as severe as in bipolar I or II	2 if manic 3 if irritable	2–3 h/d total

Specific symptoms that should be assessed in children or adolescents with suspected mania/hypomania include

1. Euphoric/expansive mood: Normal children can be extremely happy, silly, or giddy when they are very excited about a special event (eg, Christmas morning, birthday parties). Children with true mania are euphoric for no reason. Their euphoria tends to be irritating to those around them and occurs in situations when there is no good reason to be happy or silly. Manic adolescents can also become overly silly or unrealistically optimistic. During a manic phase, these patients often have no insight about the inappropriateness of their moods.

2. Irritable mood and anger: Irritability is not a symptom specific to manic children, because children and adolescents who have major depressive disorder, dysthymic disorder, or oppositional defiant disorder are also frequently irritable. Irritability is also common in children who have pervasive developmental disorder, anxiety disorders, schizophrenia, or ADHD. The child may become markedly belligerent and highly irritable with many intense outbursts of anger. An adolescent may appear extremely oppositional, belligerent, short, curt, or hostile. Manic irritability sometimes can be differentiated from other causes of irritability by its episodic and hostile nature. Manic irritability frequently leads to many outbursts of anger that are usually present more than 50% of the time when these patients are awake.

3. Decreased need for sleep: Children or adolescents experiencing mania typically report needing less sleep than usual and will not feel tired the next day despite being sleep deprived. It is important to distinguish a decreased need for sleep from initial insomnia that results in excessive somnolence the next day. It is also important to factor in developmental needs for sleep: prepubertal children need 8 to 10 hours of sleep per day, and adolescents need 10 to 12 hours per day, which they rarely get because of outside activities and after-school employment [25,26]. Manic children may sleep 3 to 4 hours and then get up and wander the house in the middle of the night, looking for things to do. They sometimes cook or wander outside to play. Manic adolescents may "crash" around 4 or 5 AM, and wake up a few hours later, grumpy, but able to function.

4. Unusual energy: There should be a distinct increase in energy level from baseline when the child is manic or hypomanic. For example, children with ADHD are seemingly always active and restless, whereas bipolar children are more active when manic but less active when depressed.

5a. Increase in goal-directed activity: Children, when manic, may draw a lot, build different things, or write short stories or graphic novels in a short period of time. Children or adolescents who are hypomanic may be fairly productive, but as their mania progresses they may become increasingly disorganized and nonproductive.

5b. Motor hyperactivity: The child or adolescent may appear very restless or motor driven and shift from activity to activity rapidly. The patient may appear hyperactive but be able to complete multiple projects they have started before moving on to another project.

6. Grandiosity: Grandiosity is one of the more difficult symptoms to ascertain, because many young children are not yet at a cognitive developmental level to recognize that they cannot actually be "Superman" or "Superwoman." By contrast, an 8-year-old child who stands up in class and asks to "please teach the class because they know the material better than the teacher" may be pathologically grandiose.

7. Accelerated, pressured, or increased amount of speech: Children or adolescents who are manic may be loud, intrusive, and difficult to interrupt. The child or adolescent may blurt out answers during class repeatedly and appear to "know it all." A child's or adolescent's speech may become very rapid and pressured to the point that it is continuous and at times unintelligible or difficult to follow.

8a. Racing thoughts: Whereas jumping from topic to topic as in flight of ideas can be observed by others, the determination of racing thoughts requires asking the child whether his thoughts seem to be going too fast. Children may describe racing thoughts with developmentally appropriate concrete phrases such as, "My brain is going 100 miles per hour," or, "My mouth can't keep up with my brain." The child or adolescent may report that they have so many great ideas they can't keep them straight or get them out fast enough. Racing thoughts are often evident in a child's pressured speech.

8b. Flight of ideas: The child or adolescent may change topics of discussion rapidly, in a manner quite confusing to anyone listening. For an interviewer unfamiliar with a child and his background, it is necessary to determine whether a parent or other knowledgeable adult can easily follow the stream of words. Younger and less verbally facile children who are talkative can be confusing to follow because of their limited ability to organize language, but this is not flight of ideas.

9. Poor judgment: The child or adolescent may become involved in pleasurable activities that have a high risk for adverse consequences. Poor judgment may manifest as hypersexual behavior, frequent fighting, increased recklessness, use of drugs and alcohol, shopping sprees, and reckless driving. It is important to rule out sexual abuse or exposure to sexually explicit materials as a possible cause of hypersexual behavior in any child, including one who has bipolar disorder. The hypersexual behavior of manic patients usually has an erotic, pleasure-seeking quality to it, whereas the hypersexual behavior of children who have been sexually abused is often anxious and compulsive in nature.

10. Distractibility: For distractibility to be considered a manic symptom, it needs to reflect a change from baseline functioning, occur in conjunction

with a manic mood shift, and not be explained exclusively by another disorder, particularly ADHD.

11. Hallucinations: Auditory or visual hallucinations are sometimes present in children who have bipolar disorder [27]. It is useful to distinguish benign perceptual distortions that are not impairing and are not considered signs of psychosis (eg, hearing one's name being called or hypnogogic [before sleep] and hypnopompic [upon awakening] perceptual phenomena) from those that are impairing and that are more serious in nature (eg, hearing voices that command the child to stab someone with a knife).

12. Delusions: Manic patients can sometimes develop grandiose delusions (eg, that they can fly or are "the savior of mankind"). Such delusions are a sign of psychosis common in bipolar disorder.

13. Mood lability: The patient's parents/caretakers often report multiple, severe mood swings daily with the intensity of mood swings being out of proportion to the provoking stimulus. It is helpful to ask about the number of severe mood swings per day and their intensity and average duration.

A number of medications and medical disorders may exacerbate or mimic bipolar symptoms, and it is important to assess these potential confounds before initiating treatment. Potential medical disorders and medications that should be evaluated before making the diagnosis of a bipolar disorder in children and adolescents are listed in Boxes 1 and 2.

Screening/diagnostic tools

Several instruments are available to screen for bipolar disorder in children and adolescents. The Young Mania Rating Scale (YMRS) is currently being used in several pediatric controlled trials of mood stabilizers and atypical anti-psychotics for bipolar disorder. Young and colleagues [28] at the Washington

---

Box 1. Medical conditions that may mimic mania in children and adolescents

1. Hyperthyroidism
2. Closed or open head injury
3. Temporal lobe epilepsy
4. Multiple sclerosis
5. Systemic lupus erythematosus
6. Fetal alcohol spectrum disorder/alcohol related neurodevelopmental disorder
7. Wilson's disease

Box 2. Medications that may increase mood cycling in children and adolescents

1. Serotonin-specific reuptake inhibitors
2. Serotonin and norepinephrine reuptake inhibitors
3. Tricyclic antidepressants
4. Aminophylline
5. Corticosteroids
6. Sympathomimetic amines (pseudoephedrine and others)

University School of Medicine created the YMRS in 1978. The YMRS is an 11-item instrument that was designed to be administered by a trained clinician during a 15- to 30-minute interview. In 1992 Fristad and colleagues [29] at Ohio State University used the YMRS to rate 11 children who had *DSM-III-R* mania and 11 children who had ADHD [29]. The mean age of these patients was 8.7 years, and the cohort included inpatients and outpatients. They reported the YMRS scores of the manic patients were 24.1 ± 8.1 versus a mean score of 7.8 ± 4.8 for the ADHD children ($P<0001$). Although scores on hyperactivity rating scales (Conners-Parent and Teacher Forms) did not differ between these two groups, YMRS scores correlated significantly with severity of mania. In an extension of their first study, Fristad and colleagues [30] used the YMRS to rate 10 inpatients who had bipolar disorder, 10 inpatients who had ADHD but not a mood disorder, and 10 outpatients who had ADHD but not a mood disorder. The 10 subjects who had bipolar disorder (mean age, 9 years) met *DSM III-R* criteria for a mixed or manic episode. The mean YMRS scores of each group were bipolar 31.0 ± 4.2; inpatient ADHD, 16.1 ± 8.8; and outpatient ADHD, 9.2 ± 4.7. Despite these excellent studies, the YMRS is less than ideal for rating children and adolescents who have manic symptoms, because the YMRS was designed for adult inpatients, some of the items are based on patient report at the low end of the scale and on observation at the high end of the scale, and it is not adequate for rating milder manic symptoms in outpatient children and adolescents. Because it was the only scale validated in children and adolescents, however, it has been widely used in industry-sponsored trials in pediatric bipolar disorder.

Another screening instrument for bipolar spectrum disorders in adults is the Mood Disorders Questionnaire (MDQ). This MDQ was developed by Hirschfeld and colleagues [31,32] and is a self-report, single-page, paper-and-pencil inventory that can be quickly and easily scored by a clinician. The MDQ screens for a lifetime history of a manic or hypomanic syndrome by including 13 "yes/no" items derived from the *DSM-IV* criteria and clinical experience. A yes/no question also asks whether several of any reported manic or hypomanic symptoms or behaviors were experienced simultaneously. A MDQ screening score of 7 or more was chosen as the optimal cutoff for adults, because it provided good sensitivity and very good specificity. Hirschfeld [32] reported that 7 of 10 people who had a bipolar spectrum disorder would be correctly identified by the MDQ, whereas 9 of 10 of those who did not have a bipolar spectrum disorder would be successfully screened out [32]. Although the MDQ was developed for and validated in adults, a version of this scale is being validated in bipolar adolescents by Karen Wagner of University of Texas Medical Branch at Galveston (Karen Wagner, personnel communication, 2005). It can be used as screening tool in older adolescents with the caveat that many adolescents do not have significant insight about their moods and behavior. A copy of the MDQ is included in Appendix 2.

Another instrument developed specifically to screen for bipolar disorders in children and adolescents is the Short Form of the General Behavior Inventory (GBI). This instrument is an adaptation of the GBI that was originally developed by Depue and colleagues [33] to identify and quantify subsyndromal mood disorder in college students and adults. Eric Youngstrom and colleagues [34] at Case Western Reserve University validated a Parent version of the GBI (P-GBI) as a 73-item instrument in a large outpatient sample of children and adolescents. Youngstrom subsequently developed a short form of the Parent-GBI (PGBI-SF) containing 10 items by selecting the items that maximally discriminated bipolar disorder from other diagnoses and that optimize the diagnostic efficiency of the resulting short-form of the GBI. The GBI-SF has recently been validated by Youngstrom and colleagues (personal communication, 2005) and can be administered to parents about their child or adolescents.

A rating scale that can be used by clinicians to assess manic symptoms in children and adolescents is the K-SADS-Mania Rating Scale (K-SADS-MRS) developed by David Axelson and colleagues [35] at Western Psychiatric Institute and Clinic in Pittsburgh. This scale was developed from the fourth edition of the K-SADS-P (Present Episode Version) [36] with 12 questions from the mania section of the K-SADS-P and two items from the psychosis section, as well as a new item that was designed to assess mood lability. This scale was found to have excellent internal consistency and inter-rater reliability [35]. A score of 12 or higher on this scale differentiated bipolar patients who had clinically significant manic symptoms from those who did not, with a sensitivity of 87% and a specificity of 81%. The *DSM-IV* criteria for mania and hypomania, as well as psychotic symptoms, are assessed as part of the K-SADS-MRS, and clinicians can easily integrate the K-SADS-MRS into a diagnostic interview. A copy of the K-SADS-MRS is presented in Appendix 1.

A useful strategy in clinical practice is to use the MDQ as a screening instrument for adolescents, to administer the short form of the P-GBI to a parent or caretaker about their child or adolescent, and to interview the patient and the parent/caretaker using the K-SADS-MRS. It is important to interview both the patient and the caretaker, because bipolar patients can report on subjective feelings such as racing thoughts and difficulty sleeping, whereas caretakers are often more objective about episodes of increased energy, activity levels, and moods. It is helpful to inquire about current symptoms as well as any periods of time when the patient was "very hyperactive" or "driven." Often this strategy can uncover past episodes of mania or hypomania that have been overlooked.

Comorbid disorders

Comorbid disorders are the rule rather than the exception among children and adolescents who have bipolar disorder. These comorbid disorders often complicate the presentation and treatment response. The most common comorbid diagnosis among children and adolescents who have bipolar disorder is ADHD. Several studies have determined that ADHD is more common in prepubertal-onset bipolar disorder than in adolescent-onset bipolar disorder [37,38]. The rate of comorbid ADHD in prepubertal children is around 60% to 90%, whereas in adolescents the rate is 30% to 40%. Children who have ADHD do not demonstrate the elated mood, grandiosity, hypersexuality, decreased need for sleep, racing thoughts, and other manic symptoms that are present in children who have mania and comorbid ADHD [39]. Another disorder frequently comorbid in children who have bipolar disorder is conduct disorder. Kovacs and Pollock [40] found a 69% rate of conduct disorder among 26 children and adolescents who had bipolar disorder. Moreover, adolescents who have bipolar disorder are four to five times more likely to develop a substance use disorder than those who do not have a bipolar disorder [41]. Children and adolescents with pervasive developmental disorders may be at increased risk for developing mania [16]. Common comorbid disorders found in patients who have pediatric bipolar disorders are listed in Table 2.

Pharmacotherapy of bipolar disorders

Although there are few controlled trials of mood stabilizers and atypical antipsychotics in children and adolescents who have bipolar disorder [42,43],

Table 2
Estimated rates of frequent comorbid disorders

Disorder	Prepubertal (%)	Adolescent (%)
Attention-deficit hyperactivity disorder	70–90	30–60
Anxiety disorders	20–30	30–40
Conduct disorders	30–40	30–60
Oppositional defiant disorder	60–90	20–30
Substance abuse	10	40–50
Learning disabilities	30–40	30–40

Table 3
Mood stabilizer dosing/monitoring in children and adolescents who have bipolar disorder

Generic name	Trade name in United States	How supplied (mg)	Starting dose	Target dose	Therapeutic serum level	Cautions
Carbamazepine	Tegretol	100, 200	Outpatients: 7 mg/kg/d (2–3 daily doses)	Based on response and serum levels	8–11 mg/L	Monitor for P-450 drug interactions
Carbamazepine XR	Tegretol XR	100, 200, 400				
Gabapentin	Neurontin	100, 300, 400	100 mg bid or tid	Based on response	Not applicable	Watch for behavioral disinhibition
Lamotrigine	Lamictal	25, 100, 200	12.5 mg qd	Increase weekly based on response	Not applicable	Monitor carefully for rashes, serum sickness
Lithium$^+$ carbonate	Lithobid	300 (& 150 generic)	Outpatients: 25 mg/kg/d (2–3 daily doses)	30 mg/kg/d (2–3 daily doses)	0.8–1.2 mEq/L	Monitor for hypothyroidism
Lithium$^+$ carbonate	Eskalith	300 or 450 controlled release				Avoid in pregnancy
Lithium$^+$ citrate	Cibalith-S	Li-Citrate 5 cm^3 = 300 mg				
Oxcarbazepine	Trileptal	150, 300, 600	150 mg bid	20–29 kg (900 mg/d) 30–39 kg (1200 mg/d) >39 kg (1800 mg/d)	Not applicable	Monitor for hyponatremia
Topiramate	Topamax	25, 100	25 mg qd	100–400 mg/d	Not applicable	Monitor for memory problems, kidney stones
Valproic acid	Depakene	125, 250, 500	20 mg/kg/d (2 daily doses)	20 mg/kg/d (2–3 daily doses)	90–120 mg/L	Monitor liver functions, for pancreatitis and polycystic ovarian syndrome
Divalproex sodium	Depakote					Avoid in pregnancy

these agents are the ones most commonly used to treat this population. Many of the psychotropic medications used to treat adults who have bipolar disorders are also used for children and adolescents. Information on dosing and clinical monitoring of the traditional and novel mood stabilizers is provided in Table 3.

Traditional mood stabilizers

Lithium

Lithium is the best studied mood stabilizer for children and adolescents who have bipolar disorder and is the only medication approved by the US Food and Drug Administration for the treatment of acute mania and bipolar disorder in adolescents (ages 12–18 years). In the only prospective, placebo-controlled, investigation of lithium in children and adolescents who have bipolar disorders (n = 25), Geller and colleagues [42] found that after 6 weeks of treatment, patients treated with lithium showed a statistically significant improvement in global assessment of functioning (46% response rate in the lithium-treated group versus 8% response rate in the placebo group). These patients also had comorbid substance abuse, and a statistically significant decrease in positive urine toxicology screens also occurred following lithium treatment. This study demonstrated the efficacy of lithium carbonate for the treatment of bipolar adolescents who have comorbid substance use disorders but did not measure the effect of lithium specifically on mood in these adolescents. Clinical factors that predict a poor lithium response in children and adolescents who have bipolar disorder include prepubertal onset and the presence of co-occurring ADHD [44]. Approximately 40% to 50% of children and adolescents who have bipolar disorder respond acutely to lithium monotherapy [45–47]. In general, lithium should be titrated to a dose of 30 mg/kg/day in two to three divided doses, which typically results in a therapeutic serum level of 0.8 to 1.2 mEq/L. Common side effects of lithium in children and adolescents include hypothyroidism, nausea, polyuria, polydipsia, tremor, acne, and weight gain. Lithium levels, renal function, and thyroid function tests should be assessed at baseline and monitored every 6 months.

Sodium divalproex

Despite the wide use of sodium divalproex in children and adolescents who have bipolar disorder, there are no published placebo-controlled studies of divalproex in this population. Open-label studies of divalproex in manic adolescents have reported response rates ranging from 53% to 82% [45,48–50]. In the only controlled maintenance study of children and adolescents who had bipolar disorder, Findling and colleagues [51] compared lithium versus divalproex monotherapy for up to 76 weeks after initial stabilization on the combination of lithium and divalproex. Results of this study suggest that there is no difference in time to mood relapse between lithium and divalproex.

In children and adolescents who have bipolar disorder, sodium divalproex can be initiated at a dose of 20 mg/kg/day, which will typically produce a serum level of 80 to 120 μg/mL. Common side effects of divalproex in children are weight gain, nausea, sedation, and tremor. There has been much debate regarding the possible association between divalproex and polycystic ovarian syndrome (PCOS). The initial reports of PCOS were in women who had epilepsy and who were treated with divalproex, particularly if they were treated before age 18 years [52]. The hypothesized mechanism for divalproex-induced PCOS is that obesity secondary to divalproex results in elevated insulin levels, which leads to increased androgen levels and ultimately to PCOS [53]; alternatively, divalproex may directly increase ovarian androgen biosynthesis [54,55]. Further investigations of the risk of developing PCOS in girls who have bipolar disorder are necessary. Until the relationship between divalproex and PCOS is clarified, clinicians should monitor females treated with divalproex for any signs of PCOS that include weight gain, menstrual abnormalities, hirsutism, or acne.

Carbamazepine

Carbamazepine has been used for seizure management in children and adolescents but less commonly in those who have bipolar disorder. There have also been several case reports and series describing the successful use of carbamazepine as monotherapy and adjunctive treatment in children and adolescents who have bipolar disorder [45,56,57]. Carbamazepine must be titrated slowly and requires frequent monitoring of blood levels because of CYP450 drug interactions. Side effects of carbamazepine include developing aplastic anemia and severe dermatologic reactions, such as Stevens-Johnson's syndrome, hyponatremia, nausea, and sedation. Carbamazepine is therefore less commonly used in children and adolescents who have bipolar disorder [58]. Carbamazepine is usually titrated to a dose of 15 mg/kg/day to produce a serum level of 7 to 10 μg/mL. It is difficult to use carbamazepine with sodium divalproex because of the CYP450 drug interaction with these two agents.

Novel antiepileptic agents

Several new antiepileptic drugs may have mood-stabilizing properties, although the data are presently limited regarding the efficacy and tolerability of these agents for the treatment of pediatric bipolar disorder. These novel antiepileptic drugs may be useful as adjuncts for the treatment of manic and hypomanic episodes.

Oxcarbazepine, an analogue of carbamazepine but without the potentially toxic epoxide metabolite, is a promising agent for acute mania in adults [59,60]. Presently, however, there are no data to support its use in children and adolescents who have bipolar disorder.

Lamotrigine has been reported effective as adjunctive treatment for children and adolescents who have bipolar disorder and in particular those who have bipolar depression [61–63]. Its use for pediatric bipolar disorder has been limited because of the risk of potentially lethal cutaneous reactions, such as Stevens-

Johnson syndrome and toxic epidermal necrolysis. The risk of a serious rash is greater in children and adolescents younger than 16 years old than in adults, but a recent more conservative dosing schedule seems to have substantially reduced the rate of serious rashes [64,65].

Gabapentin was no more effective than placebo for the treatment of acute mania in adults [66]. Gabapentin may be effective for the treatment of anxiety disorders in adults [67,68], however, and is generally well tolerated in children and adolescents. Gabapentin may be useful for treating children and adolescents who have bipolar disorder and who are also diagnosed as having a comorbid anxiety disorder, but controlled data are lacking.

Topiramate now has preliminary data from open studies [69] indicating it may be effective as an adjunctive treatment for pediatric bipolar disorder [70]. Despite four studies in adults indicating that topiramate is no more effective than placebo for the treatment of acute mania, a recent double-blind, placebo-controlled study of topiramate in children and adolescents who had mania suggests it may be more effective than in adults, although the study had an insufficient sample size, and the difference in reduction of manic symptoms between placebo and topiramate did not reach statistical significance [19]. Word-finding difficulties have been reported in up to one third of patients treated with topiramate [71]. Topiramate is associated with anorexia and weight loss [72] and therefore, may be useful as adjunctive treatment for children and adolescents who have bipolar disorder and who have gained weight as a result of treatment with other psychotropic medications.

Atypical antipsychotics

Atypical (second-generation) antipsychotic agents are efficacious for the treatment of schizophrenia, bipolar disorder, treatment-resistant depression, and posttraumatic stress disorder in adults [73–76]. In adults who have bipolar disorder, these agents have demonstrated efficacy for treatment of mania, depression, and maintenance [77,78]. Several case series and open-label reports and one double-blind, placebo-controlled study suggest that the atypical antipsychotics clozapine [79], risperidone [80,81], olanzapine [82–84], and quetiapine [85] are effective for the treatment of pediatric mania. In a double-blind, placebo-controlled trial, quetiapine plus divalproex was more efficacious for the treatment of adolescent mania than divalproex alone [85]. More recently, in a follow-up study, quetiapine monotherapy was found to be at least as effective as divalproex for the treatment of acute manic and mixed episodes in adolescents who had bipolar disorder. Clinically, these agents seem to be more efficacious than the traditional mood stabilizers in children and adolescents who have bipolar disorder. Currently, there are ongoing placebo-controlled trials of several atypical antipsychotics, including risperidone, olanzapine, and quetiapine, for the treatment of mania in children and adolescents. Information on dosing and clinical monitoring of atypical antipsychotics is provided in Table 4.

Table 4
Atypical antipsychotics in children and adolescents who have bipolar disorder

Generic name	Trade name in United States	How supplied (mg)	Pediatric starting dose	Target dose (mg/d)	Cautions
Clozapine	Clozaril	25, 100	25 bid	200–400	Monitor white blood cell count weekly
					Seizures possible at higher doses
Olanzapine	Zyprexa Zydis	2.5, 5, 7.5, 10, 15, 20 5, 10, 15, 20	2.5 bid	10–20	Monitor weight, cholesterol
Quetiapine	Seroquel	25, 100, 200, 300	50 bid	400–600	
Risperidone	Risperdal	0.25, 0.5, 1,2, 3, 4	0.25 bid	1–2	Monitor for extrapyramidal symptoms and galactorrhea
Ziprasidone	Geodon	20, 40, 60, 80	20 bid	80–120	Check baseline EKG and as dose increases
Aripiprazole	Abilify	5, 10, 15, 25	2.5–5 qhs	10–25	Monitor for PY-450 interactions (CYP3A4 and CYP2D6)

Despite the effectiveness of atypical antipsychotics, these agents possess notable side effects. Clozapine and olanzapine frequently cause significant weight gain in children and adolescents [86]. Several metabolic problems may occur as a result of increases in weight, including type II (non–insulin-dependent) diabetes mellitus, hyperlipidemia, and transaminase elevation [87,88]. Children who experience significant weight gain should be monitored especially closely for these possibilities and should be referred for exercise and nutritional counseling. Recently the American Diabetes Association in collaboration with the American Psychiatric Association published a monitoring protocol for all patients before initiating treatment with an atypical antipsychotic [89]. This protocol includes obtaining a personal and family history of obesity, diabetes, dyslipidemia, hypertension, and cardiovascular disease, measuring weight and height to calculate body mass index, measuring waist circumference (at the level of the umbilicus) and blood pressure, as well as obtaining fasting serum glucose and lipid profiles. This group recommended that the patient's weight should be reassessed at 4, 8, and 12 weeks after initiating or changing therapy with an atypical antipsychotic and quarterly thereafter at the time of routine visits. If a patient gains more than 5% of his or her initial weight at any time during therapy, consideration should be given to switching the patient to an alternative agent. Although these guidelines are extremely useful, they were not written for a pediatric population, and the 5% weight gain threshold may not be sensitive enough for children and adolescents. Ziprasidone [90] may cause QTc prolongation in children and adolescents [91]. Therefore, ziprasidone should be used with caution in children and adolescents who have bipolar disorder, and EKGs should be monitored at baseline and when dosages are increased.

Treatment strategies

The overall strategy when treating children and adolescents who have bipolar disorder is to stabilize their mood first and then treat other comorbid disorders, such as ADHD or anxiety disorders. The majority of prepubertal children who have a bipolar disorder present with mixed mania or hypomania that responds best to either a traditional mood stabilizer like divalproex or an atypical antipsychotic. The atypical antipsychotics, because of their effectiveness and ease of use, are quickly becoming first-line treatments for manic, mixed, and hypomanic episodes in children and adolescents. If a child or adolescent presents with a "classic" euphoric mania without psychotic symptoms, a trial of lithium may be helpful. Often it is difficult to maintain a child or adolescent on lithium for extended periods of time because of the associated weight gain, exacerbation of acne, and hypothyroidism. If psychotic symptoms are present as part of a child or adolescent's mania, treatment with an atypical antipsychotic agent is indicated [92].

Most children and adolescents who have bipolar disorder require combination pharmacotherapy for mood stabilization, but the data on combination treatment are limited [47,93]. In the only double-blind, placebo-controlled study of an atypical antipsychotic for the treatment of adolescents who have bipolar disorder, quetiapine in combination with divalproex resulted in a greater reduction of manic symptoms than divalproex monotherapy, suggesting that the combination of a mood stabilizer and an atypical antipsychotic is more effective than a mood stabilizer alone for the treatment of adolescent mania. In this study, quetiapine was titrated to a dose of 450 mg/day in 7 days and was well tolerated [43].

Treatment of children who have bipolar disorder and co-occurring ADHD requires mood stabilization with a traditional mood stabilizer or an atypical antipsychotic as a necessary prerequisite before initiating stimulant medications [94]. A recent randomized, controlled trial of 40 children and adolescents who had bipolar disorder and ADHD demonstrated that low-dose mixed-salts amphetamines can be used safely and effectively for treatment of comorbid ADHD symptoms after mood stabilization with divalproex [95]. Sustained-release psychostimulants may be more effective in reducing rebound symptoms in children and adolescents who have bipolar disorder. A typical dose of such stimulants for a child who has bipolar disorder and ADHD would be 36 to 54 mg/day of Concerta or Adderall XR dosed 10 to 20 mg/day.

There is limited information regarding the treatment of depression in children and adolescents who have bipolar disorder, and the role of antidepressants in the treatment of bipolar disorder depression is unclear. One retrospective study assessing treatment for depressed children and adolescents who have bipolar disorder suggested that selective serotonin reuptake inhibitors (SSRIs) may be effective treatment for acute bipolar disorder depression in children and adolescents without interfering with the acute antimanic effects of mood stabilizers. This report also suggests that SSRIs may have mood-destabilizing effects. Because too few subjects were being treated with mood stabilizers at the time when manic symptoms may have reemerged, however, the authors did not evaluate the protective effects of mood stabilizers in preventing the destabilizing effects [96]. This study indicated that depressive symptoms were seven times more likely to improve when subjects received an SSRI than when they did not. In contrast, tricyclics antidepressants, stimulants, mood stabilizers, and typical antipsychotics were not significantly associated with improvement in depressive symptomatology. Subjects in this study who were receiving a SSRI were three times more likely to develop manic symptoms at their next follow-up than subjects who were not treated with SSRIs.

Lamotrigine has been found to be effective in case series and prospective open-label studies of adolescents who have bipolar disorder [62,63] and is an emerging option for the treatment of depression in these adolescents.

Psychosocial issues

Most traditional psychotherapeutic interventions have not been systematically studied in children and adolescents who have bipolar disorder. It is necessary to educate children and adolescents and their families and teachers about bipolar illness, the importance of medication compliance, and the need for regular monitoring of mood-stabilizer serum levels and other laboratory measures. Instructing patients or their parents to keep a daily record of the level of depressive and manic symptoms (mood charting) is a tool that may help monitor symptom presence and recurrence. In a recent study, Fristad and colleagues [3] reported the efficacy of multifamily psychoeducational group therapy for the treatment of children and adolescents who have bipolar disorder and their families, and Fristad is planning to publish a manual that details this therapy.

Other useful psychosocial tactics in these patients include

- Minimizing periods of overstimulation
- Maintaining good sleep hygiene
- Addressing issues of medication nonadherence immediately
- Discussing the risk of substance abuse with the patient
- Encouraging mood charting by the patient and or parent

Patients and their families should be educated about the common and potential adverse effects of the psychotropic medications that they are prescribed, and any concerns should be addressed before the treatment is started. An excellent resource for patients and parents about the adverse effects of psychotropic medication is the book, *Helping Parents, Youth, and Teachers Understand Medications for Behavioral and Emotional Problems: A Resource Book of Medication Information Handouts*, by Dulcan and Benton [97]. Other useful print resources for parents include

1. *New Hope for Children and Teens with Bipolar Disorder: Your Friendly, Authoritative Guide to the Latest in Traditional and Complementary Solutions*, by Boris Birmaher, MD
2. *Raising a Moody Child: How to Cope with Depression and Bipolar Disorder*, by Jill S. Goldberg Arnold, MD, and Mary A. Fristad, MD
3. *Understanding and Educating Children and Adolescents with Bipolar Disorder: A Guide for Educators*, by Margot Andersen, MSW, Jane Boyd Kubisak, MS, Ruth Field, MSW, LSW, and Steven Vogelstein, MA, LCSW

In addition, several websites have been described as useful by parents whose children suffer from bipolar disorder. These include

1. Child and Adolescent Bipolar Foundation (CABF) (http://www.cabf.org). The Child and Adolescent Bipolar Foundation is a parent-led, non-profit, web-based membership organization of families raising children diagnosed with, or at risk for, early-onset bipolar disorder. The CABF website is an outstanding source of information about this disorder for patients, parents and clinicians.

2, National Alliance for the Mentally Ill (NAMI) (http://www.nami.org). NAMI is one of the best advocacy organizations in the United States for people with mental illnesses and their families.

3. Depression and Bipolar Support Alliance (DBSA) (http://www.dbsalliance. org/). The DBSA is the nation's largest patient-directed, illness-specific organization.

Summary

Pediatric bipolar disorder is increasingly recognized as a serious and prevalent mood disorder that requires early recognition and intervention. New screening and diagnostic tools are available to aid in the diagnosis of disorder in children and adolescents who have bipolar disorder. Additional data supporting the use of mood stabilizers and atypical antipsychotics in this population are also emerging. Combinations of existing psychotropics remain the most effective treatment of pediatric bipolar disorder at this point. Novel agents, particularly anticonvulsants (ie, lamotrigine), may add to the armamentarium, albeit primarily as augmenting and stabilizing agents. Bipolar disorder is a chronic disorder in children and adolescents, much like diabetes, and is best managed with supportive and educational therapies that involve the patient and the family. Several groups are developing programs that recognize this need [98–100]. Increased recognition, diagnosis, and treatment of pediatric patients who have bipolar disorder will improve the outcome for these patients and their families.

Appendix 1. K-SADS Mania Rating Scale

This scale was developed by David Axelson, MD, and Boris Birmaher, MD, at the University of Pittsburgh.

This rating scale is based on the items from the 4th Revision of the KSADS-P (Joaquim Puig-Antich, MD, and Neal Ryan, MD) and some additional descriptors from the WASH-U-KSADS (Barbara Geller, MD). The following items are to determine the severity of manic or hypomanic symptoms during a period of time prescribed by the rater/study (usually a 1-week period). At the end of the scale, the rater should note the onset and offset of the time period being rated. If any of the items are judged present, inquire in a general way to determine how the patient was behaving at the time with such questions as, "When you were this way, what kind of things were you doing? How did you spend your time?" If there have been manic periods, it is exceedingly important that they are clearly delineated.

If the subject has described only dysphoric mood, the following questions regarding the manic syndrome should be introduced with a statement such as, "I know you have been feeling (___); however, many people have other feelings mixed in or at different times too." The most difficult patients to assess are those in whom manic and depressed symptoms simultaneously coexist, superimposed on each other during the same times (mixed states). The rater should keep this possibility in mind as s/he goes through this section.

This is a semi-structured scale, so that the rater is to use his or her judgment about how many of the suggested questions will be asked for each symptom. The rater should also make additional inquiries or clarifications as indicated.

The ratings are based on all available information about the time period rated (parent and child interview, records or other reports if available). The rater is to use his or her best clinical judgment and take into account the available information about the frequency, intensity, duration, and impairment of each symptom to formulate a summary rating for each item.

1. Elation, expansive mood

Elevated mood and/or optimistic attitude toward the future which lasted at least 4 hours and was out of proportion to the circumstances. Differentiate from normal mood in chronically depressed subjects. Do not rate positive if mild elation is reported in situations (Christmas, birthdays, amusement parks) that normally overstimulate and make children very excited.

- Have (there been times when) you felt very good or too cheerful or high or terrific or great, or just not your normal self?

If unclear:

- When you felt on top of the world or as if there was nothing you couldn't do? ... That this is the best of all possible worlds? Have you felt that everything would work out just the way you wanted?
- If people saw you, would they think you were just in a good mood or something more than that?
- Did you get as if you were drunk? Did you laugh a lot, get silly? Did you feel super happy? When did this happen? (example)
  - 0 No information
  - 1 Not at all, normal, or depressed
  - 2 Slight: Good spirits, more cheerful than most people in his/her circumstances, but of only possible clinical significance
  - 3 Mild: Definitely elevated mood and optimistic outlook that is somewhat out of proportion to his/her circumstances
  - 4 Moderate: Mood and outlook are clearly out of proportion to circumstances; noticeable to others
  - 5 Severe: Quality of euphoric mood way out of proportion to circumstances
  - 6 Extreme: Clearly elated, almost constantly exalted expression, overexpansive

2. Irritability and anger

Subjective feeling of irritability, anger, crankiness, bad temper, short-tempered, resentment, or annoyance, externally directed, whether expressed overtly or not. Rate the intensity and duration of such feelings. Do not rate here if irritability is caused by depression or disruptive disorders.

- Do you get annoyed and irritated or cranky at little things?
- What kinds of things?
- Have you been feeling mad or angry also (even if you don't show it)? How angry? More than before?
- What kinds of things make you feel angry?
- Do you sometimes feel angry and/or irritable, and/or cranky and don't know why? Does this happen often?
- Do you lose you temper?
- With your family? Your friends? Who else? At school? What do you do?
- Has anybody said anything about it?
- How much of the time do you feel angry, irritable, and/or cranky? All of the time? Lots of the time? Just now and then? None of the time?
- When you get mad, what do you think about?
- Do you think about killing others? Or about hurting them or torturing them? Whom? Do you have a plan? How?
  0 No information
  1 Not at all, clearly of no clinical significance
  2 Slight and doubtful clinical significance
  3 Mild: Often (at least 3×3 hours each week) feels definitely more angry, irritable than called for by the situation relatively frequently but never very intensely; or often argumentative; quick to express annoyance; no homicidal thoughts
  4 Moderate: Most days irritable/angry or more than 50% of awake time; often shouts, loses temper; occasional homicidal thoughts
  5 Severe: At least most of the time child is aware of feeling very irritable or quite angry or has frequent homicidal thoughts (no plan) or thoughts of hurting others; or throws and breaks things around the house
  6 Extreme: Most of the time feels extremely angry or irritable, to the point s/he "can't stand it"; or frequent uncontrollable tantrums

3. Decreased need for sleep

Less need for sleep than usual in order to feel rested (average for several days when needed less sleep). (Refer to norms on insomnia.)

- Have you needed less sleep than usual to feel rested? How much sleep do you ordinarily need?

- How much do you sleep when you are feeling so good?
- When you wake up do you feel good and rested?
- When you cannot fall asleep or when you get up through the night, what types of things do you do?
- Watch TV? Read? Or do you do active things? (eg, rearrange furniture? clean house? exercise?)
- Do you have a lot of thoughts go through your mind when awake? What kinds of thoughts?
- Do you worry? About what types of things?
- How long are you awake? How often during the night? During the week?
  0 No information
  1 No change or more sleep needed
  2 Up to 1 hour less than usual
  3 Up to 2 hours less than usual
  4 Up to 3 hours less than usual
  5 Up to 4 hours less than usual
  6 4 or more hours less than usual

4. Unusually energetic

More active than his/her usual level without expected fatigue.

- Have you had more energy than usual to do things?
- Did people tell you that you were (are) non-stop?
- Did you agree with them? Did it seem like too much energy? Do you know why? Were you doing too many things? Did you feel tired?
- When did this happen? (example)
  0 No information
  1 No difference than usual or less energetic
  2 Slightly more energetic but of questionable significance
  3 Little change in activity level but less fatigued than usual
  4 Somewhat more active than usual with little or no fatigue
  5 Much more active than usual with little or no fatigue
  6 Unusually active all day long with little or no fatigue

5a. Increase in goal-directed activity

As compared with usual level. Consider changes in scholastic, social, sexual, or leisure involvement or activity level associated with work, family, friends, new projects, interests, or activities (eg, telephone calls, letter writing).

- Is there any time when you were more active or involved in things compared to the way you usually are? What about in school, at your club, scouts, church, at home, friends, hobbies, new projects or interests?

- Were you doing a lot of things?
- How much of your day has been spent in this?
- Were you trying to do so many different things that you couldn't keep up?
- When did this happen? (example)
  0 No information
  1 No change or decrease
  2 Slightly more interest or activity but of questionable significance
  3 Mild but definite increase in general activity level involving several areas
  4 Moderate generalized increase in activity level involving several areas
  5 Marked increase and almost constantly involved in numerous activities in many areas
  6 Extreme (eg, constantly active in a variety of activities from awakening until going to sleep)

5b. Motor hyperactivity

Visible manifestations of generalized motor hyperactivity which occurred during a period of abnormally elevated, expansive, or irritable mood. Make certain that the hyperactivity actually occurred and was not merely a subjective feeling of restlessness. Make sure it is not chronic but episodic hyperactivity.

- When you were (__), were there times when you were (high, feeling so good, so angry) that you were always moving, could not stay put, were unable to sit still or you always had to be moving, pacing up and down?
- Or are you always like that?
  0 No information
  1 Not at all or retarded
  2 Slight increases which is of doubtful clinical significance
  3 Mild: Unable to sit quietly in a chair
  4 Moderate: Paces about a great deal
  5 Marked: Almost constantly moving and pacing about
  6 Extreme: So hyperactive that s/he would exhaust her/himself if not restrained

6. Grandiosity

Increased self-esteem and appraisal of his/her worth, power, or knowledge (up to grandiose delusions) as compared with usual level. Persecutory delusions should not be considered evidence of grandiosity unless that subject feels the persecution results from some of his/her special attributes (eg, power, knowledge).

- Have you felt more self-confident than usual?
- Have you felt much better than others? . . . smarter? . . . stronger?

- Why?
- Have you felt that you are a particularly important person or that you had special talents or abilities?
- What about special plans?
- When did this happen? (example)
  - 0 No information
  - 1 Not at all or decreased self esteem
  - 2 Slight: Somewhat more confident about himself but of doubtful clinical significance
  - 3 Mild: Definitely overestimates or exaggerates at least two of his talents, prospects, or plans
  - 4 Moderate: Disproportionately inflated self-esteem involving several areas of functioning
  - 5 Severe: Marked, global, overevaluation of her/himself and her/his abilities, but falls short of true delusions
  - 6 Extreme: Clear grandiose delusions

7. Accelerated, pressured, or increased amount of speech

- When you were (__), were there times that you talked very rapidly or talked on and on and couldn't be stopped?
- Did people say you were talking too much?
- Could people understand you?
  - 0 No information
  - 1 Not at all or retarded speech
  - 2 Slight increase, which is doubtful clinical significance
  - 3 Mild: Noticeably more verbose than normal, but conversation is not strained
  - 4 Moderate: So verbose that conversation is strained
  - 5 Marked: So rapid that conversation is difficult to maintain
  - 6 Extreme: Talks rapidly or continuously and cannot be interrupted; conversation extremely difficult or impossible

8a. Racing thoughts

Subjective experience that thinking was markedly accelerated.

- When you were (__), were there times when your thoughts raced through your mind?
- Did you have more ideas than usual or more than you could handle?
  - 0 No information
  - 1 Not at all
  - 2 Doubtful

3 Mild: Occasional racing thoughts at least three times per week

4 Moderate: Racing thoughts at least 50% of awake time

5 Severe: Racing thoughts most of the time

6 Extreme: Almost constant racing thoughts

8b. Flight of ideas (observed or reported by informant)

Accelerated speech with abrupt changes from topic to topic, usually based on understandable associations, distracting stimuli, or play on words. In rating severity consider speed of associations and inability to complete ideas or sustain attention in a goal-directed manner. When severe, complete or partial sentences may be galloping on each other so fast that apparent sentence-to-sentence de-railment and/or sentence incoherence may also be present. An extreme example of this symptom is "You have to be quiet to be sad. Everything having to do with 's' is quiet—on the q.t.—sit, sob, sigh, sin, sorrow, surcease, sought, sand, sweet mother's love, and salvation."

- Have there been times when people could not understand you?
- When they said you did not make sense?
- Could you give me an example?
  0 No information
  1 Not at all or some other form of
  2 Slight: Occasional instances, which are of doubtful clinical significance
  3 Mild: Occasional instances of abrupt change in topics with some impairment in understandability; more than 5% of sentence to sentence transitions are abrupt
  4 Moderate: Frequent instances with moderate impairment in understand-ability (>10%)
  5 Severe: Very frequent instances with definite impairment in understand-ability (>25%)
  6 Extreme: Most speech consists of such rapid changes of topic that it is impossible to follow (>50%)

9. Poor judgment

Excessive involvement in dangerous activities without recognizing the high potential for painful consequences.

- When you were (___), did you do anything that caused trouble for you or your family ... or friends?
- What about anything that could have?
- Did you do things you normally wouldn't do (like giving away a whole lot of things or taking a whole lot of chances)?

- Did you think of what would happen before you did it?
- Was there anything that you did that you now think you should not have done?
  0 No information
  1 Not at all
  2 Slight: Of doubtful clinical significance
  3 Mild: For example, calls friends at odd hours
  4 Moderate: For example, purchases many things she/he doesn't need and can't afford or gives money away
  5 Severe: For example, on impulse, goes to places without plans or money and takes too many chances
  6 Very Severe: Attempts activities with potentially very
  dangerous consequences

10. Distractibility (observed or reported by informant)

Child presents evidence of difficulty focusing his/her attention on the questions of the interviewer, jumps from one thing to another, cannot keep track of his/her answers, and is drawn by irrelevant stimuli he cannot shut off. Not to be confused with avoidance of uncomfortable themes.

- Have you ever been told that you have trouble sticking to what you are supposed to do? Did you?
- Can you give me an example?
- Has a teacher told you that you "always" get distracted?
  0 No information
  1 Not at all
  2 Slight: Of doubtful clinical significance
  3 Mild: Present but responds to structuring and repetition
  4 Moderate: Difficult to complete interview because of child's inattentiveness, which does not respond to structure
  5 Severe: Impossible to complete interview because of child's inattentiveness

11. Hallucinations

Sometimes children, when they are alone, hear voices or see things, or smell things, and they don't quite know where they come from.

- Has this happened to you?
- Do you ever hear voices when you are alone?
- Have you ever seen things that were not there?

- When did you?
- What did you see?
- What did you hear?
- Has there been anything unusual about the way things sounded?
- How often have you heard these voices (noises)? (smell, feeling, visions) Is it some of the time, only now and then, most of the time, or all of the time?
- What do you think it is?
- Do you think it is your imagination or real?
- Did you think it was real when you (heard, saw, etc) it?
- Do you think it's real or your imagination now?
- What did you do when you (heard, saw, etc) it?
  0 No information or not applicable
  1 Not at all; absent
  2 Suspected/possible
  3 Mild: Definitely present but subject is generally aware it is his imagination and usually able to ignore it; occurs no more than once per week
  4 Moderate: Generally believes in the reality of the hallucinations, but it has little influence on his behavior or occurs at least once per week
  5 Severe: Convinced his hallucination is real and significantly effects his actions (ie, locks door to keep pursuers away) or occurs frequently
  6 Extreme: Actions based on hallucinations have major impact on him or others (eg, unable to do school work because of constant "conversations") or occurs most of the time

12. Delusions

- Do you know what imagination is? Tell me.
- Sometimes does your imagination play tricks on you? What kind of tricks? Tell me more about them.
- Do you have any ideas about things that you don't tell anyone because they might not understand? What are they?
- Do you have any secret thoughts? Tell me about them.
- Do you believe in other things that other people don't believe in? Like what? Is anybody out to hurt you?
- Does anybody control your mind or body (like a robot)?
- Is anything happening to your body?
- Do you ever feel the world is coming to an end?
- Do you ever think you are an important or great person? Who?
- Are you sure that this (. . .?) is this way?
- Could there be any other reason for it?
- Who do you know that it happens as you say?
- Any other possible explanation?

- Do you enjoy making up stories like this?
- Or is it different from making up stories?

(Interviewer might suggest other possible explanations and see how the subject reacts to them.)

- Did you ever think that this was your imagination?
- Do you think it could be your imagination?
- What did you do about ... ?
  0 No information
  1 Definitely not delusional
  2 Suspected
  3 Mild: Delusion definitely present but at times subject questions his false belief
  4 Moderate: Generally has conviction in his false belief
  5 Severe: Delusion has a significant effect on his actions (eg, often asks family to forgive his sins, preoccupied with belief that he is a new Messiah)
  6 Extreme: Actions based on delusions have major impact on him or others (eg, stops eating because believes food is poisoned)

13. Mood lability

Changeability of mood; rapid mood variation with several mood states (angry, elated, depressed, anxious, relaxed) within a brief period of time; appears internally driven without regard to circumstances or not related to anything external to the patient. Could be an exaggerated mood change in regard to minor slights, frustrations, or positive events.

  0 No information
  1 Not at all
  2 Slight: Some moodiness or mood variation possibly out of proportion to circumstances but of doubtful significance
  3 Mild: Definite mood changes, internally driven or somewhat out of proportion to circumstances, occurring several times per day; noticeable by others but does not cause significant impairment in functioning or relationships
  4 Moderate: Many mood changes throughout the day; can vary from elevated mood to anger to sadness within a couple of hours; changes in mood clearly out of proportion to circumstances and causes impairment in functioning
  5 Severe: Rapid mood swings nearly all of the time, with mood intensity way out of proportion to circumstances
  6 Extreme: Constant, explosive variability in mood, several mood changes occurring within minutes; difficult to identify a particular mood; changes in mood radically out of proportion to circumstances

Number of days during rating period with 4 hours of manic symptoms: _____

Percentage of rated time period that subject had manic symptoms: _____ %

Scoring

- Take maximum of 5a and 5b to determine score of item 5
- Take maximum of 8a and 8b to determine score of item 8
- Add scores of the 13 items
- Subtract 13 from total to zero the scale
- Total score is 0–64

General guidelines for correlation of Mania Rating Scale scores to CGI-BP Mania Severity scores

- No or minimal: Mania Rating Scale (MRS) ≤ 11
- Mild: MRS ~12–17
- Moderate: MRS ~18–25
- Marked or worse: MRS ≥ 26

(*From* Axelson D, Birmaher B, Brent D, et al. The K-SADS mania rating scale for pediatric bipolar disorder. J Child Adolesc Psychopharmacol 2003; 13(4):463–70; with permission.)

Appendix 2. The Mood Disorder Questionnaire

The Mood Disorder Questionnaire (MDQ)

This questionnaire should be used as a starting point. It is not a substitute for a full medical evaluation. Bipolar disorder is a complex illness, and an accurate, thorough diagnosis can only be made through a personal evaluation by your doctor. However, a positive screen here may suggest that you might benefit from seeking such an evaluation from your doctor. Regardless of the questionnaire results, if you or someone you know has concerns about your mental health, please contact your physician or another healthcare professional.

INSTRUCTIONS: Please answer each question as best you can.

	YES	NO
1. Has there ever been a period of time when you were not your usual self and...		
... you felt so good or so hyper that other people thought you were not your normal self or you were so hyper that you got into trouble?	O	O
... you were so irritable that you shouted at people or started fights or arguments?	O	O
... you felt much more self-confident than usual?	O	O
... you got much less sleep than usual and found that you didn't really miss it?	O	O
... you were more talkative or spoke much faster than usual?	O	O
... thoughts raced through your head or you couldn't slow your mind down?	O	O
... you were so easily distracted by things around you that you had trouble concentrating or staying on track?	O	O
... you had much more energy than usual?	O	O
... you were much more active or did many more things than usual?	O	O
... you were much more social or outgoing than usual, for example, you telephoned friends in the middle of the night?	O	O
... you were much more interested in sex than usual?	O	O
... you did things that were unusual for you or that other people might have thought were excessive, foolish or risky?	O	O
... spending money got you or your family in trouble?	O	O
2. If you checked YES to more than one of the above, have several of these ever happened during the same period of time?	O	O
3. How much of a problem did any of these cause you - like being able to work; having family, money or legal troubles; getting into arguments or fights?		

O No problem   O Minor problem   O Moderate problem   O Serious problem

	YES	NO
4.* Have any of your blood relatives (i.e. children, siblings, parents, grandparents, aunts, uncles) had manic-depressive illness or bipolar disorder?	O	O
5.* Has a health professional ever told you that you have manic-depressive illness or bipolar disorder?	O	O

*Derived from Hirschfeld RM. *Am J Psychiatry*. 2000:157(11):1873-5.

The Mood Disorder Questionnaire

How to evaluate your results

Answering "Yes" to 7 or more of the events in question #1, answering "Yes" to question #2, and answering "Moderate problem" or "Serious problem" to question #3 is considered a positive screen for bipolar disorder.

(*From* Eli Lilly and Company, Indianapolis, Indiana; with permission.)

References

[1] Lewinsohn PM, Klein DN, Seeley JR. Bipolar disorders in a community sample of older adolescents: prevalence, phenomenology, comorbidity, and course. J Am Acad Child Adolesc Psychiatry 1995;34(4):454–63.

[2] Geller B, Luby J. Child and adolescent bipolar disorder: a review of the past 10 years. J Am Acad Child Adolesc Psychiatry 1997;36(9):1168–76.

[3] Fristad MA, Goldberg-Arnold JS. Family information for early onset bipolar disorder. In: Geller B, DelBello M, editors. Child and early adolescent bipolar disorder: theory, assessment, and treatment. New York: Guilford Publications, Inc.; 2002. p. 295–313.

[4] Geller B, Bolhofner K, Craney J, et al. Psychosocial functioning in a prepubertal and early adolescent bipolar disorder phenotype. J Am Acad Child Adolesc Psychiatry 2000;39(12): 1543–8.

[5] Weinberg WA, Brumback RA. Mania in childhood: case studies and literature review. Am J Dis Child 1976;130:380–5.

[6] Akiskal HS, Downs J, Jordan P, et al. Affective disorders in referred children and younger siblings of manic-depressives. Mode of onset and prospective course. Arch Gen Psychiatry 1985;42(10):996–1003.

[7] Kashani JH, Beck NC, Hoeper EW, et al. Psychiatric disorders in a community sample of adolescents. Am J Psychiatry 1987;144(8):584–9.

[8] Jonas BS, Brody D, Roper M, et al. Prevalence of mood disorders in a national sample of young American adults. Soc Psychiatry Psychiatr Epidemiol 2003;38(11):618–24.

[9] Youngstrom EA, Duax J. Evidence-based assessment of pediatric bipolar disorder, part I: base rate and family history. J Am Acad Child Adolesc Psychiatry 2005;44(7):712–7.

[10] Wozniak J, Biederman J, Kiely K, et al. Mania-like symptoms suggestive of childhood-onset bipolar disorder in clinically referred children. J Am Acad Child Adolesc Psychiatry 1995; 34(7):867–76.

[11] Isaac G. Misdiagnosed bipolar disorder in adolescents in a special educational school and treatment program. J Clin Psychiatry 1992;53(4):133–6.

[12] DelBello MP, Geller B. Review of studies of child and adolescent offspring of bipolar parents. Bipolar Disord 2001;3:325–34.

[13] Hodgins S, Faucher B, Zarac A, et al. Children of parents with bipolar disorder. A population at high risk for major affective disorders. Child Adolesc Psychiatr Clin N Am 2002;11(3): 533–53, ix.

[14] Geller B, Zimerman B, Williams M, et al. Diagnostic characteristics of 93 cases of a prepubertal and early adolescent bipolar disorder phenotype by gender, puberty and comorbid attention deficit hyperactivity disorder. J Child Adolesc Psychopharmacol 2000;10:157–64.

[15] Findling RL, Gracious BL, McNamara NK, et al. Rapid, continuous cycling and psychiatric co-morbidity in pediatric bipolar I disorder. Bipolar Disord 2001;3:202–10.

[16] Wozniak J, Biederman J. Childhood mania: insights into diagnostic and treatment issues. J Assoc Acad Minor Phys 1997;8(4):78–84.

[17] Geller B, Zimerman B, Williams M, et al. Reliability of the Washington University in St. Louis Kiddie Schedule for Affective Disorders and Schizophrenia (WASH-U-KSADS) mania and rapid cycling sections. J Am Acad Child Adolesc Psychiatry 2001;40(4):450–5.

[18] Geller B, Tillman R, Craney JL, et al. Four-year prospective outcome and natural history of mania in children with a prepubertal and early adolescent bipolar disorder phenotype. Arch Gen Psychiatry 2004;61(5):459–67.

[19] Delbello MP, Findling RL, Kushner S, et al. A pilot controlled trial of topiramate for mania in children and adolescents with bipolar disorder. J Am Acad Child Adolesc Psychiatry 2005; 44(6):539–47.

[20] Kovacs M, Akiskal HS, Gatsonis C, et al. Childhood-onset dysthymic disorder. Clinical features and prospective naturalistic outcome. Arch Gen Psychiatry 1994;51(5):365–74.

[21] Akiskal HS. Developmental pathways to bipolarity: are juvenile-onset depressions pre-bipolar? J Am Acad Child Adolesc Psychiatry 1995;34(6):754–63.

[22] Lewinsohn P, Klein D, Seeley J. Bipolar disorder during adolescence and young adulthood in a community sample. Bipolar Disord 2000;2(3 Pt 2):281–93.

[23] Leibenluft E, Charney DS, Towbin KE, et al. Defining clinical phenotypes of juvenile mania. Am J Psychiatry 2003;160(3):430–7.

[24] Burd L, Klug MG, Martsolf JT, et al. Fetal alcohol syndrome: neuropsychiatric phenomics. Neurotoxicol Teratol 2003;25(6):697–705.

[25] Wolfson AR, Carskadon MA. Understanding adolescents' sleep patterns and school performance: a critical appraisal. Sleep Med Rev 2003;7(6):491–506.

[26] Carskadon MA, Acebo C. Regulation of sleepiness in adolescents: update, insights, and speculation. Sleep 2002;25(6):606–14.

[27] Kafantaris V, Dicker R, Coletti DJ, et al. Adjunctive antipsychotic treatment is necessary for adolescents with psychotic mania. J Child Adolesc Psychopharmacology 2001;11:409–13.

[28] Young RC, Biggs JT, Ziegler VE, et al. A rating scale for mania: reliability, validity and sensitivity. Br J Psychiatry 1978;133:429–35.

[29] Fristad MA, Weller EB, Weller RA. The Mania Rating Scale: can it be used in children? A preliminary report. J Am Acad Child Adolesc Psychiatry 1992;31:252–7.

[30] Fristad MA, Weller RA, Weller EB. The Mania Rating Scale (MRS): further reliability and validity studies with children. Ann Clin Psychiatry 1995;7:127–32.

[31] Hirschfeld RM, Calabrese JR, Weissman MM, et al. Screening for bipolar disorder in the community. J Clin Psychiatry 2003;64(1):53–9.

[32] Hirschfeld RM, Holzer C, Calabrese JR, et al. Validity of the mood disorder questionnaire: a general population study. Am J Psychiatry 2003;160(1):178–80.

[33] Depue RA, Krauss S, Spoont MR, et al. General behavior inventory identification of unipolar and bipolar affective conditions in a nonclinical university population. J Abnorm Psychol 1989;98(2):117–26.

[34] Youngstrom EA, Findling RL, Danielson CK, et al. Discriminative validity of parent report of hypomanic and depressive symptoms on the General Behavior Inventory. Psychol Assess 2001;13(2):267–76.

[35] Axelson D, Birmaher BJ, Brent D, et al. A preliminary study of the Kiddie Schedule for Affective Disorders and Schizophrenia for School-Age Children mania rating scale for children and adolescents. J Child Adolesc Psychopharmacol 2003;13(4):463–70.

[36] Puig-Antich J, Ryan N. Kiddie Schedule for Affective Disorders and Schizophrenia. Present state version. Pittsburgh (PA): Western Psychiatric Institute and Clinic; 1986.

[37] Faraone SV, Biederman J, Wozniak J, et al. Is comorbidity with ADHD a marker for juvenile-onset mania? J Am Acad Child Adolesc Psychiatry 1997;36(8):1046–55.

[38] West SA, McElroy SL, Strakowski SM, et al. Attention deficit hyperactivity disorder in adolescent mania. Am J Psychiatry 1995;152(2):271–3.

[39] Geller B, Williams M, Zimerman B, et al. Prepubertal and early adolescent bipolarity differentiate from ADHD by manic symptoms, grandiose delusions, ultra-rapid or ultradian cycling. J Affect Disord 1998;51:81–91.

[40] Kovacs M, Pollock M. Bipolar disorder and comorbid conduct disorder in childhood and adolescence. J Am Acad Child Adolesc Psychiatry 1995;34(6):715–23.

[41] Wilens TE, Biederman J, Kwon A, et al. Risk of substance use disorders in adolescents with bipolar disorder. J Am Acad Child Adolesc Psychiatry 2004;43(11):1380–6.

[42] Geller B, Cooper TB, Sun K, et al. Double-blind and placebo-controlled study of lithium for adolescent bipolar disorders with secondary substance dependency. J Am Acad Child Adolesc Psychiatry 1998;37(2):171–8.

[43] DelBello M, Schwiers M, Rosenberg H, et al. Quetiapine as adjunctive treatment for adolescent mania associated with bipolar disorder. J Am Acad Child Adol Psychiatry 2002;41(10): 1216–23.

[44] Strober M. Mixed mania associated with tricyclic antidepressant therapy in prepubertal delusional depression: three cases. J Child Adolesc Psychopharmacol 1998;8(3):181–5.

[45] Kowatch RA, Suppes T, Carmody TJ, et al. Effect size of lithium, divalproex sodium and carbamazepine in children and adolescents with bipolar disorder. J Am Acad Child Adol Psychiatry 2000;39(6):713–20.

[46] Youngerman J, Canino IA. Lithium carbonate use in children and adolescents. A survey of the literature. Arch Gen Psychiatry 1978;35(2):216–24.

[47] Findling RL, McNamara NK, Gracious BL, et al. Combination lithium and divalproex sodium in pediatric bipolarity. J Am Acad Child Adolesc Psychiatry 2003;42(8):895–901.

[48] Wagner KD, Weller E, Biederman J, et al. An open-label trial of divalproex in children and adolescents with bipolar disorder. J Am Acad Child Adolesc Psychiatry 2002;41(10):1224–30.

[49] West SA, Keck PEJ, McElroy SL, et al. Open trial of valproate in the treatment of adolescent mania. J Child Adolesc Psychopharmacol 1994;4:263–7.

[50] Papatheodorou G, Kutcher SP, Katic M, et al. The efficacy and safety of divalproex sodium in the treatment of acute mania in adolescents and young adults: an open clinical trial. J Clin Psychopharmacol 1995;15(2):110–6.

[51] Findling RL, McNamara NK, Youngstrom EA, et al. Double-blind 18-month trial of lithium versus divalproex maintenance treatment in pediatric bipolar disorder. J Am Acad Child Adolesc Psychiatry 2005;44(5):409–17.

[52] Isojarvi JI, Laatikainen TJ, Pakarinen AJ, et al. Polycystic ovaries and hyperandrogenism in women taking valproate for epilepsy. N Engl J Med 1993;329(19):1383–8.

[53] Rasgon NL, Altshuler LL, Fairbanks L, et al. Reproductive function and risk for PCOS in women treated for bipolar disorder. Bipolar Disord 2005;7(3):246–59.

[54] Nelson-DeGrave VL, Wickenheisser JK, Cockrell JE, et al. Valproate potentiates androgen biosynthesis in human ovarian theca cells. Endocrinology 2004;145(2):799–808.

[55] Nelson-Degrave VL, Wickenheisser JK, Hendricks KL, et al. Alterations in mitogen-activated protein kinase kinase and extracellular regulated kinase signaling in theca cells contribute to excessive androgen production in polycystic ovary syndrome. Mol Endocrinol 2005;19(2): 379–90.

[56] Evans RW, Clay TH, Gualtieri CT. Carbamazepine in pediatric psychiatry. J Am Acad Child Adolesc Psychiatry 1987;26(1):2–8.

[57] Puente RM. The use of carbamazepine in the treatment of behavioural disorders in children. In: Birkmayer W, editor. Epileptic seizures—behaviour—pain. Baltimore (MD): University Park Press; 1975. p. 243–52.

[58] O'Donovan C, Kusumakar V, Graves GR, et al. Menstrual abnormalities and polycystic ovary syndrome in women taking valproate for bipolar mood disorder. J Clin Psychiatry 2002; 63(4):322–30.

[59] Nassir Ghaemi S, Ko JY, Katzow JJ. Oxcarbazepine treatment of refractory bipolar disorder: a retrospective chart review. Bipolar Disord 2002;4(1):70–4.

[60] Hummel B, Stampfer R, Grunze H, et al. Acute antimanic efficacy and safety of oxcarbazepine in and open trial with on-off-on design. Bipolar Disord 2001;3(Suppl 1):43.

[61] Kusumakar V, Yatham LN. An open study of lamotrigine in refractory bipolar depression. Psychiatry Res 1997;72:145–8.

[62] Carandang CG, Maxwell DJ, Robbins DR, et al. Lamotrigine in adolescent mood disorders. J Am Acad Child Adolesc Psychiatry 2003;42(7):750–1.

[63] Saxena K, Chang KD, Howe MG. Lamotrigine as adjunct or monotherapy in the treatment of adolescents with bipolar depression or mixed states. Presented at the 51st Annual Meeting of the American Academy of Child and Adolescent Psychiatry. Washington (DC), October 20, 2004.

[64] Messenheimer JA, Guberman AH. Rash with lamotrigine: dosing guidelines. Epilepsia 2000; 41(4):488.

[65] Messenheimer J. Efficacy and safety of lamotrigine in pediatric patients. J Child Neurol 2002; 17(Suppl 2):2S34–42.

[66] McElroy SL, Keck Jr PE. Pharmacologic agents for the treatment of acute bipolar mania. Biol Psychiatry 2000;48(6):539–57.

[67] Pande AC, Davidson JR, Jefferson JW, et al. Treatment of social phobia with gabapentin: a placebo-controlled study. J Clin Psychopharmacol 1999;19:341–8.

[68] Pande AC, Pollack MH, Crockatt J, et al. Placebo-controlled study of gabapentin treatment of panic disorder. J Clin Psychopharmacol 2000;20(4):467–71.

[69] Yatham LN, Kusumakar V, Calabrese JR, et al. Third generation anticonvulsants in bipolar disorder: a review of efficacy and summary of clinical recommendations. J Clin Psychiatry 2002;6:275–83.

[70] DelBello M, Kowatch R, Warner J, et al. Topiramate treatment for pediatric bipolar disorder: a retrospective chart review. J Child Adolesc Psychopharmacology 2002;12(4):323–30.

[71] Crawford P. An audit of topiramate use in a general neurology clinic. Seizure 1998;7:207–11.

[72] McElroy SL, Suppes T, Keck PE, et al. Open-label adjunctive topiramate in the treatment of bipolar disorders. Biol Psychiatry 2000;47(12):1025–33.

[73] Miyamoto S, Duncan GE, Marx CE, et al. Treatments for schizophrenia: a critical review of pharmacology and mechanisms of action of antipsychotic drugs. Mol Psychiatry 2005;10(1): 79–104.

[74] Trivedi MH. Treatment-resistant depression: new therapies on the horizon. Ann Clin Psychiatry 2003;15(1):59–70.

[75] Glick ID, Murray SR, Vasudevan P, et al. Treatment with atypical antipsychotics: new indications and new populations. J Psychiatr Res 2001;35(3):187–91.

[76] Kapur S, Remington G. Atypical antipsychotics: new directions and new challenges in the treatment of schizophrenia. Annu Rev Med 2001;52:503–17.

[77] Keck PJ, McElroy S, Arnold L. Bipolar disorder. Med Clin North Am 2001;85:645–61.

[78] Tohen M, Ketter TA, Zarate CA, et al. Olanzapine versus divalproex sodium for the treatment of acute mania and maintenance of remission: a 47-week study. Am J Psychiatry 2003;160(7): 1263–71.

[79] Kowatch RA, Suppes T, Gilfillan SK, et al. Clozapine treatment of children and adolescents with bipolar disorder and schizophrenia: a clinical case series. J Child Adolesc Psychopharmacol 1995;5(4):241–53.

[80] Frazier J, Meyer M, Biederman J, et al. Risperidone treatment for juvenile bipolar disorder: a retrospective chart review. J Am Acad Child Adolesc Psychiatry 1999;38:960–5.

[81] Biederman J. Open label study of risperidone in children with bipolar disorder. Poster presented at the 16th European College of Neuropsychopharmacology Congress. Prague (Czechoslovakian Republic), September 20–24, 2003.

[82] Soutullo C, Sorter M, Foster K, et al. Olanzapine in the treatment of adolescent acute mania: a report of seven cases. J Affect Disord 1999;53:279–83.

[83] Khouzam H, El-Gabalawi F. Treatment of bipolar I disorder in an adolescent with olanzapine. J Child Adolesc Psychopharmacol 2000;10:147–51.

[84] Chang K, Ketter T. Mood stabilizer augmentation with olanzapine in acutely manic children. J Child Adolesc Psychopharmacol 2000;10:45–9.

[85] Delbello MP, Schwiers ML, Rosenberg HL, et al. A double-blind, randomized, placebo-

controlled study of quetiapine as adjunctive treatment for adolescent mania. J Am Acad Child Adolesc Psychiatry 2002;41(10):1216–23.

[86] Ratzoni G, Gothelf D, Brand-Gothelf A, et al. Weight gain associated with olanzapine and risperidone in adolescent patients: a comparative prospective study. J Am Acad Child Adolesc Psychiatry 2002;41:337–43.

[87] Clark C, Burge MR. Diabetes mellitus associated with atypical anti-psychotic medications. Diabetes Technol Ther 2003;5(4):669–83.

[88] Lebovitz HE. Metabolic consequences of atypical antipsychotic drugs. Psychiatr Q 2003;74(3): 277–90.

[89] American Diabetes Association, American Psychiatric Association, American Association of Clinical Endocrinologists, et al. Consensus development conference on antipsychotic drugs and obesity and diabetes. Diabetes Care 2004;27(2):596–601.

[90] Weiden P. Ziprasidone: a new atypical antipsychotic. J Psychiatr Pract 2001;7(2):145–53.

[91] Blair J, Scahill L, State M, et al. Electrocardiographic changes in children and adolescents treated with ziprasidone: a prospective study. J Am Acad Child Adolesc Psychiatry 2005;44(1): 73–9.

[92] Kafantaris V, Coletti DJ, Dicker R, et al. Adjunctive antipsychotic treatment of adolescents with bipolar psychosis. J Am Acad Child Adolesc Psychiatry 2001;4:1448–56.

[93] Kowatch RA, Sethuraman G, Hume JH, et al. Combination pharmacotherapy in children and adolescents with bipolar disorder. Biol Psychiatry 2003;53(11):978–84.

[94] Biederman J, Mick E, Prince J, et al. Systematic chart review of the pharmacologic treatment of comorbid attention deficit hyperactivity disorder in youth with bipolar disorder. J Child Adolesc Psychopharmacol 1999;9(4):247–56.

[95] Scheffer R, Kowatch R, Carmody T, et al. A randomized placebo-controlled trial of Adderall for symptoms of comorbid ADHD in pediatric bipolar disorder following mood stabilization with divalproex sodium. Am J Psychiatry 2005;162:58–64.

[96] Biederman J, Mick E, Spencer TJ, et al. Therapeutic dilemmas in the pharmacotherapy of bipolar depression in the young. J Child Adolesc Psychopharmacol 2000;10(3):185–92.

[97] Dulcan M, Benton T. Helping parents, youth, and teachers understand medications for behavioral and emotional problems: a resource book of medication information handouts. Washington (DC): American Psychiatric Press; 1998.

[98] Fristad MA, Gavazzi SM, Mackinaw-Koons B. Family psychoeducation: an adjunctive intervention for children with bipolar disorder. Biol Psychiatry 2003;53(11):1000–8.

[99] Miklowitz DJ, George EL, Axelson DA, et al. Family-focused treatment for adolescents with bipolar disorder. J Affect Disord 2004;82(Suppl 1):S113–28.

[100] Pavuluri MN, Graczyk PA, Henry DB, et al. Child- and family-focused cognitive-behavioral therapy for pediatric bipolar disorder: development and preliminary results. J Am Acad Child Adolesc Psychiatry 2004;43(5):528–37.

ELSEVIER
SAUNDERS

Child Adolesc Psychiatric Clin N Am
15 (2006) 109–133

CHILD AND
ADOLESCENT
PSYCHIATRIC CLINICS
OF NORTH AMERICA

The Schizophrenia Prodrome:
A Developmentally Informed Review and
Update for Psychopharmacologic Treatment

Lynelle E. Thomas, MD[a,b,*], Scott W. Woods, MD[a,c]

[a]PRIME Research Clinic, New Haven, CT, USA
[b]Child Study Center, Yale University School of Medicine, 230 South Frontage Road, New Haven,
CT 06520, USA
[c]Yale University School of Medicine, New Haven, CT, USA

The possibility of treatment intervention during the schizophrenia prodromal phase has a history nearly as long as its description [1]. Until recently, however, little was known about which types of treatment would be most effective, the appropriate timing and duration of interventions, or the specific risk/benefit ratio of treatment in this symptomatic, nonpsychotic, but putatively at-risk diagnostic group. Accurate identification of those likely to develop schizophrenic psychosis offers what may be the field's best hope for developing more effective treatment strategies and perhaps secondary intervention or prevention of this potentially devastating disorder. Early intervention during this prodromal phase suggests a paradigm shift in the clinical approach to schizophrenia [2].

Before the emergence of sensitive and specific prodromal diagnostic strategies, intervention studies would have been controversial at best and unlikely to affect clinical practice. Now that this at-risk population can be identified with increasingly high and reliable diagnostic accuracy, the search for beneficial treatment interventions—biologic, psychologic, and social—and for the optimal timing for such interventions has become germane and timely.

Dr. Woods has received research grant support from Bristol-Myers Squibb, Eli Lilly, Glytech Inc., and Janssen Research Foundation.

* Corresponding author. Child Study Center, Yale University School of Medicine, 230 South Frontage Road, New Haven, CT 06520.

E-mail address: lynelle.thomas@yale.edu (L.E. Thomas).

doi:10.1016/j.chc.2005.08.011
childpsych.theclinics.com

This article presents a developmentally informed practitioner review of current research examining prospective diagnostic criteria and psychopharmacologic treatment options for the prodrome of schizophrenic psychosis.

Schizophrenia and its prodrome

Etiology

Schizophrenia is considered a disorder of disrupted maturation of the central nervous system [3,4]. It is hypothesized that pathologic neurodevelopmental processes occur during a critical stage of forebrain development in gestation and affect neurons primarily in the thalamic, prefrontal and frontal cortical, and limbic regions of the brain. These processes are likely to be expressed premorbidly by subtle behavioral, cognitive, and structural vulnerability markers. In most cases, these abnormalities require specific maturational processes (ie, synaptic elimination, myelination), which occur around puberty, to unmask the vulnerability and trigger dysfunction. These later neuromaturational processes result in the development or worsening of attenuated positive symptoms (seen in the at-risk state or prodrome). Subsequently, during the psychotic phase, a diverse but specific array of impairments in social function, social cognition, neurocognitive function, olfaction, and motor function has been well established. The related stress-vulnerability model hypothesizes that these vulnerable neural circuits may be perturbed further by environmental circumstances that typically occur during adolescence, such as stressful life events or drug abuse. Such stressors may exceed the adaptive capacity of relevant circuits, producing the characteristic symptoms that signal the onset of the illness.

The notion that therapeutic intervention during this window of neurobiologic dysgeneration might delay or arrest the abnormalities before they become fulminant or irreversible provides impetus and rationale for conducting innovative psyochpharmacologic treatment intervention studies. Ongoing follow-along research studies of child and adolescent patients identified as being at risk offer unique opportunities for further elucidation of a neurodevelopmental hypothesis [5].

Natural history

The natural history of schizophrenia can be divided into three phases: premorbid, prodromal, and psychotic [6], as depicted in Fig. 1. The premorbid phase is a period of relatively stable, mild, and asymptomatic deficits beginning at birth and generally lasting until some time after puberty. Although infants and prepubertal children who are destined to become schizophrenic can be distinguished as a group from normal children, it is not yet feasible to identify individuals as preschizophrenic during the premorbid phase.

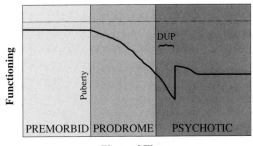

Phase of Illness

Fig. 1. Phases of schizophrenia. Model describing premorbid, prodromal, and psychotic phases of schizophrenia. The ordinate indicates age-adjusted general functional status. The dotted line indicates normal average age-adjusted functioning. The dark line indicates the path of the modal patient who has schizophrenia. DUP, duration of untreated psychosis, the period of time between onset of frank psychosis and first treatment.

The prodromal phase is the first symptomatic phase and is progressive rather than stable. It usually begins sometime after puberty and most frequently lasts 1 to a few years [6,7]. Early symptoms are relatively nonspecific: anxiety, depression, and increasing problems with attentional and other cognitive impairments, social isolation, and academic difficulties. Later in the prodrome symptoms become more specific as subsyndromal positive symptoms emerge and then crystallize into frank psychosis at the time of onset. A prototypical late-prodrome subsyndromal positive symptom might be hearing a noise that increasingly resembles a mumble or whisper. Many patients, unfortunately, may not begin treatment for months or even years after the onset of frank psychosis. The length of this period between onset and first treatment is referred to as the "duration of untreated psychosis."

Much of what is known about the schizophrenia prodrome is based on retrospective histories from patients who have developed the full disorder. Many such reports have appeared during the past century, but one of the most influential of these studies was first reported only a decade or so ago [8]. Data from retrospective studies are generally consistent with the model shown in Fig. 1. Because retrospective studies are inherently prone to recall bias, prospective methods are clearly needed as well.

Several kinds of prospective studies have been conducted, including birth-cohort, genetic high-risk, and prospective historical studies, as well as longitudinal prodromal studies. In keeping with this article's focus on recent findings and on pharmacologic treatment, these issues are addressed only briefly. The interested reader is referred to a recent more comprehensive review [9]. Birth-cohort studies identify a large number of subjects, typically 1000 to 15,000 or more, and follow them through the age of risk. Analyses then compare the 1% or so who become schizophrenic with the remaining 99% using measures that were collected prospectively. Several of these studies have "come of age" in recent years, including the 1946 British cohort [10], the 1958 United Kingdom cohort [11], the 1966 Northern Finland cohort [12,13], the 1959–1966 Philadelphia cohort [14], and the 1972–1973 Dunedin cohort [15,16].

Genetic high-risk studies are similar to birth-cohort studies but are restricted to subjects at familial risk for schizophrenia. Offspring of schizophrenic parents are at approximately 10% lifetime risk of developing schizophrenia, compared with approximately 1% of subjects in birth-cohort studies. Typically these studies have enrolled much smaller numbers of subjects, but the largest, the Copenhagen High Risk Study, enrolled 207 at-risk children. Age at enrollment has varied among these studies, with the New York Infant Development Study [17], the Jerusalem Infant Development Study [18], and the Copenhagen Obstetric High Risk Study [19] enrolling at birth, the New York High Risk Project [20] at a mean of 9 years, the Israeli High Risk Project [21] at a mean of 11 years, the Copenhagen High Risk Study [22] at a mean of 15 years, the Finnish Adoptive Study of Schizophrenia [23,24] at a mean of 16 years, and the Edinburgh High Risk Study [25,26] at a mean of 21 years. Prospective historical studies identify schizophrenic and control groups and compare them on the basis of historical data collected prospectively years previously. The types of "found data" that have been employed include draft board [27], military [28,29], school [30,31], or child-guidance clinic records [32] and childhood home movies [33,34].

Taken together, this literature has generated a remarkably detailed and consistent picture of the premorbid phase of schizophrenia, characterized by delayed milestones in infancy, motor clumsiness and social deficits in early childhood, and attentional and other cognitive deficits in later childhood and adolescence. Although findings are often quite significant statistically, the mean difference between premorbid-phase preschizophrenic children and controls is generally small, and there is substantial overlap with the control group. As a consequence, individual diagnosis during the premorbid phase is not yet feasible. For example, one of the strongest findings from the 1946 British birth-cohort study was delayed walking in the infants destined to become schizophrenic, but the mean delay compared with controls in age at walking in the preschizophrenic infants was only 1.2 months.

Unfortunately, this body of research thus far has yielded little useful information about the prodromal phase of schizophrenia. Many of the birth-cohort studies were designed to learn about childhood development generally rather than schizophrenia per se. Consequently, assessment measures or schedules of prospective assessment were sometimes not optimal for schizophrenia research aims, particularly during adolescence. There have been few published longitudinal descriptions of a prodromal phase coming from these datasets. For example, the Dunedin study assessed subjects for psychotic symptoms at 11 years, but similar data from the assessments at ages 13, 15, 18, and 21 years have not been reported. Recent exceptions include data from the Edinburgh High Risk Study, which evaluated 162 genetically predisposed subjects, aged 16 to 24 years at study entry, every 18 months for 9 years. Schizotypal symptoms at baseline increased the positive predictive value for onset of schizophrenic psychosis from approximately 10% to as high as 50% [25]. Anxiety and affective symptoms were also high at baseline among those who later converted [26]. Some of these subjects may have already entered a prodromal phase by the time of study entry. Changes in state at evaluations intermediate between baseline and conversion do not seem to have been described as yet. Another recent paper from the Finnish Adoptive Study of Schizophrenia reported on thought disorder assessments at a median age of 21 years among 75 offspring of schizophrenic mothers adopted before age 4 years and reassessed at median ages of 34 and 42 years [24]. Only six patients have converted so far, and results were somewhat inconclusive. Thus, much of what has been learned about the prodromal phase of schizophrenia comes from more recently launched longitudinal studies that enroll patients diagnosed as being at risk for schizophrenia based on recently developed diagnostic criteria.

Prospective diagnostic criteria for the schizophrenia prodrome

Early attempts

The earliest attempt to construct prodromal diagnostic criteria was the checklist in the *Diagnostic and Statistical Manual*, edition three, revised (*DSM-III-R*). This attempt did not succeed. Considerable variability in reliability was present across studies of the *DSM-III-R* prodromal symptoms assessed retrospectively in stabilized psychotic patients. Moreover, a survey of high-school students reported that the prevalence of self-report endorsement of *DSM-III-R* prodromal symptoms was very high, ranging from 10% to 50% across symptoms among older adolescents [35]. Such data resulted in the omission of the *DSM-III-R* list of prodromal symptoms in the *DSM-IV*.

Current prospective diagnostic criteria and assessment scales

In the middle and late 1990s, investigators renewed attempts to create prospective diagnostic criteria that could reliably and validly identify prodromal patients at risk for the development of schizophrenic psychosis within a time frame lending itself to intervention. The most informative early detection work has focused primarily on clarifying the features of late prodromal states. The greatest potential lies in the identification of individuals most at risk of developing psychosis in the near future, because the accuracy of true-positive case identification is believed to be higher than in the earlier prodrome. This article highlights two of the structured diagnostic interviews and diagnostic criteria resulting from these efforts and the predictive validity studies that have tested their usefulness.

Early in their study of the prodrome, investigators at the University of Melbourne, Australia, conducted a comprehensive review of descriptive work by Hafner and colleagues and other early retrospective work [36]. Their findings were consistent with the now increasingly employed model in which the early prodrome begins as nonspecific, neurotic-type symptoms (decreased concentration and attention, apathy, anergie, depressed mood, sleep disturbance, anxiety, social withdrawal, deterioration in role functioning, and irritability), with the late prodrome following with more marked deviations from normal (including more specific subthreshold forms of recognizable psychotic symptoms). Subsequently, the Melbourne group developed a structured diagnostic interview, the Comprehensive Assessment of Symptoms of At-Risk Mental States (CAARMS) that operationally defines a mental state at "ultra high risk" for conversion to psychosis [37]. The CAARMS criteria diagnose three prodromal syndromes, based on (1) attenuated positive symptoms, (2) fully psychotic but very brief and intermittent positive symptoms, and (3) a substantial recent fall in functioning along with genetic risk. Initially based on items borrowed from other measures (eg, the Brief Psychiatric Rating Scales and the Comprehensive Assessment of Symptoms and History [37]), the revised CAARMS has become a stand-alone instrument. It has been reported to demonstrate good reliability and predictive validity [38].

The authors' PRIME (Prevention through Risk Identification, Management & Education) group modified the CAARMS criteria for the three prodromal subgroups [39], primarily by emphasizing recency of onset or change in symptoms. The reader is referred to Miller and colleagues [39] for a detailed, side-by-side comparison of the two sets of criteria.

The authors' group also developed a structured diagnostic interview using probes and anchors designed specifically to assess prodromal symptoms, the Structured Interview for Prodromal Syndromes (SIPS). They demonstrated excellent inter-rater reliability with their revised criteria when using the SIPS, with 93% agreement in differentiating prodromal from nonprodromal subjects among raters at that site [40]. They also found that training was required to use the SIPS reliably across other sites [39]. In addition, they developed a rating scale to determine the current severity of prodromal symptoms, known as the Scale of Prodromal Symptoms (SOPS). Inter-rater reliability was excellent for 17 of the 19 items and was nearly excellent on the other 2 items [39].

Both the CAARMS and the SIPS criteria are fairly complex and may be more useful in research rather than clinical contexts at this point. A simplified version of the SIPS criteria may be more suited to clinical use:

1. Abnormal unusual thought content, suspiciousness, grandiosity, perceptual abnormalities, and/or disorganization of communication, all below the threshold of frank psychosis because of subsyndromal intensity, duration, or frequency

AND

2. These symptoms have begun or worsened in the past year

AND

3. These symptoms currently have occurred at least once per week during the last month

These criteria encompass the first two prodromal syndromes captured by the CAARMS and SIPS without requiring scores on the specific rating scales used in the two structured interviews. Criteria for the third syndrome (functional decline and genetic risk) are omitted, primarily because these cases are seen relatively infrequently in the absence of one of the other prodromal syndromes. In three large, descriptive samples reported to date, only 19% [41], 18% [42], and 5% [43], respectively, met criteria for the third syndrome alone. In addition, when patients with functional decline and genetic risk but no positive symptoms are followed over time, it is likely that among those progressing to psychosis, many if not most will develop subsyndromal positive symptoms and thus eventually will meet the simplified criteria before conversion.

Predictive validity

Four research groups have published data testing the predictive validity of these prodromal diagnostic criteria by following diagnosed patients over time in the absence of specific interventions: the Melbourne, Australia, PRIME, Newcastle, Australia, and Manchester, United Kingdom groups. The Melbourne group has reported on 104 patients diagnosed prospectively as prodromal using the CAARMS and followed for at least 6 months [41]. These patients had been enrolled at their PACE (Personal Assessment and Crisis Evaluation) clinic before the investigators began their clinical trial [44], or were enrolled in the control group in the trial, or declined to enter the trial. None received antipsychotic medication during follow-up. According to Kaplan-Meier estimates, 35% progressed to psychosis within 12 months. In an earlier report on a subsample of these patients, 32% of the patients who did not progress to psychosis were diagnosed at follow-up as having nonpsychotic disorders [45]. Unfortunately the authors did not measure diagnostic comorbidity at baseline, so it was difficult know whether the disorders were already present before follow-up assessment. The authors' group has analyzed data showing high rates of diagnostic comorbidity at baseline in prodromal patients [46]. In addition, no follow-up category of "still prodromal" was possible as an outcome.

The PRIME group has found that 7 of the 13 patients (54%) diagnosed prospectively as prodromal using the SIPS and who received no specific treatment progressed to psychosis within 12 months [40]. Five of the 13 prodromal patients who did not progress to psychosis (38%) were diagnosed at follow-up as still prodromal; 2 of the 13 (15%) neither progressed nor remained prodromal. Of the two patients in whom prodromal symptoms remitted, one was diagnosed as having major depression, and the other was considered healthy. None of the 16 symptomatic subjects invited for diagnostic interview but not meeting the SIPS prospective prodromal diagnostic criteria progressed to psychosis within 12 months ($P < .01$ prodromal versus nonprodromal) [40]. Another group of untreated subjects reported by the PRIME group [47] were those who were assigned to placebo in a recent clinical trial, as discussed later (Table 1). Among

Table 1
Comparison of three randomized treatment studies in prodromal patients

Study [reference]	Age range (mean) (y)	Follow-up (mo)	Innovative Treatment	Conversion rate (%)	Control Treatment	Conversion rate (%)
PACE (Melbourne, Australia) [44]	14–28 (20)	6	Risperidone/cognitive behavioral therapy	3/31 (10)	Needs based	10/28 (36)
PRIME (New Haven, CT, USA) [47,58]	12–36 (18)	12	Olanzapine	5/31 (16)	Placebo	11/29 (38)
University of Manchester (Manchester, UK) [48]	16–36 (22)	12	Cognitive behavioral therapy	2/35 (6)	Monitoring	5/26 (22)

29 such patients, 11 (38%) were known to progress to psychosis within 12 months.

Recently a group from Newcastle, Australia, has recently published a follow-up study of 74 prodromal patients diagnosed according to the CAARMS criteria and followed for a mean of 26.3 months. The mean age at intake was 17 years (range, 13–28 years). No patients received antipsychotic medication during follow-up. The rate of transition to psychosis was 50% over this period [42].

The Manchester, United Kingdom, group [48] also has published outcomes on prodromal patients assigned to a control group in a clinical trial (as discussed later and shown in Table 1), in which 5 of 26 patients (22%) converted to psychosis within 12 months.

In summary, four groups have published data on five samples consisting of 13 to 104 prodromal patients followed between one year and an average 26 months. The rates of conversion to psychosis in these samples not receiving specific treatment have been 22%, 35%, 38%, 50%, and 54%, respectively. Among symptomatic patients invited to diagnostic interview who did not meet prodromal criteria, one sample reported a zero rate of conversion at 1 year. These high positive predictive and negative predictive values are robust evidence for the predictive validity of the prodromal diagnosis based on current criteria. In addition, these high rates of development of a serious mental illness provide strong impetus for research into prevention of conversion among prodromal patients.

Psychopharmacologic treatment options

Rationale

The recent progress in prodromal classification and diagnostic accuracy justifies further investigation of potential interventions [49]. As researchers and clinicians continue to identify and gain clinical experience with prodromal patients, appreciation is growing that

1. These patients' symptoms are relatively severe compared with other patients perceived as in need of psychiatric treatment [43].
2. Prodromal patients and their families experience substantial current distress [50–52].
3. Most patients have a history of treatment-seeking behavior and have received psychiatric services previously, including medications [53].
4. Prodromal patients have shown significant signs of cognitive impairment [54].
5. Substantial current disability is suggested by relatively low baseline GAF (Global Assessment of Functioning) scores [43].

Thus, current symptoms, impairment, distress, and help-seeking provide a robust rationale for early detection and intervention research. In addition, the demonstrated risk of progression without specific treatment also highlights a compelling need for research targeting the prevention of schizophrenia.

The Institute of Medicine has outlined several types of prevention [55]. Secondary prevention can occur when a selective intervention is targeted to individuals who are determined to be at greater risk for developing a specific disorder. Early antipsychotic treatment administered before or soon after first-break psychosis can maximize treatment response, lead to better long-term outcomes, and possibly exert preventive effects [44,47,56]. Early-intervention research groups characterize their intervention strategy as illness prevention in the public health conceptualization—that is, as early intervention with the help-seeking, symptomatic individual focused on preventing a decline in functioning, as opposed to preventing the transition to psychosis per se [57]. There is no established standard of care for individuals meeting diagnostic criteria for the schizophrenia prodrome, and psychopharmacologic intervention cannot be recommended as routine for clinical practice. An established standard of care is unlikely to emerge before a substantial body of intervention research is available to inform the development of standards. Thus, although intervention during a putative prodromal phase remains controversial, intervention research need no longer be.

Antipsychotics

Two controlled trials suggest that antipsychotics may be effective in prodromal patients, and one trial suggests benefits of a cognitive-behavioral intervention. These studies are described in Table 1.

McGorry and colleagues conducted the PACE trial in Melbourne, Australia [44]. They randomly assigned prodromal patients to open-label risperidone plus cognitive behavioral therapy (CBT) versus a needs-based intervention that consisted of supportive therapy and non-neuroleptic psychotropics (see Table 1). The average age of participants was 20 years, with a range from 14 to 28 years. The average risperidone dose achieved was 1.3 mg/day. This dose is substantially lower than the minimum risperidone dose reported to be consistently effective versus placebo in exacerbated chronic patients (4 mg/day) [35]. At 6 months, 9.7% (3 of 31) of the risperidone-treated group converted to psychosis. After 6 months, risperidone was discontinued. Within the subsequent 6-month follow-up period some of the discontinued group went on to convert to psychosis. Of the control group, 36% (10 of 28) converted to psychosis. Reported follow-up information on symptom severity and adverse effects was sparse.

These findings of the Melbourne study were groundbreaking and provide intriguing evidence that atypical antipsychotic medication might prevent progression to psychosis in this at-risk group. The lack of a placebo group makes it impossible speculate on the possibility of placebo effect, however. In addition, given that biologic and somatic treatments were "bundled," it is not possible to tease out the separate effects, beneficial or otherwise, of either component. To establish the true benefits of medication, assessment of the risk/benefit ratio of the treatment alone versus placebo in larger numbers of patients would be necessary. Use of placebo controls when no standard treatment has yet been established is consistent with the World Medical Association's Declaration of Helsinki and its recent fifth revision [59].

With the Melbourne results in mind, McGlashan and colleagues and the PRIME group designed and conducted the first double-blind, placebo-controlled clinical trial of an atypical neuroleptic for the prodromal syndrome [43,60]. The clinical trial was conducted from four sites. Sixty participants were randomly assigned to receive either olanzapine or placebo. The average age of participants at enrollment was 18 years (range, 12–36 years). In line with the Melbourne study, most patients met prodromal diagnostic criteria based on attenuated positive symptoms.

Results from the first 8 weeks of the study showed that patients improved significantly more in the olanzapine group than in the placebo group on several measures, including the SOPS total score [58]. The mean modal dose over the first 8 weeks was 8.4 mg/day. This dose is slightly lower than the minimum olanzapine dose reported to be consistently effective versus placebo in exacerbated chronic patients (10 mg/day) [60]. Results from the first year showed a trend for the conversion to psychosis rate to be lower with olanzapine than with placebo [47]. These results were quite similar to those seen in the Melbourne risperidone/CBT study (see Table 1). Significant symptomatic improvement with olanzapine versus placebo was sustained from 8 weeks to 6 months or more. Weight gain was a significant adverse effect in the olanzapine group.

Perhaps at this point the most pressing question relating to antipsychotic treatment of prodromal patients is how long to continue it once begun. Unfortunately, because of small initial sample sizes and attrition over time within the samples, the two available antipsychotic treatment studies together offer little information. In the risperidone/CBT study, patients took the drug for 6 months and then stopped for another 6 months. In the olanzapine study, patients took the drug for 12 months and then stopped for another 12 months. In both studies, some patients progressed to schizophrenia during follow-up after medication discontinuation.

Antidepressants

Depressed mood is a frequent symptom early in the prodrome that can persist into the later prodrome and after onset. Stress can play a role in the progression of schizophrenia, and antidepressant medications protect the central nervous system from the adverse effects of stress. There is thus a strong rationale for investigating the possible treatment benefits of antidepressants in prodromal patients. Unfortunately, no controlled studies of antidepressants have yet been mounted successfully. The randomized trial comparing risperidone plus CBT with a needs-based control treatment [44] permitted antidepressant treatment as needed in either arm. The transition rate did not differ significantly among patients in the needs-based control group, whether or not antidepressants were employed.

Novel medications

Antipsychotic medications were tried first for prodromal patients. A part of the concern about prodromal intervention is that even the new atypical antipsychotics can have worrisome side effects, including weight gain. Many of these side effects can be more prominent in adolescents than in adults [61,62]. Although it makes sense that antipsychotic medications would be tried first for prodromal patients, the prodrome may involve neurotoxic or degenerative processes that are distinct from the neurobiology associated with the chronic stages of schizophrenia. Other medications, perhaps only weakly effective for chronic patients, could influence the potentially unique neurobiology of the prodromal phase and might thereby improve prodromal symptoms or prevent schizophrenia from developing.

There are numerous examples throughout medicine in which a treatment can be fully effective and even curative when given early in the course of illness but less effective or even completely ineffective later in the course of illness after the pathophysiology has changed. A familiar example is neonatal hypothyroidism (cretinism). This condition is asymptomatic at birth because the fetus has developed normally as the result of maternal thyroid hormone. If the illness is detected by screening shortly after birth, early thyroid hormone supplementation allows fully normal postnatal neurologic development. If the illness is not detected until neurologic symptoms develop, later thyroid hormone supplementation corrects thyroid hormone levels but does not restore normal neurologic functioning, and the child remains chronically developmentally disabled.

Some research groups are beginning to investigate medications that are not fully antipsychotic in chronic patients as possible treatments for prodromal patients [63]. These novel treatments include omega-3 essential fatty acids, which may target abnormal phospholipid metabolism in the schizophrenic central nervous system, as well as lithium and glycine. Glycine is an amino acid neurotransmitter that binds to a site on the N-methyl-D-aspartate receptor. Glycine reverses the effects of psychotogenic N-methyl-D-aspartate antagonists such as ketamine and PCP (phencyclidine) [64], and glycine supports long term potentiation [65], a neurobiologic process closely linked to activity-dependent synaptogenesis that may remediate cortical synaptic plasticity and deficits in dendritic complexity. Glycine has been used successfully as an adjunct to ongoing antipsychotic treatment in several studies of patients who have chronic schizophrenia [66]. The authors' group has recently completed an 8-week open-label pilot trial of glycine used alone in 10 prodromal patients [67]. Substantial improvements on the SOPS rating scale were observed. These results are promising, but a caveat must be mentioned that improvement in an active arm can be significantly lower when the trial employs a placebo arm as well [68]. A placebo-controlled trial of glycine will begin soon.

Nonbiologic treatments

There is some suggestion that the pathway from vulnerability state to psychotic experience might represent some breakdown of coping strategies and cognitive vulnerability [69] that could be responsive to nonbiologic interventions (eg, supportive, psychosocial interventions during the prodrome) [48]. These interventions also bypass consideration of false-positive participants being unnecessarily exposed to the risks of pharmacotherapeutic treatments. Recently a controlled study was published comparing CBT with no antipsychotic medication versus a monitoring condition in prodromal patients [48]. CBT was associated with a lower rate of progression to psychosis; however, interpretation of the results is complicated by two early-converting patients having been removed from the CBT group after randomization. In addition, the conversion rate in the control treatment was lower than that seen in the two previous antipsychotic studies (see Table 1), possibly suggesting that a different type of prodromal patient might have been recruited. A comparison across studies in Table 1 also raises the question whether the benefit seen in the Melbourne risperidone plus CBT study [44] was actually caused by the CBT rather than the risperidone. Other nonpharmacologic treatments that could be considered for study in prodromal patients include cognitive remediation [70].

Risks and benefits of prodromal intervention

What is a reasonably level trade-off of adverse effect and efficacy in intervention during the prodromal phase? Recent opinions continue to differ on this point. For example, a group recently believed that, given the current level of knowledge about risk factors and predictive accuracy, the risk–benefit assessment of biologic interventions during the prodrome is still called to question [73]. On the other hand, some investigators, whose research focuses on nontreatment questions related to the prodrome, either routinely provide medication treatment to some prodromal patients or work closely with affiliated clinicians who provide treatment to some patients based primarily on clinical judgment.

The two issues of greatest theoretic and ethical concern are the potential for false-positive and for false-negative identification, in the latter circumstance, the resulting risk for psychosis among those whose disease was undetected [49]. Patients are also potentially at risk of being stigmatized by treatment or research participation. In addition, the potential for known and yet-undiscovered negative consequences following the initiation of standard and atypical antipsychotic medications continues to create controversy concerning early interventions for putatively psychotic patients.

Of these issues of concern, the thorniest is the potential for false-positive case identification. From a risk–benefit point of view, the risk of false-negative cases with early detection is no higher than if early evaluation was not done at all. Stigmatization is always a risk, but most workers in the field believe it can be minimized by careful psychoeducational work with the patient and family.

Treatment of false-positive prodromal cases exposes patients who would never develop psychosis to the risk of antipsychotic side effects. The risk/benefit ratio for such patients would clearly be tilted toward risk. There is a possibility that such patients might benefit from relief of symptoms anyway, but this possibility is speculative and likely to remain so for some time. Clinicians contemplating clinical treatment of prodromal patients cannot know beforehand which prodromal patients are truly at risk and which are the false positives. On the other hand, the criteria, as they currently stand, confer a high enough accuracy of prediction that there now exists a substantial risk in ignoring them or in assuming that patients should be protected from awareness of the reality that they are at risk. In addition, it is possible that intervention during the prodrome, for those truly at risk and for treatment-seeking patients, might alter the risk of conversion to psychosis and improve long-term prognosis as well as addressing current symptoms and functional impairment. Thus the clinician contemplating clinical treatment of prodromal cases is currently caught between the proverbial rock and hard place.

The way out of this difficult dilemma is for clinical research to provide more information than is presently available on risks and benefits of intervention during the prodromal phase. The entire array of considerations suggests that prodromal patients constitute a clinical population whose needs warrant intervention research to provide the evidence base allowing the development of an appropriate standard of care [6].

Complicating the risk–benefit assessment is the lack of information about the specific risks of medication in this diagnostic group. In general there is limited information on adverse events in children and adolescents who are prescribed antipsychotics, although recent efforts have begun to address this gap in information. One recent analysis of adverse-event complaints to the Food and Drug Administration suggested that the low risk of extrapyramidal symptoms associated with olanzapine in adults may be comparable for children and adolescents. It also was suggested, however, that weight gain (with its attendant cardiovascular and diabetes risk) and sedation may occur more frequently in youth [74].

The case of childhood schizophrenia

Definitions

Early literature, early research, and eventually the *DSM II* conceptualized that childhood schizophrenia was, like infantile autism, part of a related spectrum of childhood psychoses, each defined by developmental delays in maturation of language, perception, and motility [75]. Subsequent research strongly supports the existence of childhood schizophrenia as a separate entity [76,77]. The consensus of available evidence suggests that schizophrenia with onset before age 13 years (early-onset schizophrenia or EOS) and later-onset schizophrenia are contiguous, and that, with appropriate developmental adjustments, conclusions regarding etiology and neurobiology can be extrapolated to children and adolescents from adult schizophrenia data [77–81]. The *DSM III* established that a diagnosis of schizophrenia in childhood and adolescence (onset before the age of 18 years) be made using the criteria used for adult schizophrenia [82]. Studies looking to evaluate these diagnostic criteria have reported mixed conclusions [83]. Some groups advocate that nosology should make distinct those cases with onset before age 13 years, that is, very early-onset schizophrenia (VEOS), from those that occur between the ages 13 and 18 years, because some evidence exists that these VEOS cases may represent a more severe form of the disease continuum [76,79]. Childhood-onset cases are generally observed to have the poorest outcome and prognosis [81,84].

Epidemiology

Adult-population studies report the prevalence of schizophrenia generally as between 0.5% and 1%. The few investigational studies of the prevalence of childhood schizophrenia have little reliability because they have used a wide array of definitions and methodologies [76]. The earliest retrospective descriptions of schizophrenia onset reported that up to 5% of adult sufferers have experienced their first episode of illness before the age of 15 years [85]. Onset under age 15 years has been reported as 50 times less common than onset in adulthood [76,84]. VEOS has been described in children as young as 4 years old [86].

Although the lifetime risk of schizophrenia is only slightly higher for males [87], the peak incidence of onset is earlier in males [88,89]. Age at onset does not necessarily differ across gender in VEOS prepubescent patients. This variance in age of onset underscores the ongoing debate over the degree (if any) puberty (eg, the biology of the changing hormonal milieu or its resulting social influences) plays in mediating (or protecting against) the neurobiology of transition to psychosis across gender. In a small VEOS sample, earlier puberty among girls was associated with earlier onset [90], but in an adult-onset sample [91], early female puberty was associated with later onset. In the VEOS sample, only 1 of 14 girls who had VEOS had prepubertal onset [90], whereas 7 of 14 boys underwent onset of psychosis prepubertally. In the adult-onset sample there were no prepubertal onsets.

An additional developmentally linked limitation related to early identification research to date and its ability to elucidate effects of puberty is that many studies report mere chronologic age, as opposed to assessment of secondary sex characteristics or a specific index of pubertal status. Chronologic age is at best a crude and at worst an inaccurate measure of true sexual development. Norms for age of pubertal onset in industrial countries decreased during the middle of the last century [92]. The rate of decline in age of puberty then slowed [93] and now seems to have stabilized during the past 2 decades [94]. Future research should determine whether similar temporal trends in age at onset of schizophrenia have been observed.

Developmental considerations in diagnosing childhood schizophrenia

Despite their similar phenomenology, a number of features of schizophrenia presenting in childhood and early adolescence seem to be qualitatively different from those of adult-onset schizophrenia. For example, classic Schneiderian first-rank symptoms are less commonly experienced in youth. Delusions and hallucinations, although common, are less complex and systematized. Visual hallucinations seem to be reported more often in EOS [95]. The presence of disorganized speech and behavior is common to a variety of disorders of childhood onset (eg, communication disorders, pervasive developmental disorders, attention-deficit hyperactivity disorder) [96] and can make accurate diagnosis in this age group especially challenging.

Hallucinatory experiences in childhood may be relatively common and may not carry a poor prognosis. The Dunedin birth-cohort study [15] reported that 14% of 761 unselected subjects endorsed psychotic symptoms at age 11 years, including 8% who endorsed hallucinations [97]. The majority of these youth are nonpathologic, carry no *DSM* diagnosis, and require no treatment. Although their risk was elevated when compared with children who did not endorse psychotic symptoms, only a small percentage (~11%) developed a schizophreniform disorder later in life [15]. In another study of adolescents who had hallucinations, among 80 subjects whose mean age was 12.9 years (range, 8–19 years), only 13 (16%) were delusional at any time in the next 3 years, although 50% were receiving psychiatric care [98]. EOS may have a more insidious onset, which might often make it difficult to distinguish between premorbid personality/cognitive abnormalities and the diagnosis of the disorder that has been termed "multidimensionally impaired disorder." Children with this disorder meet *DSM-IV* criteria for psychotic disorder, not otherwise specified, and display early behavioral and cognitive difficulties and early onset of psychotic symptoms, but their psychotic symptoms improve over time [99].

Deciphering whether childhood-reported experiences, beliefs, unusual thought content, magical thinking, or incoherent thought process/speech represent a developmentally expected immaturity of cognitive maturation or are pathologic or markers of risk in the clinical "real world" often remains a function of art more than science. Given the challenges to diagnostic accuracy and grim prognosis of EOS and VEOS, clinicians are understandably reluctant to make the diagnosis. Identified children often carry a provisional diagnosis of psychotic disorder, not otherwise specified, until the course of the illness over time allows diagnostic clarity.

Developmental considerations in diagnosing the schizophrenia prodrome

To date, researchers interested in the schizophrenia prodrome have used the same prodromal diagnostic criteria and assessment instruments (face and predictive validity described previously) in both adolescent and adult populations [72,77], with the presumption that elements and patterns essential to diagnosing the prodrome are the same in these two developmental stages. There are theoretic reasons to suspect that this practice may be valid. With increasing age, the symptomatology of youth schizophrenic patients becomes increasingly similar to that of adult patients, along with the increasing developmental and maturational capacity to express and be assessed for such symptoms. It is a logical corollary that the same would be true for prodromal symptoms. There has been, thus far, relatively limited empiric research to test whether this logical corollary holds in actual practice by examining the age-dependent phenomenologic contiguity of the prodrome. Two studies investigated the effects of age at prodromal diagnosis among 74 prodromal patients aged 13 to 28 years (mean, 17.3 years) and among 104 prodromal patients aged 14 to 28 years (mean, 19.4 years). Both studies found no significant effect of age on rate of transition to psychosis [41,42].

It is yet undetermined whether definitions, operational diagnostic criteria, or assessment tools and instruments carry the same accuracy in middle and early childhood [77,100]. There has been no specific examination of face validity and predictive validity of the SIPS or the CAARMS for the school-aged population. The age cohort of 13-year-olds and under has generally been excluded from participation in prodromal early-identification and follow-along studies.

Theoretic considerations suggest that the unmodified prodromal assessment instruments designed for adolescents and adults are unlikely to be useful or valid tools in assessing patients who may be prodromal for VEOS. Developmentally linked challenges to accurately diagnosing those at putative risk for childhood schizophrenia are analogous to the considerations relevant to assessing and diagnosing psychosis in a child or young adolescent. Investigators seeking to clarify the experience of and ultimately symptom expression in at-risk youth must take into account principles of cognitive developmental theory. Fundamentally, a child's appraisal of what is real and not real evolves over the course of normal development; the complete adult capacity to distinguish reality from fantasy is not achieved until adolescence [83]. Much of the disparity in a young person's conscious symptom appraisal and attributions and the possibility of eliciting and assessing the nature of their experience during a diagnostic assessment depends upon their language and cognitive development [15,95] and the proficiency of the assessment tool and interviewer.

Second, early-identification research for VEOS must be informed by knowledge of social-emotional developmental theory that characterizes the transition from latency to early adolescence as a developmental stage particularly marked by desire to be "normal" and to "belong." Assessment for prodromal symptoms should anticipate that a school-aged child developing early anomalous, prepsychotic experiences and beliefs might chose to rationalize or conceal symptoms rather than acknowledge experiencing distress or seeking help [15].

In addition to these theoretic considerations, a number of empiric findings concerning pre-onset features of schizophrenia presenting in childhood suggest that the prodromal phase of VEOS may appear qualitatively and quantitatively different from the prodromal phase preceding adult onset. It has been suggested that VEOS is associated with a lower premorbid IQ relative to adult-onset cases [85]. In addition there is substantial other evidence that the premorbid adjustment and impairments vary inversely with age of onset, that is, those of VEOS and EOS are typically more severe than in adult-onset cases, particularly with regard to peer relationships, school performance, and interests [85]. These considerations suggest that the boundary between premorbid and prodromal phases may be even less distinct in VEOS than in adult cases, compounding other difficulties associated with prodromal diagnosis in middle or early childhood.

One empiric study has attempted to conduct prodromal diagnostic evaluations in middle-childhood patients. Their results are consistent with the themes already discussed. The Colorado Childhood-Onset Psychosis Research Program completed structured interviews of 130 subjects 12 years and younger (some as young as 3 years old), who were referred for putative psychotic or prepsychotic symptoms [100]. Their experience raised several potential diagnostic confounds related to the application of adult-standardized prodromal criteria and assessment tools to the school-aged population. First, they observed that a child's difficulty in understanding a question might result in an inaccurate response, highlighting the influence of evolving cognitive development and maturation. Second, they found that a youngster's discomfort in speaking to an unknown adult might lead to underreporting. Third, their findings also support the premise that age-dependent variance in symptom patterns might make current identification criteria inapplicable. The authors propose that, as is standard with any child or adolescent psychiatric assessment, information regarding potential prodromal symptoms be collected from the caretaker as well as from the identified patient. They speculate that allowing the worst symptom reported by either source to be the severity level of record might make currently used criteria more applicable and valid in child populations.

Taken together, these data may suggest that the operational prodromal diagnostic criteria function similarly across the adolescent and young-adult developmental range studied but probably warrant further developmentally informed empiric evaluation, especially for younger children.

Developmental considerations in treating the prodrome

The standard of care for treatment of adult-onset schizophrenia is well established [71]. Although the American Academy of Child and Adolescent Psychiatrists has published practice parameters for childhood schizophrenia [72], the literature on schizophrenia in youth and data on clinical treatment issues are scarce. Only a few studies have been conducted examining intervention in EOS or VEOS. Although there is clear consensus that antipsychotic treatment should commence as soon as first-episode psychotic symptoms are recognized, the rational and practice for prescribing neuroleptics during the prodromal phase is less clearly established, emphatically so for children younger than 13 years.

Two studies suggest that antipsychotic medications may be helpful for prodromal patients [44,47,58]. Both of these study samples included prodromal adolescents as well as young adults (see Table 1). Neither study has yet investigated whether response to treatment differs by age in these groups. Although the data suggesting contiguity of the prodrome across adolescent and young-adult samples reviewed earlier would suggest that response to treatment also should be similar across this developmental range, future empiric investigation is needed.

There have been suggestions that antipsychotic doses lower than those employed for chronic schizophrenia may be sufficient for prodromal patients. Published data related to this issue are limited, and consequently data from young-adult first-episode and EOS patients are useful to consider as well. Studies in acutely exacerbated chronic adult patients suggest that the minimum consistently effective antipsychotic dose in these patients has been 4 mg/day for risperidone and 10 mg/day for olanzapine [60]. Similar or slightly lower doses have been used in late adolescent and young-adult first-episode patients. In one study, 555 first-episode psychosis patients aged 16 to 45 years were randomly assigned to risperidone or haloperidol and were followed for up to 4 years [101]. The risperidone mean modal dose was 3.3 mg. In another study, 263 patients aged 16 to 40 years (mean age, 23.8 years) who had first-episode psychosis were randomly assigned under double-blind conditions to receive haloperidol or olanzapine and were followed for up to 104 weeks [102]. The acute-phase mean modal dose for olanzapine was 9.1 mg/day. Recently, a randomized study restricted to psychotic youth has been published [103]. Fifty adolescents aged 8 to 19 years (mean age, 14.8 years) were randomly assigned to risperidone, olanzapine, or haloperidol for 8 weeks. The mean age at first psychotic symptoms was 12.4 years. Mean doses achieved at study end were 4.0 mg/day for risperidone and 12.3 mg/day for olanzapine. In the two published antipsychotic studies of adolescent and young-adult prodromal patients, a very low mean dose of risperidone (1.3 mg/day) was used in one [44], and a higher dose of olanzapine (8.4 mg/day) was use in the other [47,58]. It is interesting to speculate whether the CBT that was given along with medication in the risperidone study permitted doses to be minimized. Most of the doses reported in the other studies were near the minimum consistently effective antipsychotic dose in chronic patients. When antipsychotic treatment is considered for adolescent or young-adult prodromal patients, fully antipsychotic doses should not be avoided if patients have not completely remitted at lower doses and are tolerating treatment well.

Consideration of treatment of school-aged children who seem to be prodromal is a very different undertaking from such consideration in the prodromal adolescent or young adult. Difficulties in making a prodromal diagnosis in preadolescent children, together with the reported high frequency of nonpathologic psychoticlike symptoms and the complete lack of intervention research in this age group, should give pause to the prudent clinician. Antipsychotic treatment in this age range currently is probably best reserved for patients who clearly meet criteria for VEOS or other established disorders in which treatment guidelines support the practice. It would be useful, however, to follow younger patients who seem to meet prodromal diagnostic criteria to investigate the predictive validity of the methods in this age group.

Summary

In recent years substantial strides have been made in recognizing the prodrome for schizophrenia as a prospective entity in adolescents and young adults. Because these patients are symptomatic, often already have degrees of cognitive and functional impairment, and are at high risk of getting worse, they should be of substantial interest to practicing child and adolescent psychiatrists. Preliminary data suggest that atypical antipsychotic medications may improve symptoms and delay or prevent progression to schizophrenia; however, substantial additional research is needed before the balance of long-term risks and benefits can be confidently assessed. Other medications or psychotherapies could potentially benefit these patients as well.

Some centers are beginning to focus efforts on examining if and how currently used prodromal diagnostic strategies and intervention studies might inform recognition and treatment of the prodrome with high and reliable diagnostic accuracy in early adolescence and perhaps middle childhood. At present, antipsychotic treatment of younger children who seem to be prodromal should be undertaken with great caution and, ideally, in the context of a center specializing in psychotic prodrome diagnosis, treatment, and research. To inform child and adolescent clinical psychiatric practice, ongoing research must expand the developmentally considered sophistication of already-validated diagnostic criteria, assessment tools, and treatment intervention to enhance the short-term and long-term outcomes for the youngest patients and families afflicted with this disabling disorder.

References

[1] Sullivan HS. The onset of schizophrenia. Am J Psychiatry 1927;7:105–34.
[2] Simon AE, Ferrero FP, Merlo MCG. Prodromes of first-episode psychosis: how can we challenge nonspecificity? Compr Psychiatry 2001;42(5):382–92.
[3] Fish B, Marcus J, Hans SL, et al. Infants at risk for schizophrenia: sequelae of a genetic neurointegrative defect. A review and replication analysis of pandysmaturation in the Jerusalem Infant Development Study. Arch Gen Psychiatry 1992;49:221–35.
[4] McClellan J, McCurry C. Early onset psychotic disorders: diagnostic stability and clinical characteristics. Eur Child Adolesc Psychiatry 1999;8(Suppl 1):13–9.

[5] Yung AR, McGorry PD. The prodromal phase of first-episode psychosis: past and current conceptualizations. Schizophr Bull 1996;22(2):353–70.

[6] Woods SW, Miller TJ, McGlashan TH. The prodromal patient: both symptomatic and at risk. CNS Spectr 2001;6:223–32.

[7] McGee R, Williams S, Poulton R. Hallucinations in nonpsychotic children. J Am Acad Child Adolesc Psychiatry 2000;39(1):12–3.

[8] Hafner H, Maurer K, Loffler W, et al. The influence of age and sex on the onset and early course of schizophrenia. Br J Psychiatry 1993;162:80–6.

[9] Cannon M, Tarrant CJ, Huttenen MO, et al. Childhood development and later schizophrenia: evidence from genetic high-risk and birth cohort studies. In: Murray RM, Jones PB, Susser E, et al, editors. The epidemiology of schizophrenia. Cambridge (UK): Cambridge University Press; 2003. p. 100–23.

[10] Jones P, Rodgers B, Murray R, et al. Child developmental risk-factors for adult schizophrenia in the British 1946 birth cohort. Lancet 1994;344(8934):1398–402.

[11] Crow TJ, Done DJ, Sacker A. Childhood precursors of psychosis as clues to its evolutionary origins. Eur Arch Psychiatry Clin Neurosci 1995;245(2):61–9.

[12] Isohanni M, Jones PB, Moilanen K, et al. Early developmental milestones in adult schizophrenia and other psychoses. A 31-year follow-up of the northern Finland 1966 birth cohort. Schizophr Res 2001;52(1–2):1–19.

[13] Isohanni M, Murray GK, Jokelainen J, et al. The persistence of developmental markers in childhood and adolescence and risk for schizophrenic psychoses in adult life. A 34-year follow-up of the northern Finland 1966 birth cohort. Schizophr Res 2004;71(2–3):213–25.

[14] Rosso IM, Bearden CE, Hollister JM, et al. Childhood neuromotor dysfunction in schizophrenia patients and their unaffected siblings: a prospective cohort study. Schizophr Bull 2000;26(2): 367–78.

[15] Poulton R, Caspi A, Moffitt TE, et al. Children's self-reported psychotic symptoms and adult schizophreniform disorder: a 15-year longitudinal study. Arch Gen Psychiatry 2000;57(11): 1053–8.

[16] Cannon M, Caspi A, Moffitt TE, et al. Evidence for early-childhood pan-developmental impairment specific to schizophreniform disorder: results from a longitudinal birth cohort. Arch Gen Psychiatry 2002;59(5):449–57.

[17] Fish B. Neurobiologic antecedents of schizophrenia in children. Evidence for an inherited, congenital neurointegrative defect. Arch Gen Psychiatry 1977;34(11):1297–313.

[18] Hans SL, Auerbach JG, Styr B, et al. Offspring of parents with schizophrenia: mental disorders during childhood and adolescence. Schizophr Bull 2004;30(2):303–15.

[19] Mednick SA, Parnas J, Schulsinger F. The Copenhagen high-risk project, 1962–86. Schizophr Bull 1987;13(3):485–95.

[20] Erlenmeyer-Kimling L, Rock D, Roberts SA, et al. Attention, memory, and motor skills as childhood predictors of schizophrenia-related psychoses: The New York high-risk project. Am J Psychiatry 2000;157(9):1416–22.

[21] Mirsky AF, Kugelmass S, Ingraham LJ, et al. Overview and summary: twenty-five-year followup of high-risk children. Schizophr Bull 1995;21(2):227–39.

[22] Mednick SA, Parnas J, Schulsinger F. The Copenhagen high-risk project, 1962–86. Schizophr Bull 1987;13(3):485–95.

[23] Tienari P. Interaction between genetic vulnerability and family environment: the Finnish adoptive family study of schizophrenia. Acta Psychiatr Scand 1991;84(5):460–5.

[24] Metsanen M, Wahlberg KE, Saarento O, et al. Early presence of thought disorder as a prospective sign of mental disorder. Psychiatry Res 2004;125(3):193–203.

[25] Johnstone EC, Ebmeier KP, Miller P, et al. Predicting schizophrenia: findings from the Edinburgh high-risk study. Br J Psychiatry 2005;186:18–25.

[26] Owens DGC, Miller P, Lawrie SM, Jet al. Pathogenesis of schizophrenia: a psychopathological perspective. Br J Psychiatry 2005;186:386–93.

[27] Davidson M, Reichenberg A, Rabinowitz J, et al. Behavioral and intellectual markers for schizophrenia in apparently healthy male adolescents. Am J Psychiatry 1999;156(9):1328–35.

[28] Zammit S, Allebeck P, David AS, et al. A longitudinal study of premorbid iq score and risk of developing schizophrenia, bipolar disorder, severe depression, and other nonaffective psychoses. Arch Gen Psychiatry 2004;61(4):354–60.

[29] Lewis G, David AS, Malmberg A, et al. Non-psychotic psychiatric disorder and subsequent risk of schizophrenia. Cohort study. Br J Psychiatry 2000;177:416–20.

[30] Fuller R, Nopoulos P, Arndt S, et al. Longitudinal assessment of premorbid cognitive functioning in patients with schizophrenia through examination of standardized scholastic test performance. Am J Psychiatry 2002;159(7):1183–9.

[31] Cannon M, Jones P, Huttunen MO, et al. School performance in Finnish children and later development of schizophrenia–a population-based longitudinal study. Arch Gen Psychiatry 1999;56(5):457–63.

[32] Cannon M, Walsh E, Hollis C, et al. Predictors of later schizophrenia and affective psychosis among attendees at a child psychiatry department. Br J Psychiatry 2001;178:420–6.

[33] Walker E, Lewine RJ. Prediction of adult-onset schizophrenia from childhood home movies of the patients. Am J Psychiatry 1990;147(8):1052–6.

[34] Schiffman J, Walker E, Ekstrom M, et al. Childhood videotaped social and neuromotor precursors of schizophrenia: a prospective investigation. Am J Psychiatry 2004;161(11):2021–7.

[35] McGorry PD, McFarlane C, Patton GC, et al. The prevalence of prodromal features of schizophrenia in adolescence: a preliminary survey. Acta Psychiatr Scand 1995;92(4):241–9.

[36] Yung AR, McGorry PD. The prodromal phase of first-episode psychosis: past and current conceptualizations. Schizophr Bull 1996;22(2):353–70.

[37] Yung AR, Phillips LJ, McGorry PD, et al. Prediction of psychosis. A step towards indicated prevention of schizophrenia. Br J Psychiatry 1998;172(33 Suppl):14–20.

[38] Schaffner KF, McGorry PD. Preventing severe mental illnesses—new prospects and ethical challenges. Schizophr Res 2001;51(1 Special Issue SI):3–15.

[39] Miller TJ, McGlashan TM, Rosen JL, et al. Prodromal assessment with the structured interview for prodromal syndromes and the scale of prodromal symptoms: predictive validity, inter-rater reliability, and training to reliability. Schizophr Bull 2003;29(4):703–15.

[40] Miller TJ, McGlashan TH, Rosen JL, et al. Prospective diagnosis of the prodrome for schizophrenia: preliminary evidence of interrater reliability and predictive validity using operational criteria and a structured interview. Am J Psychiatry 2002;159:863–5.

[41] Yung AR, Phillips LJ, Yuen HP, et al. Risk factors for psychosis in an ultra high-risk group: psychopathology and clinical features. Schizophr Res 2004;67(2–3):131–42.

[42] Mason O, Startup M, Halpin S, et al. Risk factors for transition to first episode psychosis among individuals with 'at-risk mental states'. Schizophr Res 2004;71(2–3):227–37.

[43] Miller TJ, Zipursky RB, Perkins DO, et al. A randomized double blind clinical trial of olanzapine vs placebo in patients at risk for being prodromally symptomatic for psychosis: II. Baseline characteristics of the "prodromal" sample. Schizophr Res 2003;61(1):19–30.

[44] McGorry PD, Yung AF, Phillips LJ, et al. Randomized controlled trial of interventions designed to reduce the risk of progression to first-episode psychosis in a clinical sample with subthreshold symptoms. Arch Gen Psychiatry 2002;59:921–8.

[45] Yung AR, Phillips LJ, Yuen HP, et al. Psychosis prediction: 12-month follow up of a high-risk ("prodromal") group. Schizophr Res 2003;60(1):21–32.

[46] Rosen JL, Miller TJ, D'Andrea JT, et al. Comorbid diagnoses in persons meeting criteria for the schizophrenic prodrome [abstract]. Schizophr Res 2004;67(1 Suppl 1):73.

[47] McGlashan TH, Zipursky RB, Perkins DO, et al. Olanzapine vs placebo for prodromal schizophrenia. Schizophr Res 2004;67(1 Suppl 1):6.

[48] Morrison AP, French P, Walford L, et al. Cognitive therapy for the prevention of psychosis in people at ultra-high risk. Randomized controlled trial. Br J Psychiatry 2004;184:291–7.

[49] McGlashan TH, Miller TJ, Woods SW. Pre-onset detection and intervention research in schizophrenic psychoses; current estimates of benefits and risks. Schizophr Bull 2001;27:563–70.

[50] Yung AR, McGorry PD, McFarlane CA, et al. Monitoring and care of young people at incipient risk of psychosis. Schizophr Bull 1996;22(2):283–303.

[51] Moller P, Husby R. The initial prodrome in schizophrenia: searching for naturalistic core dimensions of experience and behavior. Schizophr Bull 2000;26(1):217–32.

[52] Miller TJ, McGlashan TM. Early identification and intervention in psychotic illness. Conn Med 2000;64(6):339–41.

[53] Preda A, Miller TJ, Rosen JL, et al. Treatment histories of patients with a syndrome putatively prodromal for schizophrenia. Psychiatr Serv 2002;53(3):342–4.

[54] Hawkins KA, Addington J, Keefe RSE, et al. Neuropsychological status of subjects at high risk for a first episode of psychosis. Schizophr Res 2004;67:115–22.

[55] Institute of Medicine (IOM). Research on children and adolescents with mental, behavioral and developmental disorders. Washington (DC): National Academy Press; 1989.

[56] Falloon IRH. Early intervention for first episodes of schizophrenia: a preliminary exploration. Psychiatry 1992;55:4–15.

[57] McGorry PD, Warner R. Consensus on early intervention in schizophrenia. Schizophr Bull 2002;28(3):543–4.

[58] Woods SW, Breier A, Zipursky RB, et al. Randomized trial of olanzapine vs placebo in the symptomatic acute treatment of patients meeting criteria for the schizophrenic prodrome. Biol Psychiatry 2003;54:453–64.

[59] Carpenter Jr WT, Appelbaum PS, Levine RJ. The declaration of Helsinki and clinical trials: a focus on placebo-controlled trials in schizophrenia. Am J Psychiatry 2003;160(2):356–62.

[60] Woods SW. Chlorpromazine equivalent doses for the newer atypical antipsychotics. J Clin Psychiatry 2003;64:663–7.

[61] Woods SW, Martin A, Spector SG, et al. Effects of development on olanzapine-associated adverse events. J Am Acad Child Adolesc Psychiatry 2002;41:1439–46.

[62] Olney JW, Farber NB. Glutamate receptor dysfunction and schizophrenia. Arch Gen Psychiatry 1995;52(12):998–1007.

[63] Kane JM, Krystal J, Correll CU. Treatment models and designs for intervention research during the psychotic prodrome. Schizophr Bull 2003;29(4):747–56.

[64] Javitt DC, Balla A, Sershen H, et al. A.E. Bennett Research Award. Reversal of phencyclidine-induced effects by glycine and glycine transport inhibitors. Biol Psychiatry 1999;45(6):668–79.

[65] Lu WY, Man HY, Ju W, et al. Activation of synaptic NMDA receptors induces membrane insertion of new AMPA receptors and LTP in cultured hippocampal neurons. Neuron 2001; 29(1):243–54.

[66] Heresco-Levy U, Ermilov M, Lichtenberg P, et al. High-dose glycine added to olanzapine and risperidone for the treatment of schizophrenia. Biol Psychiatry 2004;55(2):165–71.

[67] Woods SW, Thomas LE, Tully EM, et al. Effects of oral glycine in the schizophrenia prodrome [abstract]. Biol Psychiatry 2004;55(8S):227.

[68] Woods SW, Gueorguieva RV, Baker CB, et al. Control group bias in randomized atypical antipsychotic trials for schizophrenia. Arch Gen Psychiatry 2005;62(9):961–70.

[69] Azorin JM, Naudin J. Schizophrenia: two-faced meaning of vulnerability. Am J Med Genet 2002;114(8):921–2.

[70] Fiszdon JM, Bryson GJ, Wexler BE, et al. Durability of cognitive remediation training in schizophrenia: performance on two memory tasks at 6-month and 12-month follow-up. Psychiatry Res 2004;125(1):1–7.

[71] Lehman AF, Lieberman JA, Dixon LB, et al. Practice guideline for the treatment of patients with schizophrenia, second edition. Am J Psychiatry 2004;161(2 Suppl S):1–56.

[72] McClellan J, Werry JS, Ayres W, et al. Practice parameters for the assessment and treatment of children and adolescents with schizophrenia. J Am Acad Child Adolesc Psychiatry 1997; 36(10 Suppl S):S177–93.

[73] Davidson M, Weiser M. Prodromal schizophrenia: the dilemma of prediction and early intervention. CNS Spectr 2004;9(6):578.

[74] Woods SW, Martin A, Spector SG, et al. Effects of development on olanzapine-associated adverse events. J Am Acad Child Adolesc Psychiatry 2002;41:1439–46.

[75] Fish B, Ritvo E. Psychosis of childhood. In: Noshpitz JD, editor. Basic handbook of child psychiatry. New York: Basic Books; 1979. p. 249–304.

[76] Clark AF, Lewis SW. Practitioner review: treatment of schizophrenia in childhood and adolescence. J Child Psychol Psychiatry 1998;39(8):1071–81.

[77] Asarnow JR, Tompson MC, McGrath EP. Annotation: childhood-schizophrenia: clinical and treatment issues. J Child Psychol Psychiatr 2004;45:180–94.

[78] Schizophrenia. Biological markers in relations to clinical characteristics. Am J Psychiatry 1997; 154:64–8.

[79] Hata K, Iida J, Iwasaka H, et al. Minor physical anomalies in childhood and adolescent onset schizophrenia. Psychiatry Clin Neurosci 2003;57:17–21.

[80] Schultz SC, Findlng RL, Wise A, et al. Schizophrenia—child and adolescent schizophrenia. Psychiatr Clin North Am 1998;21:43–56.

[81] Alaghband-Rad J, Hamburger MA, Giedd JN, et al. Childhood-onset schizophrenia: biological markers in relations to clinical characteristics. Am J Psychiatry 1997;154:64–8.

[82] American Psychiatric Association. Diagnostic and statistical manual of mental disorders. 3rd edition. Washington (DC): American Psychiatric Association; 1980.

[83] Volkmar FR, Tsatsanis KD. Childhood schizophrenia. In: Lewis M, editor. Child and adolescent psychiatry—a comprehensive textbook. 3rd edition. Philadephia: Lippincott Williams and Wilkins; 2002. p. 745–54.

[84] Beitchman JH. Childhood schizophrenia: a review and comparison of adult onset schizophrenia. Psychiatr Clin North Am 1985;8:793–814.

[85] Asarnow RF, Asarnow JR. Childhood-onset schizophrenia. Schizophr Bull 1994;20:591–7.

[86] Spencer EK, Campbell M. Children with schizophrenia: diagnosis, phenomenology, and pharmacotherapy. Schizophr Bull 1994;20:713–25.

[87] Aleman A, Kahn RS, Selten J-P. Sex differences in the risk of schizophrenia. Evidence from meta-analysis. Arch Gen Psychiatry 2003;60(6):565–71.

[88] Castle D, Sham P, Murray R. Differences in distribution of ages of onset in males and females with schizophrenia. Schizophr Res 1998;33(3):179–83.

[89] Hafner H, an der Heiden W, Behrens S, et al. Causes and consequences of the gender difference in age at onset of schizophrenia. Schizophr Bull 1998;24(1):99–113.

[90] Frazier JA, Alaghband-Rad J, Jacobsen L, et al. Pubertal development and onset of psychosis in childhood onset schizophrenia. Psychiatry Res 1997;70:1–7.

[91] Cohen RZ, Seeman MV, Gotowiec A, et al. Earlier puberty as a predictor of later onset of schizophrenia in women. Am J Psychiatry 1999;156(7):1059–64.

[92] Wyshak G, Frisch RE. Evidence for a secular trend in age of menarche. N Engl J Med 1982; 306(17):1033–5.

[93] Hulanicka B, Waliszko A. Deceleration of age at menarche in Poland. Ann Hum Biol 1991; 18(6):507–13.

[94] Lee PA, Guo SS, Kulin HE. Age of puberty: data from the United States of America. APMIS 2001;109(2):81–8.

[95] Caplan R, Guthrie D, Tanguay P, et al. Formal thought disorder in childhood onset schizophrenia and schizotypal personality disorder. J Child Psychol Psychiatr 1990;31:1103–14.

[96] American Psychiatric Association. Diagnostic and statistical manual of mental disorders. 4th edition. Washington (DC): American Psychiatric Association; 1994.

[97] McGee R, Williams S, Poulton R. Hallucinations in nonpsychotic children. J Am Acad Child Adolesc Psychiatry 2000;39(1):12–3.

[98] Escher S, Romme M, Buiks A, et al. Formation of delusional ideation in adolescent hearing voices: a prospective study. Am J Med Genet 2002;114:913–20.

[99] Kumra S, Jacobsen LK, Lenane M, et al. Multidimensionally impaired disorder—is it a variant of very early-onset schizophrenia. J Am Acad Child Adolesc Psychiatry 1998;37(1):91–9.

[100] Ross RG, Schaeffer J, Compagnon N, et al. Creating school-age versions of semistructured interviews for the prodrome to schizophrenia: lessons from case reviews. Schizophr Bull 2003; 29(4):729–35.

[101] Schooler N, Rabinowitz J, Davidson M, et al. Risperidone and haloperidol in first-episode psychosis: a long-term randomized trial. Am J Psychiatry 2005;162(5):947–53.

[102] Lieberman JA, Tollefson G, Tohen M, et al. Comparative efficacy and safety of atypical and conventional antipsychotic drugs in first-episode psychosis: a randomized, double-blind trial of olanzapine versus haloperidol. Am J Psychiatry 2003;160(8):1396–404.

[103] Sikich L, Hamer RM, Bashford RA, et al. A pilot study of risperidone, olanzapine, and haloperidol in psychotic youth: a double-blind, randomized, 8-week trial. Neuropsychopharmacology 2004;29(1):133–45.

ELSEVIER
SAUNDERS

Child Adolesc Psychiatric Clin N Am
15 (2006) 135–159

CHILD AND
ADOLESCENT
PSYCHIATRIC CLINICS
OF NORTH AMERICA

Treatment-Refractory Schizophrenia in Children and Adolescents: An Update on Clozapine and Other Pharmacologic Interventions

Harvey N. Kranzler, MD[a,b], Hana M. Kester, BA[c],
Ginny Gerbino-Rosen, MD[a,b], Inika N. Henderson, PsyD[b],
Joseph Youngerman, MD[a,b], Guy Beauzile, MD[d],
Keith Ditkowsky, MD[e], Sanjiv Kumra, MD[a,c],*

[a]Department of Psychiatry, Albert Einstein College of Medicine, 1300 Morris Park Avenue,
Bronx, NY 10461, USA
[b]Bronx Children's' Psychiatric Center, 1000 Waters Place, Bronx, NY 10461, USA
[c]Department of Psychiatry Research, Zucker Hillside Hospital,
North Shore—Long Island Jewish Health System, 75-59 263rd Street, Glen Oaks, NY 11004, USA
[d]Sagamore Children's Psychiatric Center, 197 Half Hollow Road, Dix Hills, NY 11746, USA
[e]Division of Child and Adolescent Psychiatry, Schneider Children's Hospital,
North Shore—Long Island Jewish Health System, 269-01 76th Avenue, New Hyde Park,
NY 11040, USA

Schizophrenia is a devastating illness, regardless of the age at which it presents, but when it occurs in childhood or adolescence the consequences are profound. Children and adolescents who have early-onset schizophrenia (EOS) have onset of psychotic symptoms by age 18 years and experience deterioration in adaptive function from an already impaired premorbid level. Despite the recent availability

This work was supported in part by a National Alliance for Research on Schizophrenia and Depression grant (to Dr. Kumra as a Lieber Investigator), National Institute of Mental Health grant MH01990 (to Dr. Kumra). Dr. Kumra is a consultant for Janssen Pharmaceuticals and has received research support for investigator-initiated studies from Pfizer, Inc., for multisite studies from Janssen Pharmaceuticals, and drug supplies for National Institute of Mental Health–sponsored and foundation studies from GlaxoSmithKline, Novartis, and Eli-Lilly. Dr. Kranzler receives unrestricted educational grants from both Eli-Lilly and Janssen Pharmaceuticals.

* Corresponding author. Department of Psychiatry Research, The Zucker Hillside Hospital, North Shore—Long Island Jewish Health System, 75-59 263rd Street, Glen Oaks, NY 11004.

E-mail address: skumra@lij.edu (S. Kumra).

doi:10.1016/j.chc.2005.08.008   *childpsych.theclinics.com* of a number of second-generation antipsychotics (eg, risperidone and olanzapine, among others), the number of children who fail to respond to standard antipsychotic treatment and who present to state hospital systems for long-term care has not changed significantly. To date, there have been few published controlled treatment trials in children and adolescents who have schizophrenia.

This article primarily reviews the prevalence of EOS, the long-term outcome of this severe form of the disorder from naturalistic studies of children primarily treated with conventional antipsychotics, and currently available pharmacologic strategies for treatment. It also discusses the pharmacologic management for children and adolescents who have treatment-refractory schizophrenia and, in particular, the use of clozapine in this population. For this article, EOS, with onset of psychotic symptoms by age 18 years, is distinguished from and childhood-onset schizophrenia (COS), with onset by age 13 years.

The prevalence, significance, and outcome of early-onset and treatment-refractory schizophrenia

Early-onset schizophrenia

As reviewed by Krausz and Muller-Thomsen [1], there are no uniform data on the prevalence of EOS. Retrospective studies of mental illness in children and adolescents often cannot identify definitive diagnoses in this age group, perhaps because clinicians fear subsequent stigmatization from an uncertain diagnosis. Clinical experience would suggest that COS is exceedingly rare [2], with adult-onset schizophrenia being almost 50 times more prevalent [3]. The prevalence of adult-onset schizophrenia versus COS is almost certainly an overestimate. On the other hand, the National Institute of Mental Health (NIMH) group [4,5] reports that a number of children who have either transient or affective psychoses are misdiagnosed as having schizophrenia. This estimate is based on the NIMH protocol of initially screening such individuals and then conducting a careful diagnostic evaluation on a psychiatric inpatient unit after a washout of all antipsychotic medications, a procedure that often is not feasible in normal clinical settings.

Another diagnostic difficulty arises in distinguishing children who have pervasive developmental disorder from those who have COS, in that both disorders are associated with early developmental abnormalities and social deficits [4]. It is thought that the occurrence of autistic-spectrum symptoms during the premorbid phase of illness in probands that have COS may reflect a nonspecific marker of early abnormal neurodevelopment or perhaps shared risk factors common to both disorders [6].

Outcome of patients with early-onset schizophrenia

Compared with adult-onset samples, children and adolescents who have EOS show evidence of a greater decline in cortical gray matter volume on anatomic brain MR imaging scans during adolescence [7] and evidence for more salient familial [8,9], and perhaps genetic, risk factors [10]. Based on these data, it has been inferred that EOS may represent a more severe form of the disorder.

Although most treatment trials present evidence of drug efficacy with reduction of psychotic symptoms during short-term trials, the effect of these therapies on long-term functional outcome is perhaps more important to the patients, their parents, and the clinicians who treat these conditions. The available data, largely collected from children and adolescents treated with conventional antipsychotics, suggest that the outcome of patients who have EOS is generally thought to be poor [1,11] and possibly is worse than that of adult-onset cases [12]. Three studies that examined outcome after an average interval of about 5 years have reported rates of remission ranging from 3% [13] to 30% [14,15]. In all three studies, treatment consisted of conventional antipsychotics. Schmidt and colleagues [16] compared the clinical and social outcomes of patients who had EOS with those of adult-onset patients after a mean follow-up period of 7.4 years. They found that more than two thirds of the 118 cases of EOS in their sample had had at least one more psychotic episode and were in need of continuing psychiatric treatment compared to those who had adult-onset schizophrenia. Social impairment was also greater for the patients who had EOS, particularly in the areas of self-care and social contacts. In two studies [11,17] with longer follow-up periods (averaging 15–16 years), the reported rates of full remission were 5% and 20%, respectively, with the majority of patients experiencing continuous symptoms. Eggers and Bunk [18] have reported the longest follow-up data (42 years) with a small sample (n = 44) of EOS cases. They found that 50% of the patients had continuous symptoms, and 25% were in partial remission. Poor premorbid function, insidious onset, and onset of psychotic symptoms before age 12 years have also been reported to predict poorer outcome [18–20].

Cognitive deficits have been widely reported in adolescents who have EOS [21,22]. Patients with adolescent-onset schizophrenia (onset of psychotic symptoms between the ages of 13 and 18 years) do not seem to differ from those with COS in patterns of neuropsychologic test performance [23]. It has not been demonstrated using a longitudinal design, however, whether cognitive deficits are predictive of later functional outcome, as has been shown repeatedly in adult samples [24]. A better understanding of how cognitive performance may be related to community outcome in adolescents who have EOS is important, particularly because new pharmacologic agents are being developed that may specifically target these deficits in schizophrenia.

Treatment-refractory schizophrenia

Currently accepted criteria for treatment resistance in adult studies require that persons be persistently ill with schizophrenia and have undiminished positive symptoms (such as hallucinations or delusions) despite adequate antipsychotic drug treatment [25]. In most adult treatment studies, adequate antipsychotic drug treatment has been defined as two failures of antipsychotic treatment lasting at least 4 to 6 weeks, assuming that there are no severe adverse effects that would justifiably prompt drug discontinuation and shorten the length of the treatment trial. Because of the lack of fixed-dose studies and developmental variations (eg, biologic maturation and endocrinologic status) in children and adolescents, the optimal dosage and length of treatment for each antipsychotic medication remains unknown, and the decision as to whether a prior antipsychotic trial was adequate remains largely subjective. The American Academy of Child and Adolescent Psychiatry, however, suggests that a 4- to 6-week trial of an antipsychotic drug using dosages ranging from 0.5 mg to 9.0 mg/kg chlorpromazine or the equivalent daily dosage of another antipsychotic drug is adequate [26].

Why study treatment-refractory children and adolescents with schizophrenia?

Between one fifth and one third of all patients who have schizophrenia do not respond adequately to drug treatment [27]. Although it is unclear whether children and adolescents who have schizophrenia are actually less responsive to neuroleptic agents [28,29], earlier age of onset in adult patients is reported to be a predictor of poor therapeutic response [30,31]. In a large group of patients who experienced onset of schizophrenia in the second and third decades of life, Meltzer and colleagues [31] reported that relatively young age at onset (ie, 20 years or younger) was associated with greater impairment at follow-up, poorer response to treatment, and higher risk of rehospitalization, regardless of gender. Children and adolescents who have treatment-refractory schizophrenia are often highly symptomatic and may require extensive periods of hospital care. Although there has been limited services-type research in the area of adolescent-onset schizophrenia, administrative experience in the state of New York suggests that the care of this population requires a disproportionately high percentage of the total costs of treating childhood psychiatric disorders.

The optimal treatment of these patients remains an important public health challenge that has been relatively understudied. Most studies of treatment-refractory schizophrenia do not study patients under the age of 18. The mean ages of patients who had treatment-refractory schizophrenia enrolled in the Meltzer [32], Breier [33], and Lieberman [34] clozapine studies were 35, 34, and 28 years, respectively. Although children and adolescents who have psychotic disorders seem to show a clinical response to antipsychotic medications similar to that of adults [35,36], animal [37] and human studies [36,38,39] indicate that children and adults may differ in sensitivity to or tolerability for adverse effects of new-generation psychotropic agents. Specifically, these studies suggest that children and adolescents may be more sensitive to the extrapyramidal side effects (EPS) induced by neuroleptic agents, particularly parkinsonian bradykinesia and acute dystonia. To date, the assumption that atypical antipsychotics will have a decreased risk of EPS and decreased incidence of newly emergent dyskinesias remains untested in children and adolescents.

The use of antipsychotics in treatment-refractory early-onset schizophrenia

Conventional antipsychotics

Although some studies [28,29] support the use of conventional neuroleptics in the treatment of children and adolescents who have psychotic disorders, these medications are often associated with inadequate treatment response and a relative lack of efficacy against negative symptoms and cognitive dysfunction. In addition, these agents are associated with significant side effects such as tardive dyskinesia, galactorrhea, and gynecomastia [36,40]. Clozapine, risperidone, olanzapine, quetiapine, ziprasidone, and aripiprazole, are currently the only agents approved by the Food and Drug Administration (FDA), and that approval is for adults, not for children or adolescents. This article discusses the evidence from controlled treatment trials supporting the use of each medication in children and adolescents. Because of the rarity of EOS, there have been few controlled treatment trials in this population, and because of limited resources to recruit subjects nationally or to establish a network of treatment sites, it has not been possible to date to accrue an informative, homogenous sample of patients who have schizophrenia. There are, however, several ongoing controlled treatment trials comparing atypical antipsychotics directly with each other and atypical antipsychotics relative to placebo in this population. It is hoped that these trials will generate important information regarding the relative efficacy and safety of these medications in children and adolescents.

Clozapine

Clozapine, the first new-generation antipsychotic, has advantages over conventional antipsychotics in terms of lower rates of EPS [41–43] and tardive dyskinesia [34,44] and has greater effectiveness for positive symptoms in patients whose disease is refractory to conventional antipsychotics [42,45,46]. Clozapine may also produce greater benefit than conventional drugs in many other areas, including negative symptoms and the deficit state [45,47], may increase social and vocational adjustment [32,48] and medication compliance [32,49], may reduce suicidal behavior [50] and alcohol and substance abuse [24,51–53], and may prevent rehospitalization [54,55]. Also, there is some evidence that adults who do not respond to second-generation drugs respond to clozapine at a rate comparable to that seen in patients who do not respond to traditional drugs. In one study, 41% of adult patients who had treatment-resistant schizophrenia who failed to improve when receiving olanzapine in a double-blind or open trial met a priori response criteria during an 8-week open trial of clozapine [56]. Clozapine remains the only antipsychotic drug consistently found to be effective for individuals who have treatment-resistant schizophrenia, as tested in multiple double-blind trials.

Despite the broad range of benefits associated with clozapine use in adults who have treatment-refractory disease, the authors believe that this therapy remains underused in children and adolescents. This underuse may reflect the limited database in children to guide clinicians, the uneasiness on the part of physicians in managing side effects, particularly hematologic adverse events, and a reluctance on the part of patients to submit to frequent blood testing. Physicians and patients should be aware that there is a range of benefits of clozapine use in severely ill children and adolescents who have treatment-resistant schizophrenia that may be greater than the risks associated with this therapy. Also, with careful monitoring, the risks associated with clozapine can be minimized.

Most studies of second-generation antipsychotics conducted in patients who have EOS have been open clinical trials with small samples. In general, these studies support the use of clozapine in children and adolescents who have schizophrenia, and the incidence of adverse events seems to be the same as reported in adult studies [36,57–66].

Published data for 30 children and adolescents who had schizophrenia were reported from patients studied at the NIMH in either open or double-blind protocols [36]. In the NIMH cohort of patients who had schizophrenia that was nonresponsive to neuroleptic agents, the distribution of males and females was equal, with approximately two thirds having had an insidious onset. At the time of referral many of the patients had already experienced extensive hospitalization and neuroleptic exposure.

A double-blind, parallel-group comparison of haloperidol and clozapine in 21 patients who had treatment-refractory COS (mean age of symptom onset, 14.0 years) found clozapine superior to haloperidol for both positive and negative symptoms and for measures of overall improvement [36]. Clozapine doses began at 6.25 mg to 25 mg/day, depending on the patient's weight, and could be increased every 3 to 4 days by one to two times the starting dose. The mean dose of clozapine at the sixth week of treatment was 149 mg/day (range, 25–525 mg/day). Medical monitoring included weekly complete blood cell counts with differential, liver function tests, an electroencephalogram, and an EKG before drug initiation and at week six of treatment. Given the typical slow titration schedule for clozapine in children and adolescents, a 6-week interval probably underestimated the potential benefit of this therapy in this population, and longer treatment trials are needed. At the completion of the 6-week clozapine trial, many of these patients were able to return to a less restrictive setting because of the dramatic improvement in clinical symptomatology and the reduction of aggressive outbursts [36]. Several studies of adults who have schizophrenia have reported that clozapine is more effective than standard antipsychotic therapy in reducing violent behavior and hostility [33,67–70]. Similarly, clozapine has a significant impact on reducing aggressive behaviors in children and adolescents who have treatment-refractory schizophrenia in the state hospital system in New York [71]. Such data, which reflect the impact of treatment interventions in naturalistic treatment settings, as opposed to specialized research units, are important to provide accurate estimates of the effect size of interventions.

Thirteen of 21 patients who participated in the NIMH double-blind trial continued to receive clozapine for an additional 30 to 45 months after completion of the study, and continued benefits in overall functioning were seen at 2-year follow-up [36]. Among patients who received clozapine either in open or double-blind trials, 62% were rated as much improved or very much improved on the Clinical Global Impression scale after 6 weeks of treatment.

Unfortunately, as seen in adults, the use of clozapine is associated with serious adverse events such as blood dyscrasias and seizures. In the NIMH sample, during a 2- to 4-year observation period, 7 of 27 patients had to stop otherwise effective clozapine therapy because of serious adverse events. Two of these patients developed neutropenias (absolute neutrophil count <1500) which recurred with drug rechallenge, three patients developed persistent seizure activity despite anticonvulsant treatment, one patient developed excessive weight gain, and one patient developed a threefold elevation in liver enzymes. In each of these cases, there were no permanent or long-lasting negative consequences after drug withdrawal [36]. Two large retrospective studies of adolescents who had schizophrenia report a dropout rate of 5% to 17% because of similar adverse events [59,60]. Whether the higher dropout rate in the NIMH sample is a chance event or a reflection of a greater susceptibility to toxic effects in a population with a younger mean age cannot be determined.

The authors' group recently conducted a retrospective chart review of 172 children and adolescents who had been treated with clozapine in an open-label fashion using a flexible titration schedule at Bronx Children's Psychiatric Center [66], in whom the development of neutropenia was explored. Neutropenia (absolute neutrophil count <1500/mm^3) developed in 23 patients (13%), and agranulocytosis (absolute neutrophil count <500/mm^3) was seen in one patient (0.6%). Using survival analysis methods, the cumulative probability of developing an initial hematologic adverse event (neutropenia, agranulocytosis) at 1 year of clozapine treatment was 16.1% (95% CI, 9.7%–22.5%). Eleven (48%) of 24 patients who developed a hematologic adverse event were successfully rechallenged on clozapine. Eight (5%) of 172 patients from this sample eventually discontinued clozapine because of a hematologic adverse event (one agranulocytosis, seven neutropenia). In this population, the cumulative incidence of agranolocytosis was comparable with that reported in the adult literature, but the cumulative incidence of neutropenia was somewhat higher [72].

Current available guidelines suggest that blood counts need to be monitored on a weekly basis during the first 6 months of clozapine treatment and on a biweekly basis thereafter [26]. With these provisions, to authors' knowledge no cases of death resulting from hematologic adverse events in children and adolescents treated with clozapine have been reported. For the management of agranulocytosis, the first steps should be immediate discontinuation of clozapine and other medications that might be associated with a lowering of the white blood cell count and repeating the white blood cell count to ensure that there has not been a laboratory error. These precautions should be followed by a hematologic consultation to determine whether an inpatient hospitalization is necessary to avoid the risk of infection or whether the administration of granulocyte-macrophage colony-stimulating factor would be helpful. The decision to rechallenge a patient who has developed agranulocytosis while taking clozapine should be made on an individual basis. Some of the potential considerations in the decision-making process would be advice from a hematologist, the wishes of the parents and patient, review of past treatment response to other antipsychotic medications to determine whether a suitable therapeutic alternative is available, and consideration of the influence and necessity of other medications that the patient is currently receiving. For the management of neutropenia, these considerations remain valid, but it is important to note that some patients, particularly African Americans and Afro-Caribbeans, have a periodic lowering of their white blood cell count that may be normative and not pathologic. Although children who have developed a first episode of neutropenia seem to be at higher risk for developing a second episode, there are no good data to suggest whether or not these patients are actually at higher risk for developing agranulocytosis [66]. There is some thought that the pathophysiology of agranulocytosis and neutropenia may be different [66].

Alternatives to clozapine therapy for children who have treatment-refractory schizophrenia

As discussed previously, the available evidence most strongly supports the use of clozapine in the treatment of children and adolescents who have treatment-refractory schizophrenia. In considering options other than clozapine for this subgroup, one might consider olanzapine, quetiapine, aripiprazole, risperidone, or one of several other alternative interventions.

Olanzapine

Olanzapine has many similarities to clozapine. Olanzapine has significant affinity for 5- hydroxytryptamine 2a (5-HT2a) and D4 receptors in comparison to D2 receptors and also has significant affinity for 5-HT2c, 5-HT3, 5-HT6, D3, D1, muscarinic (especially M1), alpha1, and H1 receptors. Both clozapine and olanzapine have been shown to block ketamine-induced alterations in brain metabolism in rats [73], but a relatively high dose of olanzapine was required to block ketamine-induced brain metabolic activation in this study [73]. From a preclinical viewpoint, olanzapine is most similar to clozapine among available agents, although they are by no means identical. In clinical studies, olanzapine produces significantly fewer EPS than haloperidol [74–78]. Olanzapine may also be less likely to cause tardive dyskinesia than conventional antipsychotics [78]. As reviewed by Glazer [79], the 1-year risk of development of tardive dyskinesia was 0.52% with olanzapine treatment and was 7.45% with haloperidol treatment based on a study population of patients who participated in three separate clinical studies. (This review excludes the first 6 weeks of treatment, during which patients underwent medication changes and frequent Abnormal Involuntary Movement Scale assessments were performed).

In addition to its demonstrated efficacy in treating positive symptoms, there have been reports in adults that olanzapine is better than conventional agents in reducing negative symptoms [77,80,81], cognitive impairments [82], and rehospitalization during maintenance therapy [83]. So far, these potential advantages of olanzapine have not been demonstrated against conventional agents at low doses (most comparisons were with haloperidol averaging 15 mg/day) or other second-generation agents. Olanzapine may have some advantage over conventional drugs in patients who have treatment-refractory schizophrenia [84], particularly at higher dosages (ie, >20 mg/day) [85–90]. Preliminary data from a relevant international double-blind study of clozapine versus olanzapine in adult patients who had treatment-resistant schizophrenia (n=180) found no significant difference between treatments [85]. In this 18-week study, the final mean dose of olanzapine was 22.2 ± 3.9 mg/day, and the final mean dose of clozapine of 354.2 ± 146.1 mg/day.

One well-designed, recently published, double-blind olanzapine/chlorpromazine trial, which treated adult patients at a fixed dose of 25 mg/day of olanzapine [25], produced negative findings. In that study, only 3 (7%) of 42 patients responded to olanzapine treatment. The role of olanzapine in adult patients who have treatment-resistant disease therefore remains an open question. Although data from positron emission tomography imaging [91] would predict that higher doses of olanzapine (30 mg/day) might have a higher likelihood of EPS and prolactin elevation, dosages of 25 mg/day have been well tolerated in adult studies, and the EPS experienced by patients were reported as mild and transient [25]. The duration and dose of an adequate olanzapine trial for severely ill children and adolescents who have schizophrenia remain unclear, however. To the authors' knowledge, no published case reports of adverse effects associated with high-dose olanzapine in children and adolescents have been published [90].

Preliminary experience using olanzapine in a tertiary care setting in children and adolescents who have treatment-resistant schizophrenia suggests that some may benefit, but the proportion is not as high as with clozapine. These data are based on a small sample receiving open treatment for 8 weeks using doses of up to 20 mg/day [92]. Olanzapine doses were initiated at 2.5 mg every other day (<40 kg) or 2.5 mg every day (>40 kg), depending on the child's weight, and could be increased to 2.5 mg/day (<40 kg) or 5 mg/day (>40 kg) on day three. Thereafter, dosage was adjusted upward to a maximum of 20 mg/day (using day one of treatment as the start date) by flexible increments of 2.5 mg to 5 mg every 5 to 9 days, as determined by the treating physician. The Clinical Global Impression Scale was used to assess improvement after 8 weeks of treatment with olanzapine, as compared with clinical condition upon entry into the study. Of the 10 patients who participated in this trial, 3 were rated as being much improved, 4 as minimally improved, 1 as no change, 1 as minimally worse, and 1 as much worse [92]. The mean dose of medication at the sixth week of treatment for olanzapine was 17.5 ± 2.3 mg/day (range, 12.5–20 mg). The most frequent side effects were increased appetite and weight gain, constipation, nausea/vomiting, headache, somnolence, insomnia, difficulty concentrating, sustained tachycardia, increased nervousness, and transient elevation of liver transaminases. The incidence of these side effects is comparable to the side effect profile of adult patients who have participated in open or double-blind trials of olanzapine. No cases of neutropenia or seizures occurred with olanzapine.

Although olanzapine has a more benign side-effect profile than clozapine, preliminary data based on a comparison of 23 patients who received 6-week open trials of clozapine or olanzapine at the NIMH suggest that clozapine has superior efficacy at week six, relative to either baseline drug-free status or admission status (on admission medications), for both positive and negative symptoms in this group of severely ill children [92].

Recently, Sikich and colleagues [35] conducted a double-blind, parallel treatment trial with risperidone, olanzapine, or haloperidol for 8 weeks. Fifty patients aged 8 to 19 years, who had a broad spectrum of psychotic disorders, participated. All treatments were found to reduce psychotic symptoms, and response rate to olanzapine and risperidone in adolescents who had psychotic disorders was comparable to that observed with haloperidol [35].

Risperidone

Risperidone was the first of the second-generation drugs to follow clozapine on the market in the United States. Risperidone's atypicality is dose dependent, in that at higher doses (8 mg/day) it is clearly associated with EPS, and there seem to be fewer beneficial therapeutic effects [93–95]. Although the incidence of tardive dyskinesia seems to be lower with risperidone than with conventional drugs, similar to findings in adults [65], a series of cases of tardive dyskinesia have been reported in adults and children taking risperidone. Risperidone has shown some benefit in a portion of adult patients who have treatment-refractory disease [93,96]. A recent European multicenter trial [97] found risperidone to be equivalent to clozapine in treatment-refractory adults. This study has been criticized on a number of grounds, most importantly because the mean dose of clozapine was much lower than that used in most studies that have demonstrated clozapine's efficacy in refractory patients. In addition, the response rate to both drugs, although equivalent, was much higher than seen with clozapine after 8 weeks of treatment in other studies. In a 6-week double-blind clozapine/risperidone study of 29 adult patients who had treatment-refractory schizophrenia, clozapine was superior to risperidone for positive symptoms and EPS [98]. No significant differences were found on two measures of negative symptoms, total symptom scores, and depression scores [98]. Using 20% change in Brief Psychiatric Rating Scale total score to identify categorical responders, the investigators found that 5 (35.7%) of the 14 patients assigned to clozapine and 3 (20.0%) of the 15 patients assigned to risperidone met the response criteria ($P = .34$).

Risperidone has been associated with prolactin elevation [99], which could lead to amenorrhea, galactorrhea, and erectile and ejaculatory dysfunction, all of concern to adolescent patients. In a large, multisite, head-to-head comparison of risperidone and olanzapine, more patients had elevated serum prolactin levels in the risperidone group than in the olanzapine group [56]. The long-term effects of antipsychotic-induced prolactin elevations on pubertal development, fertility, and endocrine function in adolescents are currently unknown. (See the article by Becker and Epperson elsewhere in this issue for further exploration of this topic.)

Quetiapine

Quetiapine is an FDA-approved second-generation antipsychotic. Its antipsychotic efficacy at doses of 150 to 750 mg/day has been demonstrated in short-term comparisons with placebo, chlorpromazine, and haloperidol (12 mg) in three large, multicenter trials [100–102]. Findings with respect to negative symptom reduction were inconsistent and varied with dosage and the specific rating scale employed. In terms of side effects, this drug produces few EPS and no significant prolactin elevation. Concern has been raised about potential ophthalmologic effects of quetiapine, however. The data supporting its effectiveness in refractory adult patients are limited [103,104], and thus the exact role of quetiapine in children and adolescents who have treatment-refractory schizophrenia remains unclear.

Ziprasidone

Ziprasidone is a novel antipsychotic that has a number of attractive features for the treatment of adolescents with EOS. Ziprasidone, a benzisothizolyl piperazine, is a D2 antagonist with a more potent affinity for 5-HT-2a receptors than for D2 receptors [105]. The ratio of 5HT2a-to-D2 receptor affinities for ziprasidone is comparable to those of risperidone and clozapine, and a relationship between a high ratio of 5HT2/D2 affinity and low potential for EPS has been proposed. Other characteristics of ziprasidone include a low affinity for adrenergic and histaminergic receptors and a negligible affinity for cholinergic receptors, with a low potential for problems with hypotension and anticholinergic side effects. Ziprasidone also has a moderate inhibitory action at norepinephrine and serotonin reuptake sites, suggesting potential efficacy for anxiety and mood symptoms. In adults, ziprasidone has been shown to be effective at doses of 80 to 160 mg/day in the treatment of schizophrenia [106,107]. The superiority of ziprasidone to conventional antipsychotic agents in terms of positive and negative symptoms in schizophrenia remains unclear [108].

Ziprasidone has also been associated with a substantially lower propensity for weight gain than other antipsychotics [109], with efficacy apparently comparable to that of risperidone [110] and olanzapine [105] in short-term trials. Ziprasidone was less likely than olanzapine to affect body weight, total cholesterol, triglycerides, and low-density lipoprotein cholesterol levels negatively [105]. In adults, ziprasidone has also been shown to be less likely than other second-generation antipsychotics to induce movement disorders and elevated serum prolactin levels [108,110].

Ziprasidone, however, has also been reported to have a greater capacity than other antipsychotic drugs to prolong the QT/QTc interval, and this side effect may limit the use of ziprasidone by child psychiatrists [111]. In a preliminary 8-week, double-blind, placebo-controlled study of 28 children and adolescents who had Tourette's syndrome, ziprasidone therapy (5–40 mg/day) seemed to be effective, and most adverse effects were reported as mild and transient [112]. No EKG abnormalities were reported.

Because of emerging concerns regarding the use of other second-generation antipsychotic medications that have been associated with weight gain and emergence of insulin resistance, it is critical to test the safety and efficacy of ziprasidone more broadly in adolescents who have EOS. Unfortunately, there are no published data regarding the safety of ziprasidone in EOS and very little published pediatric data with respect to liability for cardiac side effects (eg, prolongation of QTc interval) [113], particularly at doses typically used to treat pediatric patients who have schizophrenia (>120 mg/day). There are some data suggesting that there are no significant QTc interval changes in adults exposed to high-dose ziprasidone (240–320 mg/day) [114]. Given the recent report of a sudden death in a patient who had Tourette's syndrome during a clinical trial of ziprasidone [115], large safety-monitoring studies are needed to guide clinicians concerning the optimal schedule for EKG monitoring for children and adolescents being prescribed ziprasidone.

Aripiprazole

Aripiprazole is a newly available antipsychotic agent for the treatment of schizophrenia that is a dopamine D2 receptor partial agonist with partial agonist activity at the serotonin (5-HT-1a) receptors and antagonist activity at 5-HT-2a receptors. This is the first non-D2 receptor antagonist with clear antipsychotic action [116] and thus provides child psychiatrists with another treatment option, particularly for children who have experienced weight gain, prolactin elevation, or EPS while taking other antipsychotic therapies. Like ziprasidone, studies in adults indicate that aripiprazole has less of a negative impact than olanzapine on patients' weight and plasma lipid profiles [117]. As with ziprasidone, these short-term data would indicate a potentially lower likelihood of the development of metabolic syndrome and long-term adverse cardiovascular events than seen with other second-generation antipsychotic agents. Aripiprazole has been shown to be superior to placebo in short-term trials of adults who have schizophrenia and to be equivalent to other commonly used antipsychotic medications such as olanzapine [117], risperidone [116], and haloperidol [118]. Reports of the use of aripiprazole in children and adolescents primarily have been large case series of children who have bipolar disorder [119]; the authors know of no published studies in adolescents who have schizophrenia or in adults who have treatment-refractory schizophrenia.

Weight gain, hyperglycemia, and hypertriglyceridemia associated with second-generation agents

In adult studies, second-generation antipsychotic treatment recently has been linked to obesity, hypertriglyceridemia, and diabetes, all of which are risk factors for cardiovascular diseases [120]. Increasingly, there has been a focus on the early detection and prevention of these problems for patients receiving long-term treatment with the newer atypical antipsychotics. The incidence of these side effects in children and adolescents treated with these agents is unknown, although preliminary data suggest that children and adolescents treated with atypical antipsychotics may be at particularly high risk of developing weight gain and metabolic syndrome [35,121–123].

A meta-analysis by Allison and colleagues [109] found the degree of weight gain, estimated by a random effects regression at 10 weeks of treatment, to be 9.8 lb (4.5 kg) with clozapine, 9.1 lb (4.2 kg) with olanzapine, 4.6 lb (2.1 kg) with risperidone, and 1.0 lb (0.9 kg) with ziprasidone. Wirshing and colleagues [124] conducted a retrospective analysis of 122 clinical records of 92 male patients who had schizophrenia and examined the relative weight-gain liabilities of clozapine, risperidone, olanzapine, and sertindole, compared with haloperidol. The authors concluded that clozapine and olanzapine caused the most weight gain, risperidone was intermediate, and sertindole had less associated weight gain than haloperidol. A 5-year naturalistic study of 82 adult patients (mean age, 36.4 years; SD, 7.8) treated with clozapine showed that patients experienced significant weight gain and increase in serum triglyceride levels, and 30 of 82 patients (37%) were diagnosed as having new-onset diabetes during the 5-year observation period [125]. Of interest, weight gain was not found to be a significant risk factor for developing diabetes in this study, suggesting that mechanisms other than obesity may be involved in non–insulin-dependent diabetes associated with clozapine [125]. The authors suggest that potential risk factors for the development of diabetes might include increasing age, race, genetic factors, lack of physical activity, or dietary factors, and that the potential mechanism by which clozapine produces diabetes could involve suppression of insulin, insulin resistance, or impairment of glucose use [125]. Similarly, in a study of 21 patients, Leadbetter and colleagues [126] found that during 16 weeks of clozapine treatment, 38% of the patients experienced marked weight gain, and 29% had moderate weight gain. As reviewed by Miller [127], data from naturalistic studies suggest that the longer the duration of clozapine treatment, the greater the weight gain.

Similarly, as summarized by Conley [128], increased appetite was more common in olanzapine- than in haloperidol-treated adult patients in four clinical trials of olanzapine. Weight gain in the amount of 4.4 to 6.6 lb (2–3 kg) was seen in adult patients taking olanzapine in comparison with both placebo and haloperidol during the 6-week acute phases of the clinical trials; the most significant weight increases occurred in patients who were the most underweight before beginning treatment with olanzapine [75]. Premarketing data also showed that, during long-term treatment trials, 56% of olanzapine-treated patients reported a weight gain of 7% or more of their body weight, which is the commonly accepted starting point for clinically significant weight-related problems [129]. Some unpublished data suggest that adolescents treated with olanzapine might be particularly sensitive to weight gain [128]. In addition, there have been case reports of adults who have developed hyperglycemia [130], new-onset diabetes [130], and diabetic ketoacidosis [131,132] in association with olanzapine treatment.

It is possible that weight gain after the initiation of clozapine or olanzapine treatment may exacerbate subclinical diabetes or promote glucose abnormalities. Goldstein and colleagues [133] have reported on seven patients who developed new-onset diabetes between 5 weeks and 17 months after starting olanzapine treatment. Five of these patients required hospitalization to manage hyperglycemia, three had a definite family history of diabetes, and four continued to require medical treatment for diabetes. Increased plasma triglyceride levels, which have been frequently reported in patients taking olanzapine, may precipitate or exacerbate diabetes [134]. Sheitman and colleagues [135] reported on nine chronically institutionalized patients whose fasting plasma lipid levels and weight were measured before starting treatment with olanzapine and again after 6 months of treatment. With a mean dose of 19 mg/day of olanzapine, mean triglyceride levels increased from 170 to 240 mg/dL (normal range, 25–200 mg/dL). After 12 weeks of treatment with olanzapine (mean dose, 13.8 ± 4.4 mg/day), fasting triglycerides levels increased a mean of 60 mg/dL in 25 adult patients. (See the article by Correll elsewhere in this issue for further exploration of this topic.)

Potential augmentation strategies to antipsychotics

Approximately 50% of adolescents do not respond or are partially responsive to clozapine or olanzapine [36,92]. These adolescents who have schizophrenia represent a major clinical problem. Various augmentation strategies have been studied in adults who have schizophrenia and do not respond to neuroleptics. Lithium, anticonvulsants, benzodiazepines, beta-blockers, electroconvulsive therapy, antidepressants, and antipsychotic combinations have each been reported to have some benefit in adults who have treatment-resistant schizophrenia [27,136]. None of these alternative therapies has been studied in youth with EOS, however, and their potential for side effects and lack of documented efficacy in this age group need to be weighed when considering their use. At present, there is considerable controversy regarding the use of antipsychotic polypharmacy or augmentation, although clinically it is a widespread practice used to accelerate clinical response in inpatient settings because of managed-care constraints regarding length of hospital stay and also, perhaps, because of potentially complementary receptor occupancy profiles. Most experts, however, would advise child psychiatrists to consider long-term trials of a sequence of atypical antipsychotic monotherapies at maximal therapeutic doses before adding another agent [137].

Lithium

Adjunct lithium therapy may have benefit for some patients who have treatment-resistant schizophrenia [136,138–140], but more recent controlled studies do not find substantial added benefit [141–143]. Also, there exists the danger of potential delirium, encephalopathy, and neurotoxicity when using lithium in combination with conventional antipsychotics [144,145].

Anticonvulsants

Although carbamazepine and valproic acid are often considered as an adjunct therapy in patients who have schizophrenia, the published controlled data for carbamazepine [146] had relatively few subjects, and the recorded efficacy was modest. There have been no controlled trials evaluating valproic acid as an augmentation therapy in treatment-refractory schizophrenia. There is, however, some evidence that treatment with divalproex in combination with an atypical antipsychotic in hospitalized adults who have schizophrenia results in earlier improvement in psychotic symptomatology [147] and in reductions in hostility during the first week of treatment [148].

Lamotrigine

Recent preclinical and clinical evidence suggests that lamotrigine may be a promising augmentation strategy for children and adolescents who do not respond to clozapine therapy. The occurrence of potentially severe drug rashes associated with lamotrigine use, particularly in children, has limited its use. Lamotrigine is an anticonvulsant with neuroprotective properties which blocks voltage-sensitive sodium channels and reduces the release of excitatory amino acids [149]. There is increasing evidence to suggest that the glutamate system represents a logical target for initial clozapine augmentation studies [150,151]. First, both phencyclidine and ketamine induce a syndrome closely resembling schizophrenia in humans. These drugs are believed to block the ion channel in the N-methyl-D-aspartate (NMDA) receptor complex, resulting in diminished glutamatergic neurotransmission at this receptor complex. Recent data show that both dopaminergic and glutamatergic terminals converge on the spines of pyramidal neurons in the cortex, indicating a common site of action for both dopamine agonists and phencyclidine. Although the nature of dopamine modulation of glutamatergic transmission is not understood fully, it has been hypothesized that modulation of glutamate release by D1 receptors might mediate some of the effects of dopamine on psychosis [152]. Second, maturational changes in the brain's response to NMDA antagonists correspond to the typical age of schizophrenia onset. Specifically, a high percentage of adults display psychotic symptoms upon awakening from ketamine anesthesia, whereas children show little or no susceptibility. Third, agonists or partial agonists of the glycine modulatory site of the glutamatergic NMDA receptors that enhance glutamatergic transmission improve negative symptoms of schizophrenia [153]. Also, glutamate levels and the activity of the enzyme glutaminase have been found to be increased in the dorsolateral prefrontal cortex of patients who have schizophrenia [154]. Together, these observations have led to a hypothesis that a putative NMDA receptor dysfunction or dysregulation may contribute to the pathophysiology of schizophrenia [152,155].

If a dysfunction/dysregulation of the NMDA receptor occurs in schizophrenia, this defect could result in a loss of GABAergic inhibitory control over the major excitatory projections to the cerebral cortex. The moderately increased neurotransmitter release and associated overstimulation of postsynaptic neurons could explain the cognitive and behavioral symptoms in schizophrenia and over time could trigger injury throughout many corticolimbic regions. Glucocorticoids and stress can increase glutamatergic tone in the hippocampus [152], and hippocampal atrophy has been observed in patients who had EOS during adolescence [156]. Rodent studies indicate that lamotrigine can prevent the neurotoxic consequences of NMDA receptor dysfunction. Similar effects have also been seen in humans. In a challenge study of 16 healthy, normal volunteers, the administration of lamotrigine before administration of subanesthetic doses of ketamine significantly decreased ketamine-induced symptoms resembling positive and negative symptoms of schizophrenia, perceptual alterations, and impairments in memory and learning [157]. Also, in two pilot studies of clozapine in adult patients who had treatment-resistant schizophrenia, a significant improvement in psychotic symptoms was seen with the addition of lamotrigine over a 12-week period, suggesting that lamotrigine interacts with the glutamatergic system in a different way than does clozapine [150,158].

Lamotrigine is a safe, effective, FDA-approved drug that has been successfully used as monotherapy and as add-on treatment for partial seizures in children [159], with fewer untoward cognitive effects and less weight gain than seen with other antiepileptic drugs. Lamotrigine has also been shown to be effective in the treatment of adults who have bipolar disorder. These data provide a rationale for considering the use of lamotrigine in combination with clozapine for adolescents who have treatment-refractory EOS.

Benzodiazepines

Although some controlled data support the use of adjunct benzodiazepines in treatment-resistant schizophrenia [160,161], there is no firm evidence for a specific adjunct antipsychotic effect with these agents.

Beta-blockers

Although some data support the use of beta-blockers in refractory schizophrenia [162], no available controlled studies used current diagnostic criteria, and there is very limited evidence that long-term therapy with these agents is beneficial.

Electroconvulsive treatment

There have been no controlled studies of electroconvulsive treatment in patients who have treatment-resistant schizophrenia. Although some data support the use of electroconvulsive treatment in poorly responsive patients who have schizophrenia [163], issues of persistence of the therapeutic effect and long-term maintenance have not yet been determined.

Neuroleptic combinations

In clinical practice, the combination of novel antipsychotics and traditional drugs is quite popular. To the authors' knowledge there have been no controlled trials evaluating whether the addition of a typical neuroleptic to ongoing risperidone or olanzapine treatment is beneficial in poorly responsive patients. Recent treatment recommendations from a panel of experts have discouraged the use of polypharmacy in children and adolescents who have serious psychiatric disorders, particularly because the available evidence does not support the usefulness of this practice [164]. Specifically, in a recent study of 30 adults who had schizophrenia and who were partially responsive to clozapine, adjunctive risperidone treatment did not significantly reduce psychopathology during a 6-week period [165]. Given the potential for worsening of metabolic side effects associated with combinations of antipsychotic medications, it is imperative for physicians to complete cross-tapers of antipsychotic medications and periodically to re-evaluate the need for continuing multiple medications in patients who have treatment-refractory schizophrenia.

Future directions

This article has summarized evidence for treatment approaches in children and adolescents who have treatment-refractory schizophrenia. Recent evidence suggests that several of these agents show promise in terms of short-term therapeutic effect and are better tolerated and thus more acceptable to children and their families than previous conventional antipsychotic medications. It is possible that this increased satisfaction in terms of both drug efficacy and tolerability will result in better rates of long-term compliance. Despite the availability of second-generation antipsychotic medications, it seems that early-onset of schizophrenia is still associated with a particularly malignant long-term course and severe disability in functional outcome. Understanding the mechanism of the emergence of disability in adolescent-onset schizophrenia remains an important research priority. Although the newer antipsychotic medications seem to provide less exposure risk to the development of tardive dyskinesia, the long-term morbidity of these newer agents because of increased weight gain, the emergence of diabetes, and cardiovascular disorders remains unclear. Because clinical experience suggests that most children and adolescents who have schizophrenia are not stabilized with the use of antipsychotic monotherapy, additional controlled studies are needed to evaluate potential augmentation strategies for antipsychotic medications. It is hoped that evidence supporting the use of specific augmentation strategies will lead to the development of evidence-based treatment algorithms to maximize treatment response and long-term outcome in this population.

References

[1] Krausz M, Müller-Thomsen T. Schizophrenia with onset in adolescence: an 11-year followup. Schizophr Bull 1993;19(4):148–53.
[2] McClellan J, Werry J. Practice parameters for the assessment and treatment of children and adolescents with schizophrenia. J Am Acad Child Adolesc Psychiatry 1994;33(5):616–35.
[3] Beitchman JH. Childhood schizophrenia: a review and comparison with adult-onset schizophrenia. Psychiatric Clin North Am 1985;8(4):793–8.
[4] McKenna K, Gordon CT, Lenane M, et al. Looking for childhood-onset schizophrenia: the first 71 cases screened. J Am Acad Child Adolesc Psychiatry 1994;33(5):636–44.
[5] Stayer C, Sporn A, Gogtay N, et al. Looking for childhood schizophrenia: case series of false positives. J Am Acad Child Adolesc Psychiatry 2004;43:1026–9.
[6] Sporn AL, Addington AM, Gogtay N, et al. Pervasive developmental disorder and childhood-onset schizophrenia: comorbid disorder or a phenotypic variant of a very early onset illness? Biol Psychiatry 2004;55:989–94.
[7] Thompson PM, Vidal C, Giedd JN, et al. Mapping adolescent brain change reveals dynamic wave of accelerated gray matter loss in very early-onset schizophrenia. Proc Natl Acad Sci USA 2001;98:11650–5.
[8] Asarnow RF, Neuchterlein KH, Subotnik KL, et al. Neurocognitive impairments in non-psychotic parents of children with schizophrenia and attention-deficit/hyperactivity disorder: the University of California, Los Angeles Family Study. Arch Gen Psychiatry 2002;59: 1053–60.
[9] Gochman PA, Greenstein D, Sporn A, et al. Childhood onset schizophrenia: familial neuro-cognitive measures. Schizophr Res 2004;71(1):43–7.
[10] Addington AM, Gornick M, Duckworth J, et al. GAD1 (2q31.1), which encodes glutamic acid decarboxylase (GAD(67)), is associated with childhood-onset schizophrenia and cortical gray matter volume loss. Mol Psychiatry 2005;10(6):581–8.
[11] Maziade M, Gingras N, Rodrigue C, et al. Long-term stability of diagnosis and symptom dimensions in a systematic sample of patients with onset of schizophrenia in childhood and early adolescence. I: nosology, sex and age of onset. Br J Psychiatry 1996;169:361–70.
[12] Hollis C. Adult outcomes of child- and adolescent-onset schizophrenia: diagnostic stability and predictive validity. Am J Psychiatry 2000;157:1652–9.

[13] Werry JS, McClellan JM, Chard L. Childhood and adolescent schizophrenic, bipolar, and schizoaffective disorders: a clinical and outcome study. J Am Acad Child Adolesc Psychiatry 1991;30:457–65.

[14] Russell AT. The clinical presentation of childhood-onset schizophrenia. Schizophr Bull 1994; 20:631–46.

[15] Asarnow JR. Annotation: child-onset schizophrenia. J Child Psychol Psychiatry 1994;35(8): 1345–71.

[16] Schmidt M, Blanz B, Dippe A, et al. Puberty and the onset of psychosis. Schizophr Res 1995; 10(1):7–14.

[17] Eggers C. Course and prognosis in childhood schizophrenia. J Autism Child Schizophr 1978; 8:21–36.

[18] Eggers C, Bunk D. The long-term course of childhood-onset schizophrenia: a 42-year follow up. Schizophr Bull 1997;23(1):105–17.

[19] Werry JS, McClellan JM. Predicting outcome in child and adolescent (early onset) schizophrenia and bipolar disorder. J Am Acad Child Adloesc Psychiatry 1992;31(1):147–50.

[20] Amminger GP, Resch F, Mutschlechner R, et al. Premorbid adjustment and remission of positive symptoms in first-episode psychosis. Eur Child Adolesc Psychiatry 1997;6(4):212–8.

[21] McClellan J, Prezbindowski A, Breiger D, et al. Neuropsychological functioning in early onset psychotic disorders. Schizophr Res 2004;68:21–6.

[22] Oie M, Rund BR. Neuropsychological deficits in adolescent-onset schizophrenia compared with attention deficit hyperactivity disorder. Am J Psychiatry 1999;156:1216–22.

[23] Rhinewine J, Lencz T, Thaden E, et al. Neurocognitive profile in adolescents with early-onset schizophrenia: clinical correlates. Biol Psychiatry 2005 Jul 13 [Epub ahead of print].

[24] Green MF, Kern RS, Heaton RK. Longitudinal studies of cognition and functional outcome in schizophrenia: implications for MATRICS. Schizophr Res 2004;71(1):41–51.

[25] Conley RR, Kelly DL, Gale EA. Olanzapine response in treatment-refractory schizophrenic patients with a history of substance abuse. Schizophr Res 1998;33:95–101.

[26] Practice parameters for the assessment and treatment of children and adolescents with schizophrenia. J Am Acad Child Adolesc Psychiatry 2001;40(7 Suppl):4S–23S.

[27] Conley RR, Buchanan RW. Evaluation of treatment-resistant schizophrenia. Schizophr Bull 1997;23(4):663–74.

[28] Pool D, Bloom W, Mielke D, et al. A controlled evaluation of loxitane in seventy-five adolescent schizophrenic patients. Curr Ther Res 1976;19:99–104.

[29] Spencer EK, Kafantaris V, Padron-Gayol MV, et al. Haloperidol in schizophrenic children: early findings from a study in progress. Psychopharmacol Bull 1992;28:183–6.

[30] Lieberman JA, Safferman AZ, Pollack S. Clinical effects of clozapine in chronic schizophrenia: response to treatment and predictors of outcome. Am J Psychiatry 1994;151:1744–52.

[31] Meltzer HY, Rabinowitz J, Lee MA, et al. Age at onset and gender of schizophrenia patients in relation to neuroleptic resistance. Am J Psychiatry 1997;154:475–82.

[32] Meltzer HY. Treatment of the neuroleptic nonresponsive schizophrenic patient. Schizophr Bull 1992;18:515–42.

[33] Breier A, Buchanan RW, Kirkpatrick B, et al. Effects of clozapine on positive and negative symptoms in outpatients with schizophrenia. Am J Psychiatry 1994;151(1):20–6.

[34] Lieberman JA, Saltz BL, Johns CA, et al. The effects of clozapine on tardive dyskinesia. Br J Psychiatry 1991;158:503–10.

[35] Sikich L, Hamer RM, Bashford RA, et al. A pilot study of risperidone, olanzapine, and haloperidol in psychotic youth: a double-blind, randomized, 8-week trial. Neuropsychopharmacology 2004;29:133–45.

[36] Kumra S, Frazier JA, Jacobsen LK, et al. Childhood-onset schizophrenia: a double-blind clozapine-haloperidol comparison. Arch Gen Psychiatry 1996;53:1090–7.

[37] Teicher MG, Barber NI, Gelbard HA, et al. Developmental differences in acute nigrostriatal and mesocorticolimbic system response to haloperidol. Neuropsychopharmacology 1993;9(2): 147–56.

[38] Lewis R. Typical and atypical antipsychotics in adolescent schizophrenia: efficacy,

tolerability, and differential sensitivity to extrapyramidal symptoms. Can J Psychiatry 1998; 43:596–604.

[39] Mandoki M. Risperidone treatment of children and adolescents: increased risk of extrapyramidal side effects? J Child Adolesc Psychopharmacol 1995;5:49–67.

[40] Campbell M, Grega D, Green W, et al. Neuroleptic-induced dyskinesias in children. Clin Neuropharmacol 1995;6:207–22.

[41] Claghorn J, Honigfeld G, Abuzzahab Sr FS, et al. The risks and benefits of clozapine versus chlorpromazine. J Clin Psychopharmacol 1987;7(6):377–84.

[42] Kane J, Honigfeld G, Singer J, et al, Clozaril Collaborative Study Group. Clozapine for the treatment-resistant schizophrenia: a double-blind comparison with chlorpromazine. Arch Gen Psychiatry 1988;45:789–96.

[43] Casey DE. Clozapine: neuroleptic-induced EPS and tardive dyskinesia. Psychopharmacology (Berl) 1989;99(Suppl):S47–53.

[44] Kane JM, Woerner MG, Pollack S, et al. Does clozapine cause tardive dyskinesia? J Clin Psychiatry 1993;54(9):327–30.

[45] Pickar D, Owen RR, Litman RE, et al. Clinical and biologic response to clozapine in patients with schizophrenia. Crossover comparison with fluphenazine. Arch Gen Psychiatry 1992;49(5): 345–53.

[46] Kane JM. Tardive dyskinesia: epidemiological and clinical presentation. In: Borroni E, Kupfer DJ, editors. Psychopharmacology: the fourth generation of progress. New York: Raven Press; 1995. p. 1485–96.

[47] Meltzer HY. Clozapine: is another view valid? Am J Psychiatry 1995;152:821–5.

[48] Lindstrom LH. The effect of long-term treatment with clozapine in schizophrenia. Acta Psychiatr Scand 1988;77:524–9.

[49] Lindstrom LH. Long-term clinical and social outcome studies in schizophrenia in relation to the cognitive and emotional side effects of antipsychotic drugs. Acta Psychiatr Scand 1994;89: 74–6.

[50] Meltzer HY, Alphs L, Green AI, et al, International Suicide Prevention Trial Study Group. Clozapine treatment for suicidality in schizophrenia: International Suicide Prevention Trial (InterSePT). Arch Gen Psychiatry 2003;60(1):82–91.

[51] Albanese MJ, Khantzian EJ, Murphy SL, et al. Decreased substance use in chronically psychotic patients treated with clozapine. Am J Psychiatry 1994;151(5):780–1.

[52] Buckley P, Thompson P, Way L, et al. Substance abuse among patients with treatment-resistant schizophrenia: characteristics and implications for clozapine therapy. Am J Psychiatry 1994; 151(3):385–9.

[53] Marcus P, Snyder R. Reduction of comorbid substance abuse with clozapine. Am J Psychiatry 1995;152(6):959.

[54] Essock SM, Hargreaves WA, Dohm FA, et al. Clozapine eligibility among state hospital patients. Schizophr Bull 1996;22(1):15–25.

[55] Pollack S, Woerner M, Kane J. Clozapine reduces rehospitalization among schizophrenic patients. Poster presented at the 37th Annual Meeting of the New Clinical Drug Evaluation Unit Meeting. Boca Raton (FL), May 27–30, 1997.

[56] Conley RR, Tamminga CA, Kelly DL, et al. Treatment-resistant schizophrenic patients respond to clozapine after olanzapine non-response. Biol Psychiatry 1999;46:73–7.

[57] Towbin KE, Dykens EM, Pugliese RG. Case study: clozapine for early developmental delays with childhood-onset schizophrenia: protocol and 15-month outcome. J Am Acad Child Adoles Psychiatry 1994;33:651–8.

[58] Siefen G, Remschmidt H. Treatment results with clozapine in schizophrenic adolescents. Z Kinder Jugenpsychiatr 1986;14(3):245–57.

[59] Remschmidt H, Schulz E, Martin M. An open trial of clozapine in thirty-six adolescents with schizophrenia. J Child Adolesc Psychiatry 1994;4:31–41.

[60] Schmidt M, Trott G, Blanz B, et al. Clozapine medication in adolescents. In: Psychiatry: a world perspective. Proceedings of the VIII World Congress of Psychiatry. Amsterdam: Elsevier Publishing Co.; 1989. p. 1100–4.

[61] Mozes T, Toren P, Chernauzan N. Case study: clozapine treatment in very early onset schizophrenia. J Am Acad Child Adolesc Psychiatry 1994;33:65–70.

[62] Grcevich SJ, Findling RL, Rowane WA. Risperidone in the treatment of children and adolescents with schizophrenia: a retrospective study. J Child Adolesc Psychopharmacol 1996; 6(4):251–7.

[63] Armenteros JL, Whitaker AH, Welikson M, et al. Risperidone in adolescents with schizophrenia: an open pilot study. J Am Acad Child Adolesc Psychiatry 1997;36(5):694–700.

[64] Jacobsen LK, Walker M, Edwards J, et al. Clinical effects of clozapine in the treatment of a young adolescent with schizophrenia. J Am Acad Child Adolesc Psychiatry 1994;33: 645–60.

[65] Correll CU, Leucht S, Kane JM. Lower risk for tardive dyskinesia associated with second-generation antipsychotics: a systematic review of 1-year studies. Am J Psychiatry 2004; 161(3):414–25.

[66] Gerbino-Rosen G, Roofeh D, Tompkins DA, et al. Hematological adverse events in clozapine-treated children and adolescents. J Am Acad Child Adolesc Psychiatry 2005;44(10):1024–31.

[67] Ratey JJ, Leveroni C, Kilmer D, et al. The effects of clozapine on severely aggressive psychiatric inpatients in a state hospital. J Clin Psychiatry 1993;54(6):219–23.

[68] Volavka J, Zito JM, Vitrai J, et al. Clozapine effects on hostility and aggression in schizophrenia. J Can Psychopharmacol 1993;13(4):287–9.

[69] Cohen SA, Underwood MT. The use of clozapine in a mentally retarded and aggressive population. J Clin Psychiatry 1994;55(10):440–4.

[70] Bellus SB, Stewart D, Kost PP. Clozapine in aggression. Psychiatr Serv 1995;46(2):187.

[71] Kranzler H, Roofeh D, Gerbino-Rosen G, et al. Clozapine: its impact on aggressive behavior among children and adolescents with schizophrenia. J Am Acad Child Adolesc Psychiatry 2005;44(1):55–63.

[72] Alivir JM, Lieberman JA. Agranulocytosis: incidence and risk factors. J Clin Psychiatry 1994; (Suppl B):137–8.

[73] Duncan GE, Miyamoto S, Leipzig JN, et al. Comparison of the effects of clozapine, risperidone and olanzapine on ketamine induced alterations in regional brain metabolism. JPET 2000; 293:8–14.

[74] Beasley Jr CM, Tollefson G, Tran P, Satterlee, et al for the Olanzapine HGAD Study Group. Olanzapine versus placebo and haloperidol. Acute phase results of the North American double-blind olanzapine trial. Neuropsychopharmacology 1996;14:111–23.

[75] Beasley Jr CM, Hamilton SH, Crawford AM, et al. Olanzapine versus haloperidol: acute phase results of the international double-blind olanzapine trial. Eur Neuropsychopharmacol 1997; 7(2):125–37.

[76] Tran PV, Dellva MA, Tollefson GD, et al. Extrapyramidal symptoms and tolerability of olanzapine versus haloperidol in the acute treatment of schizophrenia. J Clin Psychiatry 1997; 58(5):205–11.

[77] Tollefson GD, Beasley Jr CM, Tran PV, et al. Olanzapine versus haloperidol in the treatment of schizophrenia and schizoaffective and schizophreniform disorders: results of an international collaborative trial. Am J Psychiatry 1997;154(4):457–65.

[78] Tollefson GD, Beasley Jr CM, Tamura RN, et al. Blind, controlled, long-term study of the comparative incidence of treatment-emergent tardive dyskinesia with olanzapine or haloperidol. Am J Psychiatry 1997;154:1248–54.

[79] Glazer WM. Review of incidence studies of tardive dyskinesia associated with typical anti-psychotics. J Clin Psychiatry 2000;61(Suppl 4):15–20.

[80] Beasley Jr CM, Sanger T, Satterlee W, et al for the Olanzapine HGAP Study Group. Olanzapine versus placebo: results of a double-blind, fixed-dose olanzapine trial. Psychopharmacology (Berl) 1996;124:159–67.

[81] Tollefson GD, Sanger TM. Negative symptoms: a path analytic approach to a double-blind, placebo-and haloperidol-controlled clinical trial with olanzapine. Am J Psychiatry 1997;154(4): 466–74.

[82] Purdon SE, Jones BD, Stip E, et al. Neuropsychological change in early phase schizophrenia

during 12 months of treatment with olanzapine, risperidone or haloperidol. The Canadian Collaborative Group for research in schizophrenia. Arch Gen Psychiatry 2000;57(3):249–58.

[83] Fulton B, Goa KL. Olanzapine. A review of its pharmacological properties and therapeutic efficacy in the management of schizophrenia and related psychoses. Drugs 1997;53(2):281–98.

[84] Breier A, Hamilton SH. Comparative efficacy of olanzapine and haloperidol for patients with treatment resistant schizophrenia. Biol Psychiatry 1999;45(4):403–11.

[85] Beuzen JN, Birkett MA, Kiesler GM, et al. Olanzapine vs. clozapine: an intermediate double-blind study in the treatment of resistant schizophrenia. Presented at the 39th Meeting of the New Clinical Drug Evaluation Unit. 1999.

[86] Dursun SM, Gardner DM, Bird DC, et al. Olanzapine for patients with treatment-resistant schizophrenia: a naturalistic case-series outcome study. Can J Psychiatry 1999;44:701–4.

[87] Fanous A, Lindenmayer JP. Schizophrenia and schizoaffective disorder treated with high doses of olanzapine. J Clin Psychopharmacol 1999;19:275–6.

[88] Mountjoy CQ, Baldacchino AM, Stubbs JH. British experience with high-dose olanzapine for treatment-refractory schizophrenia. Am J Psychiatry 1999;156:158–9.

[89] Reich J. Use of high-dose olanzapine in refractory psychosis. Am J Psychiatry 1999;156:661.

[90] Heimann SW. High-dose olanzapine in an adolescent. J Am Acad Child Adolesc Psychiatry 1999;38:496–7.

[91] Kapur S, Zipursky RB, Remington G, et al. 5-HT2 and D2 receptor occupancy of olanzapine in schizophrenia: a PET investigation. Am J Psychiatry 1998;155:921–8.

[92] Kumra S, Jacobsen LK, Lenane M, et al. Childhood-onset schizophrenia: an open-label study of olanzapine in adolescents. J Am Acad Child Adolesc Psychiatry 1998;37:377–85.

[93] Marder S, Meibach R. Risperidone in the treatment of schizophrenia. Am J Psychiatry 1994; 151:825–35.

[94] Chouinard G, Jones B, Remington G, et al. A Canadian multicenter placebo-controlled study of fixed doses of risperidone and haloperidol in the treatment of chronic schizophrenia patients. J Clin Psychopharmacol 1993;13:25–40.

[95] Wirshing DA, Marshall BD, Green MF, et al. Risperidone in treatment-refractory schizophrenia. Am J Psychiatry 1999;156:1374–9.

[96] Flynn SW, MacEwan GW, Altman S, et al. An open comparison of clozapine and risperidone in treatment-resistant schizophrenia. Pharmacopsychiatry 1998;31(1):25–9.

[97] Bondolfi G, Dufour H, Patris M, et al. Risperidone versus clozapine in treatment-resistant chronic schizophrenia: a randomized double-blind study. The Risperidone Study Group. Am J Psychiatry 1998;155(4):499–504.

[98] Breier A, Berg PH. The psychosis of schizophrenia: prevalence, response to atypical antipsychotics, and prediction of outcome. Soc Biol Psychiatry 1999;46:361–4.

[99] Kleinberg DL, Davis JM, de Coster R, et al. Prolactin level and adverse events in patients treated with risperidone. J Clin Psychopharmacol 1999;19:57–61.

[100] Arvanitis LA, Miller BG for the Seroquel Trial 13 Study Group. Multiple fixed doses of "Seroquel" (quetiapine) in patients with acute exacerbation of schizophrenia: a comparison with haloperidol and placebo. Biol Psychiatry 1997;42:233–46.

[101] Small JG, Hirsch SR, Arvanitis LA, et al for the Seroquel Study Group. Quetiapine in patients with schizophrenia. Arch Gen Psychiatry 1997;54:549–57.

[102] Peuskens J, Link CG. A comparison of quetiapine and chlorpromazine in the treatment of schizophrenia. Acta Psychiatr Scand 1997;96(4):265–73.

[103] Sacchetti E, Panariello A, Regini C, et al. Quetiapine in hospitalized patients with schizophrenia refractory to treatment with first-generation antipsychotics: a 4-week, flexible-dose, single-blind, exploratory, pilot trial. Schizophr Res 2004;69:325–31.

[104] Pierre JM, Wirshing DA, Wirshing WC, et al. High-dose quetiapine in treatment refractory schizophrenia. Schizophr Res 2005;73(2–3):373–5.

[105] Simpson GM, Glick ID, Weiden PJ, et al. Randomized, controlled, double-blind multi-center comparison of the efficacy and tolerability of ziprasidone and olanzapine in acutely ill patients with schizophrenia or schizoaffective disorder. Am J Psychiatry 2004;161(10): 1837–47.

[106] Keck Jr PE, Reeves KR, Harrington EP for the Ziprasidone Study Group. Ziprasidone in the short-term treatment of patients with schizoaffective disorder: results from two double-blind, placebo-controlled, multicenter studies. J Clin Psychopharmacol 2001;21(1):27–35.

[107] Daniel DG, Zimbroff DL, Potkin SG, et al. Ziprasidone 80 mg/day and 160 mg/day in the acute exacerbation of schizophrenia and schizoaffective disorder: a 6-week placebo-controlled trial. Ziprasidone Study Group. Neuropsychopharmacology 1999;20(5):491–505.

[108] Goff DC, Posever T, Herz L, et al. An exploratory haloperidol-controlled dose-finding study of ziprasidone in hospitalized patients with schizophrenia or schizoaffective disorder. Clin Psychopharmacol 1998;18(4):296–304.

[109] Allison DB, Mentore JL, Heo M, et al. Antipsychotic-induced weight gain: a comprehensive research synthesis. Am J Psychiatry 1999;156(11):1686–96.

[110] Addington DE, Pantelis C, Dineen M, et al. Efficacy and tolerability of ziprasidone versus risperidone in patients with acute exacerbation of schizophrenia or schizoaffective disorder: an 8-week, double-blind, multicenter trial. J Clin Psychiatry 2004;65(12):1624–33.

[111] Labellarte MJ, Crosson JE, Riddle MA. The relevance of prolonged QTc measurement to pediatric psychopharmacology. J Am Acad Child Adolesc Psychiatry 2003;42(6):642–50.

[112] Sallee FR, Kurlan R, Goetz CG, et al. Ziprasidone treatment of children and adolescents with Tourette's syndrome: a pilot study. J Am Acad Child Adolesc Psychiatry 2000;39(3): 292–9.

[113] Blair J, Scahill L, State M, et al. Electrocardiographic changes in children and adolescents treated with ziprasidone: a prospective study. J Am Acad Child Adolesc Psychiatry 2005; 44(1):73–9.

[114] Levy WO, Robichaux-Keene NR, Nunez C. No significant QTc interval changes with high-dose ziprasidone: a case series. J Psychiatr Pract 2004;10(4):227–32.

[115] Scahill L, Blair J, Leckman JF, et al. Sudden death in a patient with Tourette syndrome during a clinical trial of ziprasidone. J Psychopharmacol 2005;19(2):205–6.

[116] Potkin SG, Saha AR, Kujawa MJ, et al. Aripiprazole, an antipsychotic with a novel mechanism of action, and risperidone vs placebo in patients with schizophrenia and schizoaffective disorder. Arch Gen Psychiatry 2003;60(7):681–90.

[117] McQuade RD, Stock E, Marcus R, et al. A comparison of weight change during treatment with olanzapine or aripiprazole: results from a randomized, double-blind study. J Clin Psychiatry 2004;65(Suppl 18):47–56.

[118] Kane JM, Carson WH, Saha AR, et al. Efficacy and safety of aripiprazole and haloperidol versus placebo in patients with schizophrenia and schizoaffective disorder. J Clin Psychiatry 2002;63(9):763–71.

[119] Biederman J, McDonnell MA, Wozniak J, et al. Aripiprazole in the treatment of pediatric bipolar disorder: a systematic chart review. CNS Spectr 2005;10(2):141–8.

[120] Kane JM, Barrett EJ, Casey DE, et al. Metabolic effects of treatment with atypical antipsychotics. J Clin Psychiatry 2004;65(11):1447–55.

[121] Correll CU, Malholtra AK. Pharmacogenetics of antipsychotic-induced weight gain. Psychopharmacol 2004;174(4):477–89.

[122] Bloch Y, Vardi O, Mendlovic S, et al. Hyperglycemia from olanzapine treatment in adolescents. J Child Adolesc Psychopharmacol 2003;13(1):97–102.

[123] Ratzoni G, Gothelf D, Brand-Gothelf A, et al. Weight gain associated with olanzapine and risperidone in adolescent patients: a comparative prospective study. J Am Acad Child Adolesc Psychiatry 2002;41(3):337–43.

[124] Wirshing DA, Wishing WC, Kysar L, et al. Novel antipsychotics: comparison of weight gain liabilities. J Clin Psychiatry 1999;60:358–63.

[125] Henderson DC, Cagliero E, Gray C, et al. Clozapine, diabetes mellitus, weight gain, and lipid abnormalities: a five year naturalistic study. Am J Psychiatry 2000;157(6):975–81.

[126] Leadbetter R, Shutty M, Pavalonis D, et al. Clozapine-induced weight gain: prevalence and clinical relevance. Am J Psychiatry 1992;149:68–72.

[127] Miller DD. Review and management of clozapine side effects. J Clin Psychiatry 2000; 61(Suppl 8):14–7.

[128] Conley RR, Meltzer HY. Adverse events related to olanzapine. J Clin Psychiatry 2000; 61(Suppl 8):26–9 [discussion: 30].

[129] Physicians' desk reference. Montvale (NY): Medical Economics Data Production Co; 2000.

[130] Ober SK, Hudak R, Rusterholtz A. Hyperglycemia and olanzapine [letter]. Am J Psychiatry 1999;165:970.

[131] Wirshing DA, Spellberg BJ, Erhart SM, et al. Novel antipsychotics and new onset diabetes. Biol Psychiatry 1998;44:778–83.

[132] Lindenmayer JP, Patel R. Olanzapine-induced ketoacidosis with diabetes mellitus [letter]. Am J Psychiatry 1999;156:1471–2.

[133] Goldstein LE, Sporn J, Brown S, et al. New onset diabetes mellitus and diabetic ketoacidosis associated with olanzapine treatment. Psychosomatics 1999;40:438–43.

[134] Grundy SM. Hypertriglyceridemia, atherogenic dyslipidemia, and the metabolic syndrome. Am J Cardiol 1998;81(4A):18B–25B.

[135] Sheitman BB, Bird PM, Binz W, et al. Olanzapine-induced elevation of plasma triglyceride levels. Am J Psychiatry 1999;156(9):1471–2.

[136] Wolkowitz OM. Rational polypharmacy in schizophrenia. Ann Clin Psychiatry 1993;5:79–90.

[137] Stahl SM, Grady MM. A critical review of atypical antipsychotic utilization: comparing monotherapy with polypharmacy and augmentation. Curr Med Chem 2004;11(3):313–27.

[138] Small JG, Kellams JJ, Milstein V, et al. A placebo-controlled study of lithium combined with neuroleptics in chronic schizophrenic patients. Am J Psychiatry 1975;132:1315–7.

[139] Growe GA, Crayton JW, Klass D, et al. Lithium in chronic schizophrenia. Am J Psychiatry 1979;136:454–5.

[140] Carmen JS, Bigelow LB, Wyatt RJ. Lithium combined with neuroleptics in chronic schizophrenic and schizoaffective patients. J Clin Psychiatry 1981;42:124–8.

[141] Levinson DF, Umapathy C, Musthaq M. Treatment of schizoaffective disorder and schizophrenia with mood symptoms. Am J Psychiatry 1999;156:1138–48.

[142] Terao T, Oga T, Nozaki S, et al. Lithium addition to neuroleptic treatment in chronic schizophrenia: a randomized double-blind, placebo-controlled, cross-over study. Acta Psychiatr Scand 1995;92:220–4.

[143] Schulz SC, Thompson PA, Jacobs M, et al. Lithium augmentation fails to reduce symptoms in poorly responsive schizophrenia outpatients. J Clin Psychiatry 1999;60:366–72.

[144] Cohen WJ, Cohen NH. Lithium carbonate, haloperidol and irreversible brain damage. JAMA 1974;230:1283–7.

[145] Miller F, Menninger J. Lithium-neuroleptic neurotoxicity is dose-dependent. J Psychopharmacol 1987;7:89–91.

[146] Simhandl C, Meszaros K. The use of carbamazepine in the treatment of schizophrenia and schizoaffective psychosis: a review. J Psychiatry Neurosci 1992;17:1–14.

[147] Casey DE, Daniel DG, Wasseff AA, et al. Effect of divalproex combined with olanzapine or risperidone in patients with an acute exacerbation of schizophrenia. Neuropsychopharmacology 2003;28(1):182–92.

[148] Citrome L, Casey DE, Daniel DG, et al. Adjunctive divalproex and hostility among patients with schizophrenia receiving olanzapine or risperidone. Psychiatr Serv 2004;55(3):290–4.

[149] Calabrese JR, Trisha S, Charles BI, et al. A double-blind, placebo-controlled, prophylaxis study of lamotrigine in rapid-cycling bipolar disorder. J Clin Psychiatry 2000;61(11):841–50.

[150] Tiihonen J, Hallikainen T, Ryynanen OP, et al. Lamotrigine in treatment-resistant schizophrenia: a randomized placebo-controlled crossover trial. Biol Psychiatry 2003;54(11):1241–8.

[151] Kremer I, Vass A, Gorelik I, et al. Placebo-controlled trial of lamotrigine added to conventional and atypical antipsychotics in schizophrenia. Biol Psychiatry 2004;56(6):441–6.

[152] Duchowny M, Pellock JM, Graf WD, et al. A placebo-controlled trial of lamotrigine add–on therapy for partial seizures in children. Neurology 1999;46:240–2.

[153] Duchowny M, Pellock JM, Graf WD, et al. A placebo-controlled trial of lamotrigine add-on therapy for partial seizures in children. Neurology 1999;53:1724–31.

[154] Dursun SM, McIntosh D, Milliken H. Clozapine plus lamotrigine in treatment-resistant schizophrenia. Arch Gen Psychiatry 1999;56(10):950.

[155] Gilman JT, Duchowny MS, Messenheimer JA, et al. Long-term tolerability of lamotrigine (Lamictal) in pediatric patients. Ann Neurol 2001;(Suppl 1):S92.

[156] Anand A, Charney DS, Oren DA, et al. Attenuation of the neuropsychiatric effects of ketamine with lamotrigine: support for hyperglutamatergic effects of N-methyl-D-aspartate receptor antagonists. Arch Gen Psychiatry 2000;57(3):270–6.

[157] Glauser TA. Expanding first-line therapy options for children with partial seizures. Neurology 2000;55(3):S30–7.

[158] Goff DC, Coyle JT. The emerging role of glutamate in the pathophysiology and treatment of schizophrenia. Am J Psychiatry 2001;158(9):1367–77.

[159] Goff DC, Evins AE. Negative symptoms in schizophrenia- neurobiological models and treatment response. Harv Rev Psychiatry 1998;6(2):59–77.

[160] Lingjaerde O, Engstrand E, Ellingsen P, et al. Antipsychotic effect of diazepam when given in addition to neuroleptics in chronic psychotic patients: a double-blind clinical trial. Current Therapeutic Research 1979;26:505–12.

[161] Wolkowitz OM, Turetsky N, Reus VI, et al. Benzodiazepine augmentation of neuroleptics in treatment-resistant schizophrenia. Psychopharmacol Bull 1992;28(3):291–5.

[162] Christison GW, Kirch DH, Wyatt RJ. When symptoms persist: choosing among alternative somatic treatments for schizophrenia. Schizophr Bull 1991;17(2):217–45.

[163] Friedel RO. The combined use of neuroleptics and ECT in drug resistant schizophrenic patients. Psychopharmacol Bull 1986;22(3):928–30.

[164] Pappadopulos E, Macintyre II JC, Crimson ML, et al. Treatment recommendations for the use of antipsychotics for aggressive youth (TRAAY), Part II. J Am Acad Child Adolesc Psychiatry 2003;42(2):145–61.

[165] Anil Yagcioglu AE, Kivircik Akdede BB, Turgut TI, et al. A double-blind controlled study of adjunctive treatment with risperidone in schizophrenic patients partially responsive to clozapine: efficacy and safety. J Clin Psychiatry 2005;66(1):63–72.

ELSEVIER
SAUNDERS

Child Adolesc Psychiatric Clin N Am
15 (2006) 161–175

CHILD AND
ADOLESCENT
PSYCHIATRIC CLINICS
OF NORTH AMERICA

An Update on Pharmacologic Treatments for Autism Spectrum Disorders

Bryan H. King, MD[a], Jeff Q. Bostic, MD, EdD[b],*

[a]Children's Hospital and Regional Medical Center, University of Washington, Seattle, WA, USA
[b]Harvard Medical School, Massachusetts General Hospital, Yawkey 6926,
55 Fruit Street, Boston, MA 02114-3139, USA

Autism spectrum disorders (ASDs) are a heterogeneous group of conditions that include autism, Asperger disorder, Rett disorder, childhood disintegrative disorder, and sometimes less severe or otherwise atypical presentations currently diagnosed as pervasive developmental disorder (PDD) not otherwise specified. By definition, the diagnosis of an ASD indicates that the affected individual will experience significant difficulty in reciprocal social interactions and communication and will exhibit repetitive or nonfunctional stereotyped behaviors or preoccupations. Affected individuals commonly avoid eye contact, do not develop normal social relationships appropriate for their age, do not seem to show interest in others' thoughts or feelings, and have difficulty understanding or seeing the world through the perspective of others. Affected individuals may have restricted speech or even be nonverbal, may use language unusually (invert pronouns, repeat phrases over and over), and frequently have difficulty sustaining conversations with others. Persons who have autism are often quite concrete and may be preoccupied with parts of objects or use objects in unusual ways. They may have routines that cannot be disrupted without conflict (eg, lining up toys in a certain way) and may exhibit unusual motor behaviors such as hand flapping, body twisting, or even head banging.

Dr. King has received research funding, honoraria, or consultant fees from the National Institute of Mental Health, National Institute of Child Health and Human Development, Cure Autism Now, Abbott, and Forest pharmaceuticals. Dr. Bostic has received research funding, honoraria, consulting fees, and speaker bureau funding from Abbott, Forest, GlaxoSmithKline, Lilly, and Pfizer Pharmaceuticals.

* Corresponding author.
E-mail address: roboz@adelphia.net (J.Q. Bostic).

doi:10.1016/j.chc.2005.08.005
childpsych.theclinics.com

With growing awareness, and certainly with a broader diagnostic net, the number of persons identified who have ASD has increased markedly during the past 20 years [1–3], from approximately 1 in 4000 to more recent epidemiologic estimates of as many as 1 in 400 [4], or greater when the broader phenotype is included [5,6], and sevenfold differences in identification rates persist among the states in the United States [7]. Although there is no consensus explanation for this international increase in the prevalence of autism, the search for environmental and genetic factors is intense.

No medical test is currently available for accurate detection of autism. Medical conditions that may explain ASD symptoms are found in fewer than 5% of cases [8]. Rather, the diagnosis is based upon the history and presence of clinical symptoms. Screening surveys such as the Checklist for Autism in Toddlers [9] are encouraged among primary care physicians working with pediatric populations to improve early identification of children who have PDD. In research settings, more structured interviews are used to identify both parent/guardian observations of the child's daily behaviors and symptoms apparent to the examiner when the patient is presented with a series of cognitive, social, and emotional tasks. These latter interviews often require several hours to administer and, although ensuring some consistency with the diagnosis and thus relative homogeneity for research purposes, may still fall short of allowing a satisfyingly precise diagnosis for some individuals at the diagnostic border.

Knowledge of the cause of ASD remains elusive, but the variety of genetic factors that have been linked to autism support the conclusion that ASDs are heterogeneous and multifactorial in origin. For example, the *FMR1* gene in the fragile X syndrome, the genes responsible for tuberous sclerosis, and a host of other very different gene candidates have already been identified [10,11]. Similarly, anomalies in brain formation have been recognized [12,13], including accelerated brain growth during the first 6 months of life, decreased formation of Purkinje cells in the cerebellum, and uneven growth in amygdala, thalamus, and cerebellar regions. Even specific symptoms, such as diminished eye contact, seem to be related to abnormalities in the superior temporal sulcus [14], fusiform, and amygdala regions [15]. Meanwhile, mitochondrial or cell respiratory abnormalities have been increasingly recognized [16], perhaps in as many as 7% of patients who have autism [17]. Despite such advances, these disparate findings have yet to be successfully coalesced to provide a specific neurologic or biochemical explanation for any of the ASD phenotypes or to yield specific targets for existing pharmacotherapies. Moreover, the multiplicity of neurobiologic findings associated with ASDs continues to suggest nonspecific but perhaps common pathway phenomena such as problems with connectivity or cerebral organization [18–20].

In recent years, the only pharmacotherapeutic treatment specific to ASD to arouse popular interest was secretin. Observations by Horvath and colleagues [21] of patients receiving secretin for gastrointestinal symptoms suggested that secretin might improve communication and social relatedness. Fifteen controlled studies followed but failed to support this original case report [22].

Virtually every psychotropic medication available has been examined in patients who have ASD. Although none of the psychotropic agents specifically treats ASD or has a Food and Drug Administration indication in this population, these agents have been used to target prominent symptoms. Indeed, the most common symptoms bringing patients who have ASD to the attention of child psychiatrists are disruptive behaviors such as aggression and self-injury, repetitive behaviors, hyperactivity, and mood, anxiety, and sleep problems [23]. The identification of agents from classes useful for these symptoms typically has followed the extrapolation of their use for a symptom common in a different disease state (eg, irritability in depression, hyperactivity in attention-deficit hyperactivity disorder [ADHD], or repetitive behaviors in obsessive-compulsive disorder). ADHD symptoms have been reported in more than half of children who have ASD [24]. Although ADHD symptoms are so common in autism that an ASD diagnosis actually pre-empts that of ADHD, none of these behaviors are regarded as core symptoms of ASD.

Thus, pharmacotherapy of patients who have PDD has focused on detecting the primary emotional and behavioral target symptoms and matching these targets with the medications most likely to be helpful [25]. Although the current pool of evidence to guide this practice with respect to autism might be characterized as relatively shallow, recent efforts to study the effect of common medications for common behaviors in this population are encouraging.

Research Units on Pediatric Psychopharmacology network

In the fall of 1997, the National Institute of Mental Health funded five university-affiliated medical centers with expertise in the treatment of autism to constitute the Research Units on Pediatric Psychopharmacology (RUPP) autism network [26]. The charge to the group was to investigate the safety and efficacy of drugs that are being used widely in the treatment of autism or that may hold particular promise. Thus far, the network has chosen to study risperidone and methylphenidate.

The case for risperidone was made on the strength of a number of converging findings relating to the population that has ASD. Specifically, abnormalities in both the serotonergic and dopaminergic systems have long been described in autism, and risperidone and related newer antipsychotic drugs effectively bridge these neurotransmitter systems in interesting ways [27]. In addition to experience with first-generation neuroleptic agents in children who have autism and severe behavioral disturbance, there existed ample case reports describing the potential benefit for risperidone in patients who have autism and other developmental disabilities [26,28].

The behavioral targets identified for the initial risperidone trial included impaired social behavior, interfering repetitive phenomena, and aggressive, self-injurious, and destructive behavior. Potential safety concerns included the possibility of extrapyramidal side effects associated with neuroleptic treatment, prolactin elevation, hepatotoxicity, and, perhaps most importantly, weight gain. Concerns about side effects are particularly salient where pharmacotherapy of behavioral disturbance in autism is concerned because of the potential chronicity of medication exposure.

The results of the RUPP risperidone trial were published in 2002 and may ultimately contribute to risperidone getting a specific indication for the treatment of behavioral disturbance in autism. The network enrolled 101 subjects aged 8.8 ± 2.7 years and, using the Aberrant Behavior Checklist irritability subscale as a primary outcome measure, found that behavioral symptoms including aggression, hyperactivity, and irritability all improved significantly on risperidone dosed from 0.5 mg/day to 2.5 or 3.5 mg/day (for children weighing above 45 kg) over a period of 8 weeks [29]. Treatment responders, as defined by at least a 25% decrease in the irritability score and a rating of much improved or very much improved on the Clinical Global Impressions improvement scale, was 69% in the risperidone group and 12% in the placebo group. In 23 of the 34 responders, these improvements remained during an extension phase of 6 months. With respect to side effects, receipt of risperidone was associated with a statistically significant average weight gain of 2.7 ± 2.9 kg, compared with 0.8 ± 2.2 kg in the placebo controls. Increased appetite, fatigue, drowsiness, dizziness, and drooling were also statistically more common in the risperidone-treated subjects than in those who received placebo.

Recently, Shea and colleagues [30] replicated the RUPP results in an 8-week, randomized, double-blind, placebo-controlled trial in which risperidone or placebo solution was administered to 79 children aged 5 to 12 years. Children who were taking risperidone (mean dosage, 1.17 mg/day; maximum allowable dose = 0.06 mg/kg/day) showed significant improvement in behaviors including aggression, self-injury, and tantrums, and 87% of risperidone-treated subjects showed global improvement in their condition, compared with 40% of subjects treated with placebo. Somnolence was the most frequently reported adverse event and was observed in 72.5%, versus only 7.7% of subjects taking placebo. Mirroring the RUPP trial, risperidone-treated subjects experienced statistically significantly greater increases in weight (2.7 versus 1.0 kg) and also experienced increases in pulse rate and systolic blood pressure. Extrapyramidal symptoms scores were not different between groups.

In subsequent follow-up reports from the RUPP network [31], weight gain was examined prospectively over 6 months of treatment with risperidone. Children and adolescents experienced an average weight gain of 0.88 kg/month (5.8 kg over 6 months), but this rate was significantly lower than the initial rate of 1.4 kg/month seen during the acute (8-week) treatment interval. The propensity to weight gain did not correlate with serum leptin levels in this population. Additional studies attempting to identify other markers for treatment response or liability to side effects, particularly genetic polymorphisms, are currently underway.

The RUPP network has recently completed a second large, randomized, controlled trial of methylphenidate in children who have both PDD and ADHD. Preliminary results indicate that methylphenidate may be helpful for some children but that the percentage of responders is less than that reported for children who have ADHD alone. Because of concerns about the possibility of exacerbation of behavioral problems associated with stimulant use in this population, the investigators enrolled only subjects who tolerated the drug in a preliminary exposure. Because of this precaution, the reported rate of response may slightly overestimate the rate of response that might be expected for the general population that has PDD.

Additional studies that are in progress in the RUPP network include the first large study (n = 120) of combined drug and behavioral treatment in this population. Specifically, participants will be randomly assigned to receive risperidone plus parent management training or risperidone alone for 24 weeks. Participants showing deterioration at week four will be offered an alternative atypical neuroleptic agent, aripiprazole. These participants will still remain in their original treatment group (either medication-alone or medication plus parent management training). After 6 months of treatment, participants who are deemed responders will have their medication gradually discontinued to learn if the response can be sustained without continued medication treatment. Both adaptive and behavioral outcomes are assessed throughout the study and at a 1-year follow-up visit.

Studies to Advance Autism Research and Treatment network

With the passage of the Children's Health Act of 2000, Congress enacted legislation that mandated the creation of a new autism research network, specifically the creation of at least five centers of excellence in autism research. Each of these centers was mandated to include at least one treatment project within its overall program. In response to this mandate, the five institutes of the National Institutes of Health Autism Coordinating Committee (specifically, the National Institute of Mental Health, the National Institute of Child Health and Human Development, the National Institute of Neurological Disorders and Stroke, the National Institute on Deafness and Other Communication Disorders, and the National Institute of Environmental Health Sciences) implemented the Studies to Advance Autism Research and Treatment (STAART) network program. A total of eight centers were selected with the charge to contribute to the autism research base in the areas of causes, diagnosis, early detection, prevention, and treatment.

The initial pharmacologic target identified in several STAART sites was repetitive behavior and affective and anxiety disturbance in children who have autism. Given the widespread use of serotonin reuptake inhibitors (SSRIs) in general clinical practice and the absence of much of an evidence base that speaks to the efficacy and safety of these drugs when used in this clinical context, studies of SSRIs are critical.

Several of these sites are currently collaborating on a trial exploring the use of citalopram for children who have autism and high levels of repetitive behavior.

The study is partially modeled after the RUPP protocol with an initial 12-week efficacy determination phase and a subsequent 16-week maintenance phase, with doses of citalopram ranging from 2.5 mg to 20 mg daily. Thus far, the centers have enrolled approximately 90 subjects on the way to a total of 144 children between 5 and 17 years of age.

A second multisite study, still in development, proposes to explore the potential benefit of early and prolonged treatment with fluoxetine (over the course of 1 year) on developmental outcomes in young children who have autism. This study will be of particular interest to the field because it attempts to measure the impact of early drug treatment on core features of autistic disorder over time.

Clinical implications for medication classes

These autism network investigations, coupled with recent independent studies, provide additional guidance for contemporary clinical practice. Important recent findings are presented by each medication class (ie, antidepressants, neuroleptics, cholinergic agents, GABAergic agents, mood stabilizers, N-methyl-D-aspartate (NMDA) agents, noradrenergic agents, opioidergic agents, and stimulants).

Antidepressants

All of the SSRI antidepressants have been explored for patients who have ASD. Liquid formulations, allowing the administration of very low doses, are now available for fluoxetine, sertraline, fluvoxamine, paroxetine, citalopram, and escitalopram. At least some of these antidepressants seem to improve repetitive thoughts and behaviors. Controlled trials with fluoxetine [32] and fluvoxamine [33] in adults who have PDD showed significant benefits over placebo, and findings from a controlled trial in children and adolescents support the effectiveness of fluoxetine in reducing repetitive behaviors in children who have PDD [34]. On the other hand, a controlled trial of fluvoxamine in juveniles who have PDD revealed a much less robust response that perhaps was eclipsed by the emergence of significant side effects including behavioral activation [35]. A recent open-label study with low-dose fluvoxamine found a significant response in only 17% of treated children [36]. Sertraline has open-trial support now in both adults [37] and juveniles [38]. Paroxetine has positive case reports in juveniles [39], and citalopram [40,41] and escitalopram [42] have open trials reporting benefit for anxiety, aggression, stereotypy, and preoccupation symptoms for juveniles who have PDD.

Mirtazapine was examined in 26 juveniles and young adults who have PDD who experienced improvement on target symptoms of aggression, self-injury, irritability, hyperactivity, anxiety, depression, and insomnia [43].

Dosing parameters may differ for patients who have ASD. Hollander and colleagues [34] found liquid fluoxetine at low doses (9.9 mg/day $\pm$ 4.35 mg) effective in reducing repetitive behavior symptoms in children and adolescents who have ASD. The finding seems to hold true for other antidepressants, because Hollander [44] determined response to venlafaxine occurred in children who have ASD at one third to one tenth of the usual adult dose.

The increased use of antidepressants, particularly SSRIs [45,46], has increased concerns about side effects with their use in children. Several investigators have reported symptoms of behavioral activation in their clinical experience, and there have also been concerns about the potential induction of mania. Moreover, many of the symptoms of mania and behavioral activation clearly overlap. DeLong and colleagues [47] observed that 5 of 129 patients who had ASD and were treated with fluoxetine developed mania. All these patients had responded well to fluoxetine, and mania evolved in some cases after 3 years of successful treatment, such that addition of mood-stabilizing medication, rather than SSRI discontinuation, seemed more clinically appropriate. Owley and colleagues [42] were able to manage symptoms of behavioral activation associated with escitalopram through gradual initiation of treatment and dose reduction when necessary. Although rare, extrapyramidal side effects have also emerged in patients who have ASD treated with SSRIs [48].

Antipsychotics/neuroleptics

Other atypical neuroleptics may hold some promise for this population based on non–placebo-controlled trials. Olanzapine was superior to haloperidol in one small, open trial [49], and olanzapine significantly improved irritability, hyperactivity, and inappropriate speech in another open trial with 25 juveniles. Significant improvements based on the Clinical Global Impressions scale occurred in only 3 of 23 patients completing the trial, however [50].

In two open trials, quetiapine was effective in fewer than one third of juveniles after up to 12 weeks of treatment [51,52]. More recently, Corson and colleagues [53] found quetiapine to be modestly effective when used openly in patients who had PDD and severe behavioral disturbance.

Ziprasidone seems to b promising based on a case series of only 12 patients [54] and may be less likely to induce weight gain than risperidone, olanzapine, and quetiapine. An open switch study of adults (mean age, 43 years) who had ASD and who converted from another antipsychotic because of side effects such as weight gain or hyperprolactinemia, provided preliminary support for this strategy [55].

A recent study reporting the effects of aripiprazole in five children who had PDD noted that all of these subjects responded well and that aripiprazole may be less likely to cause substantial weight gain [56,57].

Despite some potential important differences among the antipsychotic agents, weight gain remains a troubling concern for patients who have ASD and who are treated with antipsychotics. In an open trial, the anticonvulsant topiramate was titrated up to 0.6 to 2.9 mg/kg/day in 10 patients aged 8 to 19 years who had ASD of whom 8 were receiving risperidone. Only six patients were able to sustain treatment with this agent; four of those had variable weight loss, and two gained weight [58].

Side effects of prolactinemia have emerged in juvenile patients who have ASD treated with atypical antipsychotics, most notably risperidone [59]. Over 12 weeks, patients experienced significant increases in serum prolactin, from 166 to 504 ng/mL, at doses of 0.75 to 2 mg/day.

Cholinergic agents

Donepezil, a cholinesterase inhibitor indicated for dementia of the Alzheimer type, seemed to be somewhat effective in one small, retrospective chart review of eight patients, aged 7 to 19 years, who had PDD [60]. Irritability and hyperactivity symptoms improved in half of the subjects, but no benefits in speech, repetitive behaviors, or lethargy were detected. Galantamine, another cholinesterase inhibitor, was reported to increase verbal fluency in three adults who had autism, according to caregiver reports [61]. One of the three patients developed a rash, and the medication was discontinued; the other two patients' medication was slowly titrated to a maximum of 12 mg, with reported improvement following each dosage increase. Recently, positive effects associated with open-label treatment with rivastigmine were reported by Chez and colleagues [62]. Thirty-two subjects, 3 to 12 years of age, who had autism and who were treated for 12 weeks showed improvement in both expressive speech and overall autistic behavior as measured by the Childhood Autism Rating Scale.

GABA-ergic agents

It has long been known from clinical experience that the benzodiazepines may exacerbate behavioral disturbance in patients who have autism. Marrosu and colleagues [63] reported a series of seven children who have autism in whom parenteral administration of the GABA agonist, diazepam, resulted in paradoxical increases in manifest anxiety with significant aggression. Barron and Sandman [64] similarly reported an association between the likelihood of such paradoxical responses and the presence of stereotyped behavior and self-injurious behavior (presumably likely to include individuals who have autism) in a population that has severe mental retardation. In one trial involving two subjects who had autism, a GABA antagonist, flumazenil, was administered in a randomized, placebo-controlled pilot [65]. The effects of drug were subtle and relatively transient, but the investigators were sufficiently encouraged to suggest the need for larger trials. Topiramate is considered to produce its antiepileptic effect through several mechanisms, including enhancement of GABA-mediated chloride fluxes into neurons [66]. In a retrospective chart review of patients treated with topiramate for behavioral disturbance, Hardan and colleagues [67] observed that eight of the 15 patients were significantly improved, particularly with respect to hyperactivity, inattention, and conduct symptoms. Concerns about cognitive dulling, observed in two of these patients, seem to have limited the widespread use of topiramate in children who have ASD, but controlled trials may help clarify this risk.

Mood stabilizers

Because of the common co-occurrence of epilepsy and autism and growing concerns that occult seizure activity during sleep may affect learning and language development, anticonvulsant drugs remain attractive. Many of these anticonvulsants are also considered for their mood-stabilization effects, and there is also a literature suggesting a role in the treatment of aggression and impulsivity. Valproate is currently being studied in a trial sponsored by the National Institute of Mental Health specifically looking at behavioral improvements (as assessed by the Aberrant Behavior Checklist) as the primary efficacy measure.

Glutamatergic agents

Amantadine, a noncompetitive NMDA receptor antagonist that modulates glutamatergic activity, showed limited efficacy in a recent controlled trial of 39 juveniles who had PDD [68]. Specific improvements were observed in hyperactivity and inappropriate speech. Clinicians were more likely than parents to detect significant benefits of amantadine over placebo in these patients, but none of these effects reached statistically significant separation from placebo. Lamotrigine also modulates glutamate release and was examined in a controlled trial. No significant differences emerged over placebo, even with serum levels averaging 4.2 mg/L (therapeutic level for seizure control is 0.5 mg/L–4.5 mg/L), and higher doses did not correlate with improvement [69]. The partial NMDA agonist, D-cycloserine, was recently explored by Posey and colleagues [70], who observed a dose-related, significant improvement in symptoms of social withdrawal and social responsiveness in a single-blind design involving 10 children treated with the drug for 8 weeks.

Noradrenergic agents

Because of a predisposition of children who have PDD to exhibit stereotyped movements and because of their frequently limited diets and sleep difficulties—problems that may be exacerbated by receipt of stimulant medications—nonstimulant alternatives are of particular interest in ASD/ADHD. There are as yet no published studies regarding atomoxetine in patients who have ASD. Adrenergic drugs, such as guanfacine and clonidine, may be useful in patients who have ASD and who also have notable ADHD symptoms. Posey and colleagues [71] have suggested that guanfacine may have a role in the treatment of symptoms of hyperactivity and inattention in PDD. Rates of response ranged from one in four to one in three children treated openly with this drug in a large clinical sample. Clonidine, in doses of 0.05 to 0.2 mg, has also seemed to be useful for sedation before obtaining an electroencephalogram in children who have autism [72].

Opioidergic agents

Interest in the endogenous opioid system and its relationship to autism derives from a number of observations that involve manipulations of this system with resultant effects on affiliative and stereotyped behaviors. Panksepp and colleagues [73] suggested that opioidergic abnormalities may be at the core of the disorder, but subsequent studies examining the effects of opioid antagonists, chiefly naltrexone, have produced mixed results [74]. Naltrexone has also been explored in the treatment of self-injurious behaviors in autism and other disabilities. When used for this indication, results have also been mixed.

Stimulants

Stimulant medications remain the most effective agents in the treatment of inattention and hyperactivity and have been used increasingly in patients who have ASD. Because stimulants can exacerbate ticlike behaviors or stereotypies, the risk–benefit ratio of stimulants in these patients must always be carefully examined and discussed with families. Indeed, Di Martino and colleagues [75] found that, with a single test dose of methylphenidate (0.4 mg/kg), approximately one third of patients experienced increased hyperactivity, stereotypies, dysphoria, or motor tics, so titration was not attempted. In low doses (0.3–0.6 mg/kg/day), many patients show improvement in hyperactivity but not in any of the core symptoms of ASD [76].

Vitamins

Vitamin deficiencies have been reported in patients who have ASD, although benefits from supplementation remain unclear, even when significant serum level changes are detected [77].

Pharmacotherapy practice in patients who have autism spectrum disorders

Pharmacologic treatment of patients who have ASD still relies on careful detection of symptoms most impairing to the patient and most likely to respond to existing agents. At this point, antidepressants (SSRIs and atypical antidepressants such as venlafaxine or mirtazapine) seem to be most helpful for patients who have anxiety symptoms, repetitive behaviors as seen in patients who have obsessions or compulsions, and perhaps social avoidance/withdrawal. Neuroleptics seem to be most useful for irritability, hyperactivity, and aggression. NMDA antagonists such as amantadine and perhaps memantine may be useful in some cases of social withdrawal, hyperactivity, and inappropriate speech, and D-cycloserine, an NMDA partial agonist, shows some potential to improve social responsiveness. The opioidergic agents may have a role revealed for self-injurious behaviors, but accumulating research has highlighted the problems with treating such a complex and heterogeneous problem with a single agent. Cholinergic drugs similarly may emerge an alternative treatment for patients who have significant irritability. Stimulant medications may improve inattention and hyperactivity symptoms in patients who have ASD, albeit at lower doses and with careful monitoring. Mood stabilizers are currently being investigated as well.

Regardless of the agent selected, patients who have ASD often cannot directly collaborate and invest in the pharmacotherapy process. Indeed, pill taking itself or the taste of liquid formulations constrains pharmacotherapy in many patients who have ASD. Behavioral treatments to accomplish pill swallowing have been reported effective [78], but clinicians should inquire about the strategies that families use for administering medication, both to be able to pass ideas along to others and to ensure that the medication is being administered safely and reliably.

Summary

ASD has become more commonly recognized, but causative mechanisms remain elusive. Psychopharmacologic treatments can improve symptoms and functioning among patients who have ASD, particularly when the patient's constellation of symptoms is matched with agents likely to improve those specific symptoms. Consideration of the benefit–risk ratio remains a high priority in this population, given an increased risk for seizures and other untoward effects. In addition, the sometimes exquisite sensitivity of patients who have ASD requires careful initiation, titration, and monitoring of any psychopharmacologic regimen.

References

[1] Newschaffer CJ, Falb MD, Gurney JG. National autism prevalence trends from United States special education data. Pediatrics 2005;115(3):e277–82.

[2] Merrick J, Kandel I, Morad M. Trends in autism. Int J Adolesc Med Health 2004;16(1):75–8.

[3] Jick H, Kaye JA. Epidemiology and possible causes of autism. Pharmacotherapy 2003;23(12): 1524–30.

[4] Honda H, Shimizu Y, Imai M, et al. Cumulative incidence of childhood autism: a total population study of better accuracy and precision. Dev Med Child Neurol 2005;47(1):10–8.

[5] Lauritsen MB, Pedersen CB, Mortensen PB. The incidence and prevalence of pervasive developmental disorders: a Danish population-based study. Psychol Med 2004;34(7):1339–46.

[6] Fombonne E. Epidemiological surveys of autism and other pervasive developmental disorders: an update. J Autism Dev Disord 2003;33(4):365–82.

[7] Mandell DS, Thompson WW, Weintraub ES, et al. Trends in diagnosis rates for autism and ADHD at hospital discharge in the context of other psychiatric diagnoses. Psychiatr Serv 2005;56(1):56–62.

[8] Challman TD, Barbaresi WJ, Katusic SK, et al. The yield of the medical evaluation of children with pervasive developmental disorders. J Autism Dev Disord 2003;33(2):187–92.

[9] Baron-Cohen S, Wheelwright S, Cox A, et al. Early identification of autism by the CHecklist for Autism in Toddlers (CHAT). J R Soc Med 2000;93(10):521–5.

[10] Cohen D, Pichard N, Tordjman S, et al. Specific genetic disorders and autism: clinical contribution towards their identification. J Autism Dev Disord 2005;35(1):103–16.

[11] Wassink TH, Brzustowicz LM, Bartlett CW, et al. The search for autism disease genes. Ment Retard Dev Disabil Res Rev 2004;10(4):272–83.

[12] Courchesne E, Pierce K. Brain overgrowth in autism during a critical time in development: implications for frontal pyramidal neuron and interneuron development and connectivity. Int J Dev Neurosci 2005;23(2–3):153–70.

[13] Courchesne E, Carper R, Akshoomoff N. Evidence of brain overgrowth in the first year of life in autism. JAMA 2003;290(3):337–44.

[14] Pelphrey KA, Morris JP, McCarthy G. Neural basis of eye gaze processing deficits in autism. Brain 2005;128(Pt 5):1038–48.

[15] Dalton KM, Nacewicz BM, Johnstone T, et al. Gaze fixation and the neural circuitry of face processing in autism. Nat Neurosci 2005;8(4):519–26.

[16] Filipek PA, Juranek J, Nguyen MT, et al. Relative carnitine deficiency in autism. J Autism Dev Disord 2004;34(6):615–23.

[17] Oliveira G, Diogo L, Grazina M, et al. Mitochondrial dysfunction in autism spectrum disorders: a population-based study. Dev Med Child Neurol 2005;47(3):185–9.

[18] Barnea-Goraly N, Kwon H, Menon V, et al. White matter structure in autism: preliminary evidence from diffusion tensor imaging. Biol Psychiatry 2004;55(3):323–6.

[19] Belmonte MK, Cook Jr EH, Anderson GM, et al. Autism as a disorder of neural information processing: directions for research and targets for therapy (1). Mol Psychiatry 2004; 9(7):646–63.

[20] McAlonan GM, Cheung V, Cheung C, et al. Mapping the brain in autism. A voxel-based MRI study of volumetric differences and intercorrelations in autism. Brain 2005;128(Pt 2):268–76.

[21] Horvath K, Stefanatos G, Sokolski KN, et al. Improved social and language skills after secretin administration in patients with autistic spectrum disorders. J Assoc Acad Minor Phys 1998; 9(1):9–15.

[22] Sturmey P. Secretin is an ineffective treatment for pervasive developmental disabilities: a review of 15 double-blind randomized controlled trials. Res Dev Disabil 2005;26(1):87–97.

[23] King BH. Pharmacological treatment of mood disturbances, aggression, and self-injury in persons with pervasive developmental disorders. J Autism Dev Disord 2000;30(5):439–45.

[24] Goldstein S, Schwebach AJ. The comorbidity of pervasive developmental disorder and attention deficit hyperactivity disorder: results of a retrospective chart review. J Autism Dev Disord 2004;34(3):329–39.

[25] Hollander E, Phillips AT, Yeh CC. Targeted treatments for symptom domains in child and adolescent autism. Lancet 2003;362(9385):732–4.

[26] McDougle CJ, Scahill L, McCracken JT, et al. Research Units on Pediatric Psychopharmacology (RUPP) autism network. Background and rationale for an initial controlled study of risperidone. Child Adolesc Psychiatr Clin N Am 2000;9(1):201–24.

[27] Meltzer HY. The role of serotonin in antipsychotic drug action. Neuropsychopharmacology 1999;21(2 Suppl):106S–15S.

[28] Barnard L, Young AH, Pearson J, Geddes J, et al. A systematic review of the use of atypical antipsychotics in autism. J Psychopharmacol 2002;16(1):93–101.

[29] McCracken JT, McGough J, Shah B, et al. Risperidone in children with autism and serious behavioral problems. N Engl J Med 2002;347(5):314–21.

[30] Shea S, Turgay A, Carroll A, et al. Risperidone in the treatment of disruptive behavioral symptoms in children with autistic and other pervasive developmental disorders. Pediatrics 2004; 114(5):e634–41.

[31] Martin A, Scahill L, Anderson GM, et al. Weight and leptin changes among risperidone-treated youths with autism: 6-month prospective data. Am J Psychiatry 2004;161(6):1125–7.

[32] Buchsbaum MS, Hollander E, Haznedar MM, et al. Effect of fluoxetine on regional cerebral metabolism in autistic spectrum disorders: a pilot study. Int J Neuropsychopharmacol 2001;4(2): 119–25.

[33] McDougle CJ, Naylor ST, Cohen DJ, et al. A double-blind, placebo-controlled study of Lamictal in adults with autistic disorder. Arch Gen Psychiatry 1996;53(11):1001–8.

[34] Hollander E, Phillips A, Chaplin W, et al. A placebo controlled crossover trial of liquid fluoxetine on repetitive behaviors in childhood and adolescent autism. Neuropsychopharmacology 2005;30(3):582–9.

[35] McDougle CJ, Kresch LE, Posey DJ. Repetitive thoughts and behavior in pervasive developmental disorders: treatment with serotonin reuptake inhibitors. J Autism Dev Disord 2000; 30(5):427–35.

[36] Martin A, Koenig K, Anderson GM, et al. Low-dose fluvoxamine treatment of children and adolescents with pervasive developmental disorders: a prospective, open-label study. J Autism Dev Disord 2003;33(1):77–85.

[37] McDougle CJ, Brodkin ES, Naylor ST, et al. Sertraline in adults with pervasive developmental disorders: a prospective open-label investigation. J Clin Psychopharmacol 1998;18(1): 62–6.

[38] Steingard RJ, Zimnitzky B, DeMaso DR, et al. Sertraline treatment of transition-associated anxiety and agitation in children with autistic disorder. J Child Adolesc Psychopharmacol 1997; 7(1):9–15.

[39] Posey DI, Litwiller M, Koburn A, et al. Paroxetine in autism. J Am Acad Child Adolesc Psychiatry 1999;38(2):111–2.

[40] Couturier JL, Nicolson R. A retrospective assessment of citalopram in children and adolescents with pervasive developmental disorders. J Child Adolesc Psychopharmacol 2002;12(3): 243–8.

[41] Namerow LB, Thomas P, Bostic JQ, et al. Use of citalopram in pervasive developmental disorders. J Dev Behav Pediatr 2003;24(2):104–8.

[42] Owley T, Walton L, Salt J, et al. An open-label trial of escitalopram in pervasive developmental disorders. J Am Acad Child Adolesc Psychiatry 2005;44(4):343–8.

[43] Posey DJ, Guenin KD, Kohn AE, et al. A naturalistic open-label study of mirtazapine in autistic and other pervasive developmental disorders. J Child Adolesc Psychopharmacol 2001; 11(3):267–77.

[44] Hollander E, Kaplan A, Cartwright C, et al. Venlafaxine in children, adolescents, and young adults with autism spectrum disorders: an open retrospective clinical report. J Child Neurol 2000;15:132–5.

[45] Aman M, Lam KS, Van Bourgondien ME. Medication patterns in patients with autism: temporal, regional, and demographic influences. J Child Adolesc Psychopharmacol 2005;15(1): 116–26.

[46] Martin A, Scahill L, Klin A, et al. Higher-functioning pervasive developmental disorders: rates and patterns of psychotropic drug use. J Am Acad Child Adolesc Psychiatry 1999;38(7):923–31.

[47] DeLong GR, Ritch CR, Burch S. Fluoxetine response in children with autistic spectrum disorders: correlation with familial major affective disorder and intellectual achievement. Dev Med Child Neurol 2002;44(10):652–9.

[48] Sokolski KN, Chicz-Demet A, Demet EM. Selective serotonin reuptake inhibitor-related extrapyramidal symptoms in autistic children: a case series. J Child Adolesc Psychopharmacol 2004;14(1):143–7.

[49] Malone RP, Cater J, Sheikh RM, et al. Olanzapine versus haloperidol in children with autistic disorder: an open pilot study. J Am Acad Child Adolesc Psychiatry 2001;40(8):887–94.

[50] Kemner C, Willemsen-Swinkels SH, de Jonge M, et al. Open-label study of olanzapine in children with pervasive developmental disorder. J Clin Psychopharmacol 2002;22(5):455–60.

[51] Findling RL, McNamara NK, Gracious BL, et al. Quetiapine in nine youths with autistic disorder. J Child Adolesc Psychopharmacol 2004;14(2):287–94.

[52] Martin A, Koenig K, Scahill L, et al. Open-label quetiapine in the treatment of children and adolescents with autistic disorder. J Child Adolesc Psychopharmacol 1999;9(2):99–107.

[53] Corson AH, Barkenbus JE, Posey DJ, et al. A retrospective analysis of quetiapine in the treatment of pervasive developmental disorders. J Clin Psychiatry 2004;65(11):1531–6.

[54] McDougle CJ, Kem DL, Posey DJ. Case series: use of ziprasidone for maladaptive symptoms in youths with autism. J Am Acad Child Adolesc Psychiatry 2002;41(8):921–7.

[55] Cohen SA, Fitzgerald BJ, Khan SR, et al. The effect of a switch to ziprasidone in an adult population with autistic disorder: chart review of naturalistic, open-label treatment. J Clin Psychiatry 2004;65(1):110–3.

[56] Stigler KA, Posey DJ, McDougle CJ. Aripiprazole for maladaptive behavior in pervasive developmental disorders. J Child Adolesc Psychopharmacol 2004;14(3):455–63.

[57] Stigler KA, Potenza MN, Posey DJ, et al. Weight gain associated with atypical antipsychotic use in children and adolescents: prevalence, clinical relevance, and management. Paediatr Drugs 2004;6(1):33–44.

[58] Canitano R. Clinical experience with topiramate to counteract neuroleptic induced weight gain in 10 individuals with autistic spectrum disorders. Brain Dev 2005;27(3):228–32.

[59] Gagliano A, Germano E, Pustorino G, et al. Risperidone treatment of children with autistic disorder: effectiveness, tolerability, and pharmacokinetic implications. J Child Adolesc Psychopharmacol 2004;14(1):39–47.

[60] Hardan AY, Handen BL. A retrospective open trial of adjunctive donepezil in children and adolescents with autistic disorder. J Child Adolesc Psychopharmacol 2002;12(3):237–41.

[61] Hertzman M. Galantamine in the treatment of adult autism: a report of three clinical cases. Int J Psychiatry Med 2003;33(4):395–8.

[62] Chez MG, Aimonovitch M, Buchanan T, et al. Treating autistic spectrum disorders in children: utility of the cholinesterase inhibitor rivastigmine tartrate. J Child Neurol 2004;19(3):165–9.

[63] Marrosu F, Marrosu G, Rachel MG, et al. Paradoxical reactions elicited by diazepam in children with classic autism. Funct Neurol 1987;2(3):355–61.

[64] Barron J, Sandman CA. Relationship of sedative-hypnotic response to self-injurious behavior and stereotypy by mentally retarded clients. Am J Ment Defic 1983;88(2):177–86.

[65] Wray JA, Yoon JH, Vollmer T, et al. Pilot study of the behavioral effects of flumazenil in two children with autism. J Autism Dev Disord 2000;30(6):619–20.

[66] Angehagen M, Ben-Menachem E, Ronnback L, et al. Novel mechanisms of action of three antiepileptic drugs, vigabatrin, tiagabine, and topiramate. Neurochem Res 2003;28(2):333–40.

[67] Hardan AY, Jou RJ, Handen BL. A retrospective assessment of topiramate in children and adolescents with pervasive developmental disorders. J Child Adolesc Psychopharmacol 2004;14(3):426–32.

[68] King BH, Wright DM, Handen BL, et al. Double-blind, placebo-controlled study of amantadine hydrochloride in the treatment of children with autistic disorder. J Am Acad Child Adolesc Psychiatry 2001;40(6):658–65.

[69] Belsito KM, Law PA, Kirk KS, et al. Lamotrigine therapy for autistic disorder: a randomized, double-blind, placebo-controlled trial. J Autism Dev Disord 2001;31(2):175–81.

[70] Posey DJ, Kem DL, Swiezy NB, et al. A pilot study of D-cycloserine in subjects with autistic disorder. Am J Psychiatry 2004;161(11):2115–7.

[71] Posey DJ, Puntney JI, Sasher TM, et al. Guanfacine treatment of hyperactivity and inattention in pervasive developmental disorders: a retrospective analysis of 80 cases. J Child Adolesc Psychopharmacol 2004;14(2):233–41.

[72] Mehta UC, Patel I, Castello FV. EEG sedation for children with autism. J Dev Behav Pediatr 2004;25(2):102–4.

[73] Panksepp J, Najam N, Soares F. Morphine reduces social cohesion in rats. Pharmacol Biochem Behav 1979;11(2):131–4.

[74] Williams PG, Allard A, Sears L, et al. Brief report: case reports on naltrexone use in children with autism: controlled observations regarding benefits and practical issues of medication management. J Autism Dev Disord 2001;31(1):103–8.

[75] Di Martino A, Melis G, Cianchetti C, et al. Methylphenidate for pervasive developmental disorders: safety and efficacy of acute single dose test and ongoing therapy: an open-pilot study. J Child Adolesc Psychopharmacol 2004;14(2):207–18.

[76] Handen BL, Johnson CR, Lubetsky M. Efficacy of methylphenidate among children with autism and symptoms of attention-deficit hyperactivity disorder. J Autism Dev Disord 2000; 30(3):245–55.

[77] Adams JB, Holloway C. Pilot study of a moderate dose multivitamin/mineral supplement for children with autistic spectrum disorder. J Altern Complement Med 2004;10(6):1033–9.

[78] Ghuman JK, Cataldo MD, Beck MH, et al. Behavioral training for pill-swallowing difficulties in young children with autistic disorder. J Child Adolesc Psychopharmacol 2004;14(4): 601–11.

ELSEVIER
SAUNDERS

Child Adolesc Psychiatric Clin N Am
15 (2006) 177–206

CHILD AND
ADOLESCENT
PSYCHIATRIC CLINICS
OF NORTH AMERICA

Recognizing and Monitoring Adverse Events of Second-Generation Antipsychotics in Children and Adolescents

Christoph U. Correll, MD[a],[*], Julie B. Penzner, MD[b],
Umesh H. Parikh, MD[a], Tahir Mughal, MD[a],
Tariq Javed, MD[a], Maren Carbon, MD[c],
Anil K. Malhotra, MD[a],[d]

[a]*The Zucker Hillside Hospital, North Shore—Long Island Jewish Health System, 75-59 263rd Street,
Glen Oaks, NY 11004, USA*
[b]*Weill Cornell Medical College, 1300 York Avenue, New York, NY 10021, USA*
[c]*North Shore University Hospital, North Shore—Long Island Jewish Health System,
Boas Marks Biomedical Research Center, 350 Community Drive, Manhasset, NY 11030, USA*
[d]*Albert Einstein College of Medicine, Jack and Pearl Resnick Campus, 1300 Morris Park Avenue,
Bronx, NY 10461, USA*

Despite the limited availability of randomized, controlled evidence regarding the efficacy and safety of second-generation antipsychotics (SGAs) in pediatric populations [1,2], this class of medications is being prescribed in escalating rates [3–5]. Of note, SGAs are increasingly prescribed for youngsters with non-psychotic conditions that are not limited to bipolar mania [6–8]. The increased use of SGAs relative to first-generation antipsychotics (FGAs) is a result of several factors, including the reduced risk for acute [9] and chronic [10] neuro-motor side effects, greater efficacy for some symptom domains [11,12], efficacy

---

This work was supported by The Zucker Hillside Hospital National Institute of Mental Health Advanced Center for Intervention and Services Research for the Study of Schizophrenia grant MH 074543-01 and the North Shore–Long Island Jewish Research Institute National Institutes of Health General Clinical Research Center grant MO1RR018535. Christoph U. Correll has worked as a consultant or lecturer to AstraZeneca, Bristol-Myers Squibb, Eli Lilly, and Janssen Pharmaceutica. Anil K. Malhotra has worked as a consultant or lecturer to Pfizer and Genaissance Pharmaceuticals.

* Corresponding author.
E-mail address: ccorrell@lij.edu (C.U. Correll).

for broader target symptoms [13], and possibly, improved compliance [14,15]. Despite these possible advantages, SGAs as a group are more likely than FGAs to lead to weight gain and the related abnormalities in lipid and glucose metabolism. This tendency has caused much concern, as reflected by the ADA Consensus Development Conference on Antipsychotic Drugs and Obesity and Diabetes [16], because of the known associations between weight gain and obesity with diabetes, dyslipidemia, and hypertension, all of which are leading risk factors for future cardiovascular morbidity and mortality. This article reviews the available data on the most relevant adverse events of SGAs in children and adolescents with the aim of informing antipsychotic prescribing and monitoring practices in this vulnerable population. Adequate monitoring and management and, whenever possible, prevention of side effects is crucial to promote physical and psychologic health, adequate role functioning, attainment of developmental milestones, and treatment compliance.

Specific considerations about antipsychotic use in children and adolescents

Development

The fact that children and adolescents are treated at times of vast biopsychosocial development has consequences for patterns of efficacy, effectiveness, tolerability, and safety of any medical intervention. Individual differences in development and age-related differences in developmental stages are likely to interact with the pharmacodynamic and pharmacokinetic properties of medications, potentially resulting in different patterns of adverse-event frequency and severity compared with adults. Although data regarding the bioavailability and bioactivity of medications in pediatric populations are relatively sparse, drug uptake, distribution, and metabolism are affected by several factors that differ from those in adults. In children and adolescents these factors include active tissue growth, reproductive hormone release during adolescence, a higher ratio of liver organ-to-tissue mass, greater intra- and extracellular tissue water and glomerular filtration rates, and lower protein binding and reduced fat tissue mass compared with adults [17]. Clinically, these differences usually mean that higher doses per kilogram weight are required in pediatric populations than in adults to achieve similar efficacy and that more frequent dosing per day may be required in younger children, [18]. Age and development can also influence the susceptibility to side effects [19].

Assessment strategies

The wide range of development and psychopathology encountered during childhood and adolescence can affect the validity and reliability of assessments in this population. Therefore, involvement of a second informant is often essential. Moreover, questions and tasks must be age-appropriate and sometimes gender-appropriate (particularly in adolescence) and may not always be uniformly applicable. Assisted self-report has a useful role, because it affords children and parents the opportunity to provide collaborative input. In certain situations, the child's information may be considered unreliable or cannot be obtained, so that only the guardian's responses can be coded. A review of 196 pediatric psycho-pharmacology articles published over the past 22 years revealed that there was no common method used for eliciting or reporting adverse event data [20]. These inconsistencies in ascertaining and reporting data on medication safety in pediatric patients are a major current limitation.

Height, weight, body mass index (BMI), blood pressure, and pulse should always be part of regular side-effect and health monitoring in pediatric patients. Although it is relatively easy to interpret laboratory test results that are sent to clinicians by using the normal range appropriate for the age and, where relevant, gender, the interpretation of BMI, waist circumference, blood pressure, or the definition of the metabolic syndrome in childhood is less straightforward. The definition of metabolic syndrome by at least three of five clearly defined criteria is generally accepted for adults [21]. The fact that children and adolescents are at different stages of their development, however, has led to the proposal of modified criteria (Table 1) [22,25].

In this context, the BMI is a straightforward variable in adults:

$$BMI = (weight\ in\ kg)/(height\ in\ meters^2)$$

or

$$BMI = (weight\ in\ pounds \times 703)/(height\ in\ inches^2)$$

and waist circumference and blood pressure have fixed definitions (see Table 1). By contrast, during development, the BMI, waist circumference, and blood pressure change according to age and gender, requiring a comparison with age- and gender-matched norms. For BMI, growth charts are available from the Centers for Disease Control (Table 2). Alternatively, sex- and age-adjusted BMI percentiles and z-scores can be calculated from a web-based calculator based on

Table 1
Criteria for the metabolic syndrome in adults and in children and adolescents

Criteria for metabolic syndrome in adults	Criteria for metabolic syndrome in children and adolescents
Abdominal obesity (ie, waist circumference >40 inches in males and >35 inches in females)	Waist circumference ≥ 90th percentile or BMI ≥ 95th percentile (ie, "overweight")
Fasting serum triglyceride levels ≥ 150 mg/dL	Fasting serum triglyceride levels ≥ 110 mg/dL
Fasting high-density lipoprotein cholesterol <40 mg/dL in males and <50 mg/dL in females	Fasting high-density lipoprotein cholesterol <40 mg/dL in males and females
Blood pressure ≥ 130/85 mm Hg	Blood pressure ≥ 90th percentile for sex and age
Fasting glucose ≥ 110 mg/dL	Fasting glucose ≥ 110 mg/dL

Data from Refs. [21,22,25].

Table 2
Available resources to obtain sex- and age-adjusted body mass index, waist circumference, and blood
pressure for children and adolescents

Sex- and age-adjusted parameters	Available resource
BMI percentile	Growth charts: http://www.cdc.gov/growthcharts/
BMI percentile and z-scores	Web-based calculator: http://www.kidsnutrition.org/bodycomp/ bmiz2.html
Waist circumference percentile	Tables: Fernandez JR, Redden DT, Pietrobelli A, et al. Waist circumference percentiles in nationally representative samples of African-American, European-American, and Mexican-American children and adolescents. J Pediatr 2004;145(4): 439–44
Blood pressure percentiles	Tables: National High Blood Pressure Education Program Working Group on High Blood Pressure in Children and Adolescents. The fourth report on the diagnosis, evaluation, and treatment of high blood pressure in children and adolescents. Pediatrics 2004;114:555–76

data from the third National Health and Nutrition Examination Survey (1988–1994) (see Table 2). Although the use of this methodology is crucial in medium-term and long-term studies of SGA-induced weight gain, thus far, only one published pediatric study has used age- and sex-adjusted BMI z-score changes in a 6-month study of risperidone-treated youths [70]. The use of BMI percentiles also allows a categorical definition of age- and sex-inappropriate weight status. Youngsters with BMI percentiles of less than 5% are considered underweight, those with BMI percentiles between 5% and 84.9% are considered normal, those with percentiles between 85% and 94.9% are considered at risk, and youths with a BMI percentile of 95% or above are considered overweight [184]. Only recently, waist circumference percentiles have been published that allow a diagnosis of abdominal obesity during development [23]. Finally, sex- and age-adjusted blood pressure percentiles are available in the Fourth Report on the Diagnosis, Evaluation, and Treatment of High Blood Pressure in Children and Adolescents (2004) [24].

To date a clear threshold for significant weight gain in children and adolescents, who undergo developmental periods at different velocities, is lacking. Therefore, the authors propose a set of thresholds that takes the duration of treatment and baseline BMI percentile into consideration:

1. A weight increase of more than 5% compared with baseline during the first 3 months of treatment
2. Increase in BMI z-score of 0.5 SD or more at any point during the treatment to account for age- and sex-appropriate growth
3. Crossing into the "at risk" weight category (ie, ≥ 85–94.9 BMI percentile) plus presence of one other obesity-related complication, such as hypertension (ie, ≥ 90th percentile), dyslipidemia (ie, fasting cholesterol ≥ 200 mg/dL, LDL-cholesterol > 130 mg/dL, HDL-cholesterol < 40 mg/dL, or triglycerides ≥ 150 mg/dL), hyperglycemia (ie, fasting glu-

cose ≥100 mg/dL), insulin resistance (ie, fasting insulin >20 umol/L) [185], orthopedic disorders, sleep disorders, or gall bladder disease
4. The crossing into obesity (ie, ≥ 95th BMI percentile) or abdominal obesity (ie, >90th waist circumference percentile)

The relative weight gain of 5% compared with baseline weight during the first 3 months of treatment seems justified because during this relatively short period of time growth does not contribute to weight change in a relevant way. For longer observation periods, the weight change needs to be adjusted for sex- and age-adjusted norms. The authors chose 0.5 in BMI z-score based on the data by Weiss and colleagues [25], who found that this change in growth-adjusted weight increased the risk for metabolic syndrome by 55%. Finally, two other groups require close monitoring or interventions, as they are at high risk for adverse health outcomes Youngsters in the "at risk" weight category (ie, ≥ 85–94.9 BMI percentile) who already have at least one negative weight-related clinical outcome and patients with BMI or waist circumference percentiles in the overweight/obese category are at very high risk for adverse health outcomes. Therefore, these individuals require close monitoring or interventions, independent of where they start at the time of initiation of SGA treatment.

Specific side effects related to second-generation antipsychotics

Table 3 summarizes the differential side effect patterns of the six SGAs currently available in the United States. Because in many instances data are lacking or sparse in children and adolescents, results from future studies are expected to inform the field further, making modifications of this table necessary.

Weight gain

In general, psychiatric patients are likely to gain weight and to have higher rates of overweight and obesity than the general population [26]. These adverse changes in body composition and related metabolic abnormalities probably result from multiple factors, including the underlying psychiatric illness, illness-related unhealthy behaviors, and treatment [27]. Excessive weight gain is a major concern because of its association with increased cardiovascular morbidity and mortality, which are related to abnormalities of glucose and lipid metabolism, and a higher prevalence of the metabolic syndrome [16,21]. In a study of non-psychiatric children and adolescents, the risk for metabolic syndrome increased by 55% for every half age- and sex-adjusted BMI z-score (ie, a difference of 0.5 SD) [25]. Presence of the metabolic syndrome in childhood is also associated with an increased risk for the development of atherosclerotic cardiovascular disease [28,29]. Most importantly, adolescent obesity has been shown to be more strongly predictive of coronary artery disease and colorectal cancer than adult obesity [30], suggesting that some pathogenic processes are accelerated when

Table 3

Comparative overview of side-effect profiles of second-generation antipsychotic medications in children and adolescents

Side effect	Aripiprazole	Clozapine	Olanzapine	Quetiapine	Risperidone	Ziprasidone
Anticholinergic	0	+++	++	0/+	0	0
Acute EPS	+[a]	0	+[a]	0	++[a]	+[a]
Diabetes	0/+[b]	+++	+++	++	+	0/+[b]
↑ Lipids	0/+[b]	++	++	+	+	0/+[b]
Neutropenia	0/+	++	0/+	0/ +	0/+	0/+
Orthostasis	0/+	+++	++	++	+	0
↑ Prolactin	0/↓	0	+[a]	0	+ +[a]	+[a]
↑ QTc interval	0/+[c]	+[c]	0/+[c]	+[c]	+[c]	++[c]
Sedation	0/+	+++	++	++[e]	+	0/+
Seizures	0/+	++[a]	0/+	0/+	0/+	0/+
Tardive dyskinesia	0/+[b]	0	0/+[d]	0/+[d]	0/+[d]	0/+[b]
Weight gain	+	+++	+++	++	++	+

Abbreviations: ↑ , increased; ↓, decreased; 0, none; 0/+, minimal; +, mild; ++, moderate; +++, severe.

[a] Dose-related effect.

[b] Insufficient long-term data to determine the risk fully.

[c] Relevance for the development of torsade de points not established.

[d] Less than 1% per year in adults that were often pretreated with first-generation antipsychotics.

[e] More sedating at lower doses.

occurring early in life. Finally, although studies assessing these risks in youngsters are absent, excessive weight gain may also further social stigma, heighten withdrawal from the community, reduce quality of life [31,32], and encourage medication noncompliance [33,34].

In adults, SGAs are associated with a greater potential for significant weight gain than are FGAs [35]. The potential for weight gain is particularly problematic in children and adolescents who seem to be at higher risk than adults for adverse SGA-related anthropometric changes [19,36,37]. Adult data [16,35] suggest that the promotion of weight gain and metabolic syndrome is most likely to develop in association with clozapine and olanzapine, followed by quetiapine and risperidone, which are considered to have a moderate risk; aripiprazole and ziprasidone seem to share the lowest risk. Although in adults, aripiprazole and ziprasidone seem to be almost weight neutral [35,38], in pediatric populations weight gain seems to be a side effect common to all SGAs, particularly in antipsychotic-naive patients who have not yet gained weight during previous trials [39]. Nevertheless, except for a differentially higher risk for weight gain related to risperidone [36], the relative weight gain potential of SGAs still seems to follow a pattern in youths similar to that described in adults.

Although a number of studies have reconfirmed that significant weight gain occurs in pediatric populations treated with SGAs (reviewed in [1,40]), research in this area is still limited. In particular, the differences in study populations and follow-up durations in single-drug studies, coupled with the lack of head-to-head studies, limit the ability to compare the weight gain potentials of SGAs in youths. Of note, however, stimulant cotreatment dose not seem to attenuate SGA-induced weight gain [41]. To date, only two published studies, each with fewer than 50 youngsters exposed to SGAs, have prospectively compared weight gain of two SGAs in pediatric patients. In the open-label study by Ratzoni and colleagues [37], weight gain was assessed in 50 adolescent inpatients (mean age, 17.1 years), almost exclusively patients who had schizophrenia-spectrum disorders, who received treatment with olanzapine (n = 21; mean dose, 12.7 mg/day), risperidone (n = 21; mean dose, 3.2 mg/day) or haloperidol (n = 8; mean dose, 7.6 mg/day). Data were analyzed in all 50 patients who were followed for 8 to 12 weeks. In this sample, olanzapine caused significantly greater weight gain (7.2 kg) than seen with risperidone (3.9 kg) or haloperidol (1.1 kg) ($P = .02$). The 8-week double-blind, placebo-controlled study comparing the same three antipsychotics in 50 pediatric patients (mean age: 14.18 years) with a mixture of psychotic disorders found similar results, although the amount of weight gain was higher despite the shorter study duration [42]. In this randomized study, olanzapine (n = 16; mean dose, 12.3 mg/day) also caused significantly ($P = .04$) more weight gain, 7.1 kg, than did risperidone (n = 19; mean dose, 3.9 mg/day) or haloperidol (n = 15; mean dose, 5.3 mg/day), which were associated with increases in weight of 4.9 kg and 3.5 kg, respectively. Data from an ongoing, large-scale, naturalistic study in children and adolescents reconfirm that pediatric patients treated with SGAs are at high risk for adverse changes in body composition [39]. Although in the entire sample, age- and sex-adjusted BMI percentiles increased significantly only for patients on olanzapine and risperidone, in the subgroup of antipsychotic-naive youths, all body composition parameters increased significantly with the four SGAs that had sufficient numbers of treatment-naive subjects per group.

In adults, several studies reported higher rates of metabolic syndrome in patients treated with SGAs than seen in the general population [43–47]. Although the magnitude of SGA-related weight gain in youngsters would suggest at least as unfavorable results, no data are available at this point that assess the relationship between SGA treatment and metabolic syndrome in children and adolescents.

Dyslipidemia

In addition to weight gain, SGAs have been associated with adverse effects on serum lipids, such as increases in total cholesterol, low-density lipoprotein (LDL) cholesterol, and triglycerides, and decreases in high-density lipoprotein cholesterol. Consistent with the weight-related negative effect on lipid levels, olanzapine or clozapine have had the greatest risk associated with dyslipidemia in adult populations [48–50]. Except for few case reports [51–53], data regarding the risk for dyslipidemia are missing for pediatric patients. An exception is the retrospective case series [54] of 22 child and adolescent inpatients (mean age, 12.8 years) who had been treated with risperidone (mean dose, 2.7 mg) for a mean duration of 4.9 months. In this cohort, the authors found no significant changes in serum triglyceride or cholesterol levels. This finding was surprising, because the youngsters had experienced significant weight gain of 7.0 kg, and triglyceride levels and weight were strongly correlated, with weight change contributing almost 25% of the variance in triglyceride levels. This inconsistency could be explained by the retrospective nature of the study that did not assure strictly fasting blood values. In addition, the negative results could have been caused by an independent effect of lithium or divalproex treatment, because the relationship between weight change and triglyceride levels decreased to 6% when the five patients concurrently treated with these two mood stabilizers were excluded. Because of these limitations, the authors recommended regular laboratory monitoring until a clearer picture emerges regarding SGA-related lipid dysregulations in children and adolescents. These cautious recommendations seem to be supported by results from interim analyses of an ongoing, prospective safety-monitoring study in children and adolescents that found a concerning high rate of new-onset dyslipidemia after only 3 months of treatment with four SGAs [69].

Insulin resistance and diabetes

In addition to affecting body composition and lipid metabolism adversely, SGAs have the potential to induce insulin resistance and diabetes [56]. Because the mechanisms of antipsychotic-induced weight gain and glucose abnormalities are still unknown, it is still a matter of debate how much antipsychotic treatment contributes independently to the increased baseline risk of obesity and diabetes found in psychiatric patients. In nonpsychiatric pediatric populations, as in adults, overweight is clearly linked to a higher incidence of glucose abnormalities and metabolic syndrome [25,57]. It remains to be seen, however, whether antipsychotics affect insulin resistance and lipid dysregulation solely through weight gain and increased visceral adiposity or whether at least some antipsychotics have a direct adverse effect on insulin secretion or glucose transport [58–60]. Furthermore, cotreatment with antipsychotics and divalproex may increase the risk for development of diabetes and insulin resistance [61–64].

In pediatric populations, data on the adverse effect of SGAs on glucose metabolism are largely limited to case reports of new-onset diabetes [51,52,64–68]. The only prospective data available so far originate from the aforementioned prospective, naturalistic study in children and adolescents between the ages of 5 and 19 years, suggesting that adverse effects on insulin sensitivity can be observed even within the first 3 months of treatment [55]. These findings need to be confirmed and extended in a larger sample that also includes treatment-naive youngsters receiving ziprasidone before conclusions can be reached.

Prolactin-related and sexual side effects

Both FGAs and SGAs have the potential to elevate prolactin levels. Hyperprolactinemia can result in sexual side effects, such as amenorrhea or oligomenorrhea in females, erectile dysfunction in males, decreased libido, hirsutism, and breast symptoms, such as enlargement, engorgement, pain, or galactorrhea in males or females. Whether hyperprolactinemia at the levels found in response to antipsychotic treatment can adversely affect bone density or sexual maturation is currently unknown. Sexual side effects do not show a tight correlation with actual levels of prolactin [42,71,72], and not all patients with hyperprolactinemia develop these signs and symptoms [73].

Although the effect of antipsychotics on prolactin levels is common to both pediatric and adult patients, the effect may be more pronounced in children and adolescents [19,74]. Reasons may include an age-related decrease in the number of dopamine receptors [75]. Because prolactin synthesis and response are stimulated by estrogen, menstruating females and females taking the oral contraceptive pill are at highest risk for increased prolactin levels from antipsychotics [71,76,77]. The effect of SGAs on prolactin varies across agents and dose levels [78]. Emerging data in pediatric populations suggest that risperidone has the strongest likelihood of increasing prolactin levels [72,73,79–82], followed by olanzapine [71,77]. Ziprasidone seems to lead to only transient prolactin elevation [83], and prolactin abnormalities are least likely with quetiapine [71,84] and clozapine [77]. Data regarding a potential reduction in prolactin levels by the partial dopamine agonist aripiprazole that exceed placebo are available only from adult studies [85]. In children, the existing database on hyperprolactinemia is limited in that it is based mostly on cohorts of prepubertal boys treated with risperidone. The available data, however, suggest that childhood hyperprolactinemia is dose dependent [80], seems to normalize over time [72,86,87], resolves after discontinuation of treatment [78], and that the majority of children who experience drug-induced hyperprolactinemia progress normally through puberty [88]. See the article by Becker and Epperson elsewhere in this issue for further exploration of this topic.

Neuromotor side effects

SGAs are preferred over FGAs predominantly because they cause fewer acute extrapyramidal side effects (EPS) [9] and tardive dyskinesia [10]. In a systematic review of 1-year studies, the risk for tardive dyskinesia with SGAs was found to be less than 1% per year in adults and approximately 5% in the elderly, rates that are about one fifth or less those seen with FGAs [10].

Extrapyramidal side effects and akathisia

With FGAs, children and adolescents were found to be more sensitive than adults to develop EPS [89]. As in hyperprolactinemia, this sensitivity may result from an inverse relationship between dopamine receptor density and age [75]. It is unclear if the same difference is true for SGAs, particularly risperidone, which as a class can result in EPS at higher doses [90]. Several studies with SGAs have suggested that EPS may occur more frequently in children and adolescents than in adults [87,91–94], but other studies failed to reconfirm this possibility [81,86,95,96]. These inconsistencies most likely result from differences in patient populations, disease states, and dosing regimens. The only double-blind, randomized study that compared treatment with risperidone (n = 19; mean dose,

3.3 mg/day), olanzapine (n = 16; mean dose, 12.3 mg/day) and haloperidol (n = 15; mean dose, 5.3 mg/day) in children and adolescents with psychotic disorders suggests that youngsters are at particular risk for EPS, even when treated with SGAs [42]. In this trial, EPS were present in more than half of all randomized patients, with a large proportion of patients requiring anticholinergic medications (haloperidol 67%; olanzapine 56%; and risperidone 53%). In this study, rates of akathisia were also relatively high for olanzapine (12.5%). Although little information on the risk of aripiprazole for EPS in pediatric populations is available [97,98], there has been a concern about the potential for akathisia. In one retrospective study of 30 pediatric patients (mean age, 13.3 years; range, 5–19 years) treated with aripiprazole for bipolar disorder or schizoaffective disorder, bipolar type, 7 (23%) were noted to have developed akathisia [135]. Because in this sample the mean starting dose of 9 ± 4 mg was almost identical to the mean final dose of 10 ± 3 mg, lower starting doses may avoid this side effect that can result from an initially too excessive dopamine agonism. Finally, as in adults, when compared with the other SGAs, clozapine and quetiapine seem to be associated with relatively low rates of EPS in pediatric patients [1,91]. Of note, lithium cotreatment may increase the risk for EPS [99], although pediatric literature is missing.

Withdrawal dyskinesia and tardive dyskinesia

During treatment with FGAs, children and adolescents seem to be at higher risk of developing antipsychotic-related withdrawal dyskinesias, but these symptoms seem to be most often reversible [100,101,103], which is less frequently the case in adults [186]. Similar findings are emerging for SGAs but at lower rates than for FGAs. For example, during a 3-month observation period, 8 (8.4%) of 95 children and adolescents (mean age, 13.7 years) who were treated with FGAs, SGAs, or both developed withdrawal dyskinesia, and 4 (4.2%) developed probable tardive dyskinesia [102]. In this sample, dyskinesia was significantly more associated with the use of FGAs than with the use of SGAs. In a study of child outpatients who had autism (mean age, 7.1 years) and were treated with risperidone at 1.2 mg/day, none of the 13 children who completed the 6-month study developed dyskinesia, whereas 2 (15.4%) developed mild and fully reversible withdrawal dyskinesia when risperidone was discontinued [103].

Several SGA-related case reports of tardive dyskinesia have been published in children and adolescents, three of whom were naive to FGAs [104–107]. Available long-term pediatric studies that lasted at least 1 year suggest that SGAs are associated with relatively low rates of tardive dyskinesia in children and adolescents. In five prospective studies, four with risperidone (n = 741) [73,79, 86,87] and one with olanzapine (n = 20) [108], only two new cases of tardive dyskinesia were reported. These two cases were observed in the 1-year open-label study of 504 children and adolescents who had subaverage intelligence (age range, 5–14 years) and who were treated for disruptive behavior disorders with risperidone (mean dose, 1.6 mg/day) [86]. Of note, both cases of dyskinesia were fully reversible within a few weeks of discontinuation of risperidone.

Despite these encouraging results, it is possible that the failure to find any new cases of tardive dyskinesia may have been the result of the small number of patients enrolled in most of the studies, and the lack of standardized ratings in two of the five available long-term studies could underestimate the true risk of tardive dyskinesia in youth. On the other hand, the prompt reversibility of the two observed cases reconfirms a reduced risk of persistent tardive dyskinesia in youth. Nevertheless, larger long-term studies that follow individuals after the development of tardive dyskinesia are required to reconfirm the relatively low risk of chronic neuromotor side effects of atypical antipsychotics in children and adolescents.

Cardiac side effects

QTc prolongation

FGAs and SGAs have the potential to prolong the QTc interval of the EKG; the prolongation varies in both drug classes [109]. This adverse effect is worrisome for its predisposition to torsades de pointes, a potentially fatal arrhythmia [110]. Most reports of QTc prolongation derive from adult data, but reports of sudden death in children treated with tricyclic antidepressants [111] and the recent withdrawal of Adderall XR from the Canadian market in February of 2005 because of sudden cardiac death in children (http://www.fda.gov/cder/drug/InfoSheets/HCP/adderalHCP.htm) have highlighted the concern about a potentially greater risk of adverse cardiac events during development.

Measuring QTc intervals is not trivial. Automatic EKG machine readings may underestimate the QTc interval, particularly when it exceeds 460 milliseconds [109]. Because the QT interval is affected by heart rate, this interval is corrected (QTc) to account for variation in heart rate. The most commonly used correction divides the QT interval by the square root of the R-R interval [112], but in children and adolescents an additional correction factor may be more accurate [113]. Although, in general, QTc intervals shorter than 450 milliseconds are considered normal, and intervals longer than 500 milliseconds are considered a risk for the development of torsades de pointes, the sensitivity and specificity of QTc prolongation for prediction of arrhythmia is unknown [114]. Finally, it is unclear whether an absolute cut-off point or a change in QTc values from a personal baseline is more predictive of cardiac adverse events [109].

Although all SGAs prolong QTc to a certain degree in adult and pediatric populations [109], this prolongation seems to be relevant only for ziprasidone. Manufacturer-conducted studies of ziprasidone report that it prolonged the QTc by 9 to 14 milliseconds more than risperidone, olanzapine, quetiapine, and haloperidol and demonstrated an absolute prolongation of about 10 milliseconds compared with placebo [115]. The clinical relevance of this degree of QTc prolongation is unclear, however, and a review of cardiac deaths in association with ziprasidone published in 2001 found no excess of sudden deaths [116]. In pediatric populations, a prospective, open-label trial of 20 adolescents (mean age, 13.2 years) treated with ziprasidone (mean dose, 30 mg/day) for 4.6 ± 2.0 months revealed statistically significant changes from baseline in heart rate, PR interval, and QTc interval, with a mean QTc prolongation of 28 ± 26 milliseconds [117]. The QTc prolongation was unrelated to ziprasidone dose ($r = .16$, $P = .07$). QTc intervals show some degree of variability, however, and these results may overestimate the true degree of QTc prolongation, because a single baseline EKG reading was compared with the maximum QTc interval found in all of the subsequent EKGs. An earlier double-blind, placebo-controlled study of ziprasidone in 28 pediatric patients with Tourette's syndrome did not reveal any clinically significant EKG changes [83]. Even though one case of sudden death in a child who had Tourette's syndrome and who was taking ziprasidone was reported elsewhere [118], the cause of death seemed to be unrelated to ziprasidone. Finally, a review of cardiac adverse events in children taking psychotropic medications [109] did not reveal reports of sudden death or torsades de pointes in children, adolescents, or adults taking ziprasidone, indicating that this agent has a place in the treatment of pediatric populations when baseline and follow-up monitoring is in place. It seems, however, that co-administration of a second antipsychotic [119,120] or of antidepressants [121] can further prolong the QTc interval.

Myocarditis

Among the SGAs, only clozapine has been associated with a relevant risk for myocarditis, which is most prominent early in treatment [122]. In addition, in evaluating overdoses, an increased risk of sudden death in patients receiving therapeutic doses of clozapine relative to patients taking other psychotropics has been observed [123]. Although several case reports of clozapine-associated myocarditis in children have been published [124,125], the incidence seems to be low [122,126], indicating that clinical monitoring of symptoms and signs suggestive of myocarditis may be a sufficient precaution.

Sedation

Sedation is a common side effect of FGAs and SGAs alike [90]. With the potential exception of quetiapine, which seems to be most sedating at doses at or below 200 mg/day, where it exhibits its strongest antihistamine efficacy, sedation is a dose-related phenomenon, even though most patients develop at least some degree of tolerance over time.

Although a comparison across studies with different populations, dosages, and methodologies is only a crude approximation, children and adolescents seem to be more affected by somnolence and sedation than adults. In the package inserts of all six available SGAs in the United States, rates of sedation range from 3% to 8% with risperidone, 14% with ziprasidone, 18% with quetiapine, and up to 29% and 39% with olanzapine and clozapine, respectively [127]. Because these are monotherapy studies, a comparison with pediatric studies that often allow for comedications would overestimate the difference between pediatric and adult data. Results from other relevant studies indicate approximate incidence rates of sedation of 4% to 19% for aripiprazole [38,128], 21% for ziprasidone [129], 18%

to 37% for risperidone [129–131], 25% to 39% for olanzapine [128,130,132], 34% to 43% for quetiapine [133,134], and 24% to 46% for clozapine [131,132].

In contrast, rates of sedation reported in pediatric studies are higher, ranging from 0% to 33% for aripiprazole [135,136], 42% to 69% for ziprasidone [83,137], 25% to 80% for quetiapine [138–140], 29% to 89% for risperidone [42,87,141,142], 44% to 94% for olanzapine [42,143,187,188], and 46% to 90% with clozapine [144–146]. Taken together, it seems that in children and adolescents the same rank order applies for SGAs leading to sedation, albeit at a higher rate than in adults. SGAs that are most likely to be associated with sedation are clozapine, quetiapine, and olanzapine; risperidone and, possibly, ziprasidone have intermediate sedative properties [1]. Although aripiprazole seems to be less sedating in most youngsters [136], it is unclear whether this benefit holds up at higher dosages, because in adults the rate of sedation increased from 4% at 20 mg/day to 19% at 30 mg/day [38]. Clinically the reports of "activation" after initiation of aripiprazole often seem to be related to a relatively high starting dose or a fast taper and discontinuation of a more sedating and shorter half-life antipsychotic during a switch to aripiprazole.

Liver toxicity

Several studies have reported liver abnormalities in children and adolescents treated with SGAs. In a chart review of 13 psychotic children treated with risperidone, 2 boys were identified who presented with obesity, liver enzyme abnormalities, and confirmatory evidence of fatty liver. In both cases, the liver damage was reversed after discontinuation of risperidone or associated weight loss [147]. A significant increase in mean baseline to endpoint levels of aspartate aminotransferase and alanine aminotransferase was also observed in the 19 youth randomly assigned to 8 weeks of treatment with risperidone and the 15 youngsters randomly assigned to haloperidol, whereas no significant change occurred in the 16 patients taking olanzapine [42]. It is unclear, however, whether the mean change was clinically relevant. In another chart review of 38 youths (aged 5–17 years) with a variety of psychiatric diagnoses, only 1 youngster was found to have a mild and nonsignificant elevation in liver enzymes after a mean duration of risperidone treatment of 15.2 months at a mean dose of 2.5 mg/day. These data were noted in spite of weight gain and the use of numerous concomitant psychotropic medications [148]. In another study by Masi and colleagues [73], only 1 of 53 preschool children treated with risperidone was noted to develop abnormally increased liver enzymes. Cotreatment with divalproex may increase the risk for liver enzyme abnormalities. In a retrospective study of 52 children (aged 4–18 years), combination of divalproex and olanzapine (n = 12) was associated with significantly higher rates of abnormally elevated peak as well as mean levels in at least one of the liver enzymes compared with monotherapy [149]. Elevated peak enzyme levels were present during the observation period of 8 ± 6 months in 100% of the olanzapine plus divalproex group (n = 12), 59% of the olanzapine monotherapy group (n = 17), and 26% of the divalproex monotherapy group (n = 23). Elevated mean liver enzyme levels were present in 83% of the olanzapine plus divalproex group, 47% of the olanzapine monotherapy group, and 17% of the divalproex monotherapy group. Liver enzyme elevations in patients receiving divalproex did not correlate with divalproex serum levels. Further, for 42% of the patients in the olanzapine plus divalproex group, at least one enzyme level remained elevated during the periods for which enzyme levels were available, and two patients required discontinuation of the combination treatment because of pancreatitis and steatohepatitis, respectively [149].

Neutropenia and agranulocytosis

Although all antipsychotic agents are associated with varying degrees of decreases in white blood cell counts, these decreases usually are not clinically significant [150]. The exception is clozapine, which has been reported to cause potentially life-threatening agranulocytosis with an 18-month cumulative incidence of 0.9% [151]. African Americans are at higher risk for neutropenia, because of benign fluctuations and a lower baseline white cell count in some individuals; younger age seems to be an added risk factor [152,153]. Because of the risk for neutropenia and agranulocytosis, blood draws every week for the first 6 months and every other week thereafter are required for adult as well as pediatric patients treated with clozapine [154]. Lithium augmentation has been found to increase white blood cell counts and enabled clozapine rechallenge in some pediatric patients with previous neutropenia [155]. In a recent retrospective chart review of 172 pediatric patients treated with clozapine [189], neutropenia (absolute neutrophil count <1500/mm) developed in 23 (13%) patients and agranulocytosis (absolute neutrophil count <500/mm) developed in one (0.6%) patient. The cumulative one-year probability of developing an initial adverse hematologic event during clozapine treatment was 16.1% (95% confidence interval: 9.7%–22.5%). Eleven (48%) of 24 patients who had developed an adverse hematologic event were rechallenged on clozapine without a recurrence, and only 8 patients (5%) had to stop clozapine because of either agranulocytosis (n = 1), or neutropenia (n = 7).

Thyroid dysfunction

Quetiapine has been associated with a decrease in serum total T4 in some pediatric patients [156,157]. Although the mechanism of this effect is unknown, serum free thyroxine and thyroid-stimulating hormone generally remain within the normal range in adult [158] and pediatric [156] patients receiving quetiapine, suggesting no clinical relevance of this effect.

Seizures

Although all antipsychotic agents have the propensity to lower the seizure threshold, clozapine is the only SGA that is associated with a clinically relevant risk of seizures [159]. In a case series of 21 children and adolescents (mean age, 12.0 years) who had seizure disorder, the addition of risperidone to the antiseizure medication at a mean dose of 2.4 ± 3.5 mg/day for a variety of psychiatric symptoms did not increase seizure activity in any of the subjects [160]. Caution may be necessary when combining antipsychotics, as indicated by a case report in a 27-year-old woman who developed her first seizure 1 day after addition of 100 mg quetiapine to a stable dose of olanzapine (15 mg/day), although the recent discontinuation of low-dose clonazepam in this case could be an alternative explanation [161].

Neuroleptic malignant syndrome

Neuroleptic malignant syndrome (NMS), characterized by the clinical triad of fever, tachycardia, and rigidity, is a rare but potentially fatal complication of antipsychotic treatment. It has been suggested that SGAs may be associated less with NMS than are FGAs [162] and that SGAs are associated with a more benign course of NMS [163]. A recent literature review, conducted in January 2003, yielded 68 cases of NMS associated with SGA treatment [163]. Twenty-one of theses cases occurred with clozapine, indicating that a low potential for EPS does not seem to prevent the occurrence of NMS. NMS has also been described in children and adolescents. A review of 77 pediatric cases with FGA-related NMS found that low-potency neuroleptics were associated with poorer outcome, that fever was related to longer duration of illness, and that bromocriptine and anticholinergics (either added when not present or stopped when present) were effective, whereas dantrolene was not useful in this sample [164]. Since then, several case reports of SGA-related NMS in children and adolescents have been published [165–171], underscoring the need for clinicians to remain vigilant about this rare adverse event. Because of the low incidence and unknown denominator, it is unclear whether pediatric populations are at higher risk than adults for SGA-induced NMS or its sequelae.

Recommendations for health education and monitoring

As with any treatment, prescribing SGAs should be based on a careful risk–benefit evaluation that should include the patient and caregiver in the decision-making process as much as possible. Education about the potential for certain side effects is an essential component of medication management. It prepares patients and caregivers to have realistic expectations and helps them put adverse effects into perspective and make appropriate decisions either to wait for the natural abatement of these symptoms or to seek professional help in a timely manner. Furthermore, simple advice about potentially preventive and self-monitoring strategies may be useful in reducing the magnitude of weight gain and related metabolic abnormalities. These healthy-lifestyle strategies include the reduction or, ideally, cessation of sugar-containing drinks [172,173], increased intake of fiber [174], reduction of sedentary behaviors such as watching television, and regular moderate-intensity exercise, ideally for at least 30 minutes each day [175]. Finally, the simple measure of self-monitoring of weight changes that has shown to be effective in the treatment of adults with obesity [176] may be useful in minimizing antipsychotic-induced weight gain, although data in children and adolescents are lacking.

The decision about which SGA to prescribe should be guided by the literature about efficacy and safety effects of the medication and by knowledge about patient characteristics. Table 4 summarizes the suggested assessments at baseline and follow-up in children and adolescents in whom SGA treatment is initiated.

Table 4
Health monitoring in children and adolescents treated with second-generation antipsychotics

Assessments before choosing SGA	Assessments before starting SGA	Follow-up assessments	Frequency of follow-up assessments[e]
Personal and family medical history	Height and weight BMI percentile	Height and weight BMI percentile	At each visit
Dietary habits	Blood pressure and pulse	Blood pressure and pulse	Every 3 mo
Exercise habits	Neuromotor symptoms/ signs	Neuromotor symptoms/signs	During titration, then every 3 mo
Daytime sedation	Fasting blood work[b]	Dietary habits	Monthly for 3 mo, then every 3 mo
Appetite level	Morning prolactin[c]	Exercise habits	Monthly for 3 mo, then every 3 mo
Sexual symptoms/ signs		Daytime sedation	Monthly for 3 mo, then every 3 mo
Height and weight BMI percentile[a]		Appetite level	Monthly for 3 mo, then every 3 mo
Blood pressure and pulse[a]		Sexual symptoms/ signs	Monthly for 3 mo, then every 3 mo
Neuromotor symptoms/signs[a]		Fasting blood work[b]	At 3 mo, then every 6 mo
Fasting blood work[a,b]	Except for thyroid stimulating hormone	EKG[d]	During titration if taking ziprasidone
Morning prolactin[a,c]		Thyroid stimulating hormone	Annually
EKG[d]		Morning prolactin[c]	Only when symptomatic

   [a] Optional assessments to inform choice of an SGA, will depend on patient condition and appropriateness of waiting for test results.
   [b] Full blood cell count with differential, serum electrolytes, liver and kidney function, thyroid-stimulating hormone, glucose, and lipid profile.
   [c] If abnormal sexual symptoms or signs are present.
   [d] Only recommended for ziprasidone at baseline and follow-up (ie, after dose increase and at maintenance dose), unless patient is receiving clozapine and symptoms and signs develop that are suggestive of myocarditis. Do not initiate ziprasidone if baseline QTc is above 450 ms; stop ziprasidone if QTc is above 500 ms.
   [e] Earlier and/or more frequent assessments are indicated if patients develop symptoms suggestive of an abnormality.

Assessments before choosing an SGA

The following information should be obtained in addition to the regular inquiries about psychiatric symptoms and past therapeutic and side-effect response patterns. This information will help individualize the SGA treatment by taking into consideration risk factors and pre-existing abnormalities.

1. Personal and family medical history, including presence of endocrine disorders, cardiac abnormalities, and components of the metabolic syndrome (ie, thyroid disorder, long QT syndrome, heart murmur, diabetes, obesity, hypertriglyceridemia, hypercholesterolemia, arterial hypertension), as well as sudden or unexplained death in a first-degree family member
2. Dietary habits, including frequency of fast-food consumption, number of servings of fruits and vegetables per day, amount of sugared drinks per day
3. Exercise habits, including type, frequency, and duration
4. Baseline levels of sedation and appetite (eg, using a 10-point subjective intensity or visual analogue scale)
5. Depending on the pubertal stage and maturity of the patient, the presence, duration, and severity of sexual symptoms and reproductive system abnormalities (ie, menstrual cycle abnormalities, gynecomastia, galactorrhea, abnormal sexual drive, arousal, and performance)
6. EKG monitoring before SGA initiation is currently recommended only for ziprasidone; at QTc intervals of greater than 450 milliseconds at baseline, ziprasidone should not be initiated; obtain consultation before starting ziprasidone when a physical examination is significant for pulse rate lower than 60 beats/minute, blood pressure more than two SD above normal for age, or a non-innocent heart murmur [109]; baseline potassium and magnesium should be within normal limits
7. Whenever appropriate and the condition of the patient permits, results from baseline tests, such as vital signs, EPS, abnormal involuntary movements, and fasting blood work, may be obtained before choosing a specific SGA

Baseline assessments

When an SGA is prescribed, and ideally before the first dose is taken, the following baseline assessments should be obtained:

1. Height and weight to calculate BMI and BMI percentile (see Table 2): Although abdominal obesity is most predictive of metabolic syndrome [43], routine measurements of waist circumference in youths are currently not recommended, even though sex- and age-adjusted percentiles for waist circumference have recently become available [23].
2. Blood pressure and pulse: Use a blood pressure cuff size that is appropriate for age and upper-arm diameter of the patient.

3. Neuromotor signs and symptoms (EPS, akathisia, and abnormal involuntary movements): Using structured assessment tools is encouraged, such as the Simpson Angus Scale [177] or the Extrapyramidal Symptom Rating Scale (ERSRS) [178] for EPS, the Barnes Akathisia Scale [179] for akathisia, and the Abnormal Involuntary Movement Scale (AIMS) [180] or the dyskinesia subscale of the ERSRS [178] for presence of dyskinetic movements.

4. Fasting blood work: Full blood cell count with differential, serum electrolytes, liver and kidney function, thyroid-stimulating hormone, glucose, and lipid profile should be obtained. Patients and parents should be specifically instructed that fasting after midnight includes abstaining not only from food but also from all liquids except water and that chewing gum should be avoided. If fasting blood work cannot be obtained, hemoglobin A1c levels higher than 6.1% can be used to rule out hyperglycemia for the last 3 months. In case of nonfasting blood work, triglyceride and LDL cholesterol results are of little value, whereas levels of total cholesterol and high-density lipoprotein cholesterol remain fairly unaffected.

5. In case of abnormal sexual symptoms or signs: A morning prolactin test should be added to the fasting blood work. Patients and caregivers should be instructed to withhold all morning medications until after the blood test to avoid acutely affecting the prolactin level.

6. Baseline EKG: Do not initiate ziprasidone if QTc is higher than 450 milliseconds.

Follow-up assessments

1. Height and weight to calculate BMI and BMI percentile (see Table 2). Frequency: at each clinical visit.

2. Blood pressure and pulse. Frequency: at least every 3 months unless cardiac symptoms (eg, headache, blurry vision, palpitations, tachycardia, dizziness, syncope) occur.

3. Neuromotor signs and symptoms. Frequency for EPS and akathisia: during titration phase, then every 3 months after reaching maintenance dose. Frequency for abnormal involuntary movements: every 3 months.

4. Dietary habits. Frequency: monthly for the first 3 months of treatment; every 3 months thereafter.

5. Exercise habits. Frequency: monthly for the first 3 months of treatment; every 3 months thereafter.

6. Levels of sedation and appetite. Frequency: monthly for the first 3 months of treatment; every 3 months thereafter.

7. Presence, duration, and severity of sexual symptoms and reproductive system abnormalities. Frequency: monthly for the first 3 months of treatment; every 3 months thereafter.

8. EKG monitoring (currently recommended only for ziprasidone). Frequency: after dose increase and after reaching steady state of maintenance dose. Stop ziprasidone usage if QTc interval is 500 milliseconds or longer. Obtain an

EKG (to look for ST abnormalities and T-wave inversions) if patient is taking clozapine and presents with symptoms suggestive of myocarditis (ie, unexplained fatigue, dyspnea, tachypnea, fever, chest pain, palpitations, other signs of heart failure). If a patient taking ziprasidone develops diarrhea, fluid replacement should be encouraged, and cardiac monitoring as well as potassium and magnesium levels should be considered [109].

9. Fasting blood work. Full blood cell count with differential, serum electrolytes, liver and kidney function, glucose and lipid profile. Frequency: at 3 months and at least every 6 months thereafter. Obtain follow-up blood work earlier in case of significant weight gain, or in case of symptoms suggestive of new-onset diabetes (ie, unexplained weight loss, polydipsia, polyuria). Significant weight gain is operationally defined as a) > 5% weight gain during three months, or any of the following three conditions at any time during treatment: b) ≥ 0.5 increase in BMI z-score, BMI percentile ≥ 85–94.9 plus one adverse health consequence (ie, hyperglycemia, dyslipidemia, hyperinsulinemia, hypertension, orthopedic, gall bladder, or sleep disorder), or BMI ≥ 95th percentile or abdominal obesity (ie, > 90th percentile) [23]. The assessment intervals for fasting blood work are more frequent than those recommended for adults by the ADA Consensus Statement [16] or the Mount Sinai Conference [85] because children seem to be at higher risk for antipsychotic-induced weight gain, related metabolic abnormalities, and liver abnormalities.

10. Thyroid-stimulating hormone. Frequency: annually, unless patient is taking lithium (6-monthly assessment) or presents with new-onset symptoms that are suggestive of thyroid dysfunction (immediate assessment).

11. Prolactin. Measurement is necessary only if patient had abnormal baseline value or presents with new-onset sexual symptoms or reproductive system abnormalities. Frequency: every 3 months until normal in case of abnormal baseline prolactin or whenever if patient presents with new symptoms or signs suggestive of hyperprolactinemia (ie, galactorrhea, amenorrhea, gynecomastia, or abnormalities of sexual desire, arousal, or performance).

Whenever pathologic thresholds are crossed, clinicians should encourage and monitor healthy lifestyle behaviors where appropriate and, if levels continue to be abnormal, consider referring patients to a primary health care provider or appropriate specialist for further evaluation and treatment.

Areas for future research

In general, adverse events and safety are neglected areas in research. In view of the overall dearth of pediatric psychopharmacologic studies, this lack of information weighs even more heavily for children and adolescents. The disproportion is dramatic, given that prescription rates of psychotropic medications in this population have almost reached adult proportions [4] and considering the potentially greater long-term impact of side effects in developing individuals. Therefore, the number of pediatric studies and of individuals in such studies needs to increase, and study designs should resemble real-life clinical settings [181,182]. These conditions are particularly important for long-term studies that are integral for the understanding of the persistence and secondary effects of pharmacologically induced changes. Side-effect assessments should not consist merely of passive elicitation or open-ended questions. Any pediatric psychopharmacologic study should employ a standardized pediatric side-effect scale, such as the Safety Monitoring Uniform Report Form (SMURF) [183] or another, less time-consuming rating scale. See the article by Bostic and Rho elsewhere in this issue for a simplified version of the SMURF, which is more feasible for use in clinical settings. In addition, height, weight, and vital signs should be assessed regularly, and long-term studies should include measures of sexual development.

Specifically, more data are required regarding the acute and chronic effects of SGAs on body composition, lipid metabolism, insulin resistance and diabetes, sexual maturation, acute extrapyramidal side effects and tardive dyskinesia, blood dyscrasias, and cardiac conduction in youngsters. Also needed is research on the potential chronicity or reversibility of some of these side effects and on the downstream effects of adverse anthropometric changes or alterations of prolactin levels with regard to established and emerging biologic markers for future cardiovascular and malignant morbidity. Further, large-scale, simple trials that closely match clinical practice are needed to achieve greater generalizability of the results and to allow valid subanalyses that could inform clinicians about baseline risk factors and early treatment indicators that identify individuals at high risk for certain side effects. In particular, these studies need to include sufficient numbers of individuals of both genders and from varied ethnic subgroups who are at different sexual maturational stages to assure generalizability of the findings and to assess for potential baseline risk factors that could inform treatment. In general, pediatric studies have a great potential to inform adult psychiatry, because many individuals are antipsychotic-naive or early in the treatment course, thereby limiting potentially confounding effects that are unavoidable in switch studies after prolonged exposure to previous agents. Finally, treatment trials are required to minimize or prevent specific adverse effects in pediatric populations in need for treatment with antipsychotics.

Summary

Adverse effects are part of almost all pharmacologic interventions. The acuity, severity, and chronicity of adverse effects influence medication effectiveness, physical and psychologic health, compliance, and overall outcome. The available data suggest that children and adolescents are at higher risk than adults for experiencing sedation, acute EPS, withdrawal dyskinesia, and significant weight gain during treatment with SGAs. It further seems that weight gain is not a dose-related effect and is not attenuated by stimulant cotreatment, whereas divalproex cotreatment may add to the risk. Head-to-head studies of different SGAs in pediatric patients are sparse but suggest that olanzapine, as in adults, is associated with the greatest risk for weight gain. Data on clozapine in youths are too scarce to reconfirm the even higher risk for weight gain found in pretreated adults. It seems, however, that risperidone has a more negative effect on body weight in children than in adults and that ziprasidone and aripiprazole may not be as weight neutral as found in adult studies that predominantly include individuals with long previous antipsychotic exposure that potentially masks the weight gain potential. Although it would be expected that the adverse changes in body composition would be associated with higher rates of dyslipidemia and insulin resistance, two eminent risk states for future development of diabetes and cardiovascular morbidity, more data are required to reconfirm this concern. As in adults, prolactin elevations are most pronounced and frequent with risperidone treatment. Although the prolactin increase is most prominent early in treatment, is not necessarily correlated with sexual dysfunction, may normalize over 1 year (at least in prepubertal boys), and may not affect maturation, more data are required to substantiate these preliminary findings. Blood dyscrasias are most frequent with clozapine treatment but are sufficiently infrequent and reversible with appropriate monitoring so that the risk for neutropenia should not limit the use of clozapine in treatment-resistant youngsters. The same is true for the increased seizure rate at higher doses of clozapine, which can be treated successfully with addition of valproate. QTc prolongation seems to be a potential concern for pediatric patients treated with ziprasidone, although overdoses of other agents or combinations of two SGAs may also prolong QTc. No clear case of torsades de pointes has been reported to date in a ziprasidone-treated patient, however.

Especially given the widespread and increasing use of SGAs in children and adolescents for psychotic and a wide variety of nonpsychotic conditions, more and larger-scale safety monitoring studies in youngsters that parallel clinical treatment settings are needed to inform clinicians about the acute and chronic safety profiles of different antipsychotic agents. This information is required to evaluate comprehensively the risk-to-benefit profile of individual antipsychotic agents as well as to help identify patients at high risk for the development of certain adverse events early to allow treatment adjustments. Until data that will enable the development of more individualized treatment algorithms become available, clinicians should attempt to match the differential side-effect profiles of SGAs to patient factors and employ the suggested monitoring strategies to maximize the effectiveness and minimize the adverse outcomes in those vulnerable youngsters who are in need of antipsychotic treatment.

References

[1] Cheng-Shannon J, McGough JJ, Pataki C, et al. Second-generation antipsychotic medications in children and adolescents. J Child Adolesc Psychopharmacol 2004;14(3):372–94.

[2] Pappadopulos EA, Tate Guelzow B, Wong C, et al. A review of the growing evidence base for pediatric psychopharmacology. Child Adolesc Psychiatr Clin N Am 2004;13(4):817–55.

[3] Cooper WO, Hickson GB, Fuchs C, et al. New users of antipsychotic medications among children enrolled in TennCare. Arch Pediatr Adolesc Med 2004;158(8):753–9.

[4] Zito JM, Safer DJ, DosReis S, et al. Psychotropic practice patterns for youth: a 10-year perspective. Arch Pediatr Adolesc Med 2003;157(1):17–25.

[5] Patel NC, Sanchez RJ, Johnsrud MT, et al. Trends in antipsychotic use in a Texas Medicaid population of children and adolescents: 1996 to 2000. J Child Adolesc Psychopharmacol 2002;12(3):221–9.

[6] Staller JA, Wade MJ, Baker M. Current prescribing patterns in outpatient child and adolescent psychiatric practice in central New York. J Child Adolesc Psychopharmacol 2005;15(1): 57–61.

[7] Kelly DL, Love RC, MacKowick M, et al. Atypical antipsychotic use in a state hospital inpatient adolescent population. J Child Adolesc Psychopharmacol 2004;14(1):75–85.

[8] Lyons JS, MacIntyre JC, Lee ME, et al. Psychotropic medications prescribing patterns for children and adolescents in New York's public mental health system. Community Ment Health J 2004;40(2):101–18.

[9] Tarsy D, Baldessarini RJ, Tarazi FI. Effects of newer antipsychotics on extrapyramidal function. CNS Drugs 2002;16(1):23–45 [erratum: CNS Drugs 2003;17(3):202].

[10] Correll CU, Leucht S, Kane JM. Lower risk for tardive dyskinesia associated with second-generation antipsychotics: a systematic review of 1-year studies. Am J Psychiatry 2004;161(3): 414–25.

[11] Davis JM, Chen N, Glick ID. A meta-analysis of the efficacy of second-generation antipsychotics. Arch Gen Psychiatry 2003;60(6):553–64.

[12] Leucht S, Pitschel-Walz G, Abraham D, et al. Efficacy and extrapyramidal side-effects of the new antipsychotics olanzapine, quetiapine, risperidone, and sertindole compared to conventional antipsychotics and placebo. A meta-analysis of randomized controlled trials. Schizophr Res 1999;35:51–68.

[13] Buckley PF. Broad therapeutic uses of atypical antipsychotic medications. Biol Psychiatry 2001;50(11):912–24.

[14] Menzin J, Boulanger L, Friedman M, et al. Treatment adherence associated with conventional and atypical antipsychotics in a large state Medicaid program. Psychiatr Serv 2003;54(5): 719–23.

[15] Dolder CR, Lacro JP, Dunn LB, et al. Antipsychotic medication adherence: is there a difference between typical and atypical agents? Am J Psychiatry 2002;159(1):103–8.

[16] American Diabetes Association, American Psychiatric Association, American Association of Clinical Endocrinologists, North American Association for the Study of Obesity. Consensus development conference on antipsychotic drugs and obesity and diabetes. Diabetes Care 2004; 27(2):596–601.

[17] Paxton JW, Dragunow M. Pharmacology. In: Werry JS, Aman MG, editors. Practitioner's guide to psychoactive drugs for children and adolescents. New York: Plenum Medical; 1993. p. 23–55.

[18] Geller B. Psychopharmacology of children and adolescents: pharmacokinetics and relationships of plasma/serum levels to response. Psychopharmacol Bull 1991;27(4):401–9.

[19] Woods SW, Martin A, Spector SG, et al. Effects of development on olanzapine-associated adverse events. J Am Acad Child Adolesc Psychiatry 2002;41(12):1439–46.

[20] Greenhill LL, Vitiello B, Riddle MA, et al. Review of safety assessment methods used in pediatric psychopharmacology. J Am Acad Child Adolesc Psychiatry 2003;42(6):627–33.

[21] Executive Summary of the Third Report of the National Cholesterol Education Program (NCEP) Expert Panel on Detection, Evaluation, and Treatment of High Blood Cholesterol in Adults (Adult Treatment Panel III). JAMA 2001;285(19):2486–97.

[22] Cook S, Weitzman M, Auinger P, et al. Prevalence of a metabolic syndrome phenotype in adolescents: findings from the third National Health and Nutrition Examination Survey, 1988–1994. Arch Pediatr Adolesc Med 2003;157(8):821–7.

[23] Fernandez JR, Redden DT, Pietrobelli A, et al. Waist circumference percentiles in nationally representative samples of African-American, European-American, and Mexican-American children and adolescents. J Pediatr 2004;145(4):439–44.

[24] National High Blood Pressure Education Program Working Group on High Blood Pressure in Children and Adolescents. The fourth report on the diagnosis, evaluation, and treatment of high blood pressure in children and adolescents. Pediatrics 2004;114:555–76.

[25] Weiss R, Dziura J, Burgert TS, et al. Obesity and the metabolic syndrome in children and adolescents. N Engl J Med 2004;350(23):2362–74.

[26] Allison DB, Fontaine KR, Heo M, et al. The distribution of body mass index among individuals with and without schizophrenia. J Clin Psychiatry 1999;60(4):215–20.

[27] Correll CU, Malhotra AK. Pharmacogenetics of antipsychotic-induced weight gain. Psychopharmacology (Berl) 2004;174(4):477–89.

[28] Raitakari OT, Juonala M, Kahonen M, et al. Cardiovascular risk factors in childhood and carotid artery intima-media thickness in adulthood: the Cardiovascular Risk in Young Finns Study. JAMA 2003;290(17):2277–83.

[29] Li S, Chen W, Srinivasan SR, et al. Childhood cardiovascular risk factors and carotid vascular changes in adulthood: the Bogalusa Heart Study. JAMA 2003;290(17):2271–6 [erratum: JAMA 2003;290(22):2943].

[30] Must A, Jacques PF, Dallal GE, et al. Long-term morbidity and mortality of overweight adolescents. A follow-up of the Harvard Growth Study of 1922 to 1935. N Engl J Med 1992; 327(19):1350–5.

[31] Allison DB, Mackell JA, McDonnell DD. The impact of weight gain on quality of life among persons with schizophrenia. Psychiatr Serv 2003;54(4):565–7.

[32] Strassnig M, Brar JS, Ganguli R. Body mass index and quality of life in community-dwelling patients with schizophrenia. Schizophr Res 2003;62(1–2):73–6.

[33] Perkins DO. Adherence to antipsychotic medications. J Clin Psychiatry 1999;60(Suppl 21): 25–30.

[34] Weiden PJ, Mackell JA, McDonnell DD. Obesity as a risk factor for antipsychotic non-compliance. Schizophr Res 2004;66(1):51–7.

[35] Allison DB, Mentore JL, Heo M, et al. Antipsychotic-induced weight gain: a comprehensive research synthesis. Am J Psychiatry 1999;156(11):1686–96.

[36] Safer DJ. A comparison of risperidone-induced weight gain across the age span. J Clin Psychopharmacol 2004;24(4):429–36.

[37] Ratzoni G, Gothelf D, Brand-Gothelf A, et al. Weight gain associated with olanzapine and risperidone in adolescent patients: a comparative prospective study. J Am Acad Child Adolesc Psychiatry 2002;41(3):337–43.

[38] Marder SR, McQuade RD, Stock E, et al. Aripiprazole in the treatment of schizophrenia: safety and tolerability in short-term, placebo-controlled trials. Schizophr Res 2003;61(2–3):123–36.

[39] Correll CU, Parikh UH, Mughal T, et al. Body composition changes associated with second-generation antipsychotics. Biol Psychiatry 2005;57(Suppl 8):36.

[40] Stigler KA, Potenza MN, Posey DJ, et al. Weight gain associated with atypical antipsychotic use in children and adolescents: prevalence, clinical relevance, and management. Paediatr Drugs 2004;6(1):33–44.

[41] Aman MG, Binder C, Turgay A. Risperidone effects in the presence/absence of psychostimulant medicine in children with ADHD, other disruptive behavior disorders, and subaverage IQ. J Child Adolesc Psychopharmacol 2004;14(2):243–54.

[42] Sikich L, Hamer RM, Bashford RA, et al. A pilot study of risperidone, olanzapine, and haloperidol in psychotic youth: a double-blind, randomized, 8-week trial. Neuropsychopharmacology 2004;29(1):133–45.

[43] Straker D, Correll CU, Kramer-Ginsberg E, et al. Cost-effective screening for metabolic syndrome in patients treated with second-generation antipsychotic medications. Am J Psychiatry 2005;162(6):1217–21.

[44] Almeras N, Despres JP, Villeneuve J, et al. Development of an atherogenic metabolic risk factor profile associated with the use of atypical antipsychotics. J Clin Psychiatry 2004;65(4):557–64.

[45] Cohn T, Prud'homme D, Streiner D, et al. Characterizing coronary heart disease risk in chronic schizophrenia: high prevalence of the metabolic syndrome. Can J Psychiatry 2004; 49(11):753–60.

[46] Basu R, Brar JS, Chengappa KN, et al. The prevalence of the metabolic syndrome in patients with schizoaffective disorder–bipolar subtype. Bipolar Disord 2004;6(4):314–8.

[47] Heiskanen T, Niskanen L, Lyytikainen R, et al. Metabolic syndrome in patients with schizophrenia. J Clin Psychiatry 2003;64(5):575–9.

[48] Wirshing DA, Boyd JA, Meng LR, et al. The effects of novel antipsychotics on glucose and lipid levels. J Clin Psychiatry 2002;63(10):856–65.

[49] Koro CE, Fedder DO, L'Italien GJ, et al. An assessment of the independent effects of olanzapine and risperidone exposure on the risk of hyperlipidemia in schizophrenic patients. Arch Gen Psychiatry 2002;59(11):1021–6.

[50] Meyer JM. A retrospective comparison of weight, lipid, and glucose changes between risperidone- and olanzapine-treated inpatients: metabolic outcomes after 1 year. J Clin Psychiatry 2002;63(5):425–33.

[51] Domon SE, Cargile CS. Quetiapine-associated hyperglycemia and hypertriglyceridemia. J Am Acad Child Adolesc Psychiatry 2002;41(5):495–6.

[52] Domon SE, Webber JC. Hyperglycemia and hypertriglyceridemia secondary to olanzapine. J Child Adolesc Psychopharmacol 2001;11(3):285–8.

[53] Nguyen M, Murphy T. Olanzapine and hypertriglyceridemia. J Am Acad Child Adolesc Psychiatry 2001;40(2):133.

[54] Martin A, L'Ecuyer S. Triglyceride, cholesterol and weight changes among risperidone-treated youths. A retrospective study. Eur Child Adolesc Psychiatry 2002;11(3):129–33.

[55] Correll CU, Parikh UH, Mughal T, et al. Development of insulin resistance in antipsychotic-naive youngsters treated with novel antipsychotics. Biol Psychiatry 2005;57(Suppl 8):36.

[56] Newcomer JW. Metabolic risk during antipsychotic treatment. Clin Ther 2004;26(12):1936–46.

[57] Sinha R, Fisch G, Teague B, et al. Prevalence of impaired glucose tolerance among children and adolescents with marked obesity. N Engl J Med 2002;346(11):802–10 [erratum (correction of dosage error in abstract): N Engl J Med 2002;346(22):1756].

[58] Henderson DC, Cagliaro F, Copeland PM, et al. Glucose metabolism in patients with schizophrenia treated with atypical antipsychotic agents. Arch Gen Psychiatry 2005;62:19–28.

[59] Bergman RN, Ader M. Atypical antipsychotics and glucose homeostasis. J Clin Psychiatry 2005;66(4):504–14.

[60] Ader M, Kim SP, Catalano KJ, et al. Metabolic dysregulation with atypical antipsychotics occurs in the absence of underlying disease: a placebo-controlled study of olanzapine and risperidone in dogs. Diabetes 2005;54(3):862–71.

[61] Roste LS, Tauboll E, Morkrid L, et al. Antiepileptic drugs alter reproductive endocrine hormones in men with epilepsy. Eur J Neurol 2005;12(2):118–24.

[62] Pylvanen V, Knip M, Pakarinen AJ, et al. Fasting serum insulin and lipid levels in men with epilepsy. Neurology 2003;60(4):571–4.

[63] Luef G, Abraham I, Haslinger M, et al. Polycystic ovaries, obesity and insulin resistance in women with epilepsy. A comparative study of carbamazepine and valproic acid in 105 women. J Neurol 2002;249(7):835–41.

[64] Saito E, Kafantaris V. Can diabetes mellitus be induced by medication? J Child Adolesc Psychopharmacol 2002;12(3):231–6.

[65] Courvoisie HE, Cooke DW, Riddle MA. Olanzapine-induced diabetes in a seven-year-old boy. J Child Adolesc Psychopharmacol 2004;14(4):612–6.

[66] Koller EA, Cross JT, Schneider B. Risperidone-associated diabetes mellitus in children. Pediatrics 2004;113(2):421–2.

[67] Selva KA, Scott SM. Diabetic ketoacidosis associated with olanzapine in an adolescent patient. J Pediatr 2001;138(6):936–8.

[68] Bloch Y, Vardi O, Mendlovic S, et al. Hyperglycemia from olanzapine treatment in adolescents. J Child Adolesc Psychopharmacol 2003;13(1):97–102.

[69] Correll CU, Parikh UH, Mughal T, et al. New-onset dyslipidemia in antipsychotic-naive youngsters treated with atypical antipsychotics. Biol Psychiatry 2005;57(Suppl 8):36.

[70] Martin A, Scahill L, Anderson GM, et al. Weight and leptin changes among risperidone-treated youths with autism: 6-month prospective data. Am J Psychiatry 2004;161(6):1125–7.

[71] Saito E, Correll CU, Gallelli K, et al. A prospective study of hyperprolactinemia in children and adolescents treated with atypical antipsychotic agents. J Child Adolesc Psychopharmacol 2004;14(3):350–8.

[72] Findling RL, Kusumakar V, Daneman D, et al. Prolactin levels during long-term risperidone treatment in children and adolescents. J Clin Psychiatry 2003;64(11):1362–9.

[73] Masi G, Cosenza A, Mucci M, et al. A 3-year naturalistic study of 53 preschool children with pervasive developmental disorders treated with risperidone. J Clin Psychiatry 2003;64(9): 1039–47.

[74] Wudarsky M, Nicolson R, Hamburger SD, et al. Elevated prolactin in pediatric patients on typical and atypical antipsychotics. J Child Adolesc Psychopharmacol 1999;9(4):239–45.

[75] Seeman P, Bzowej NH, Guan HC, et al. Human brain dopamine receptors in children and aging adults. Synapse 1987;1(5):399–404.

[76] Kinon BJ, Gilmore JA, Liu H, et al. Hyperprolactinemia in response to antipsychotic drugs: characterization across comparative clinical trials. Psychoneuroendocrinology 2003; 28(Suppl 2):69–82.

[77] Alfaro CL, Wudarsky M, Nicolson R, et al. Correlation of antipsychotic and prolactin concentrations in children and adolescents acutely treated with haloperidol, clozapine, or olanzapine. J Child Adolesc Psychopharmacol 2002;12(2):83–91.

[78] Pappagallo M, Silva R. The effect of atypical antipsychotic agents on prolactin levels in children and adolescents. J Child Adolesc Psychopharmacol 2004;14(3):359–71.

[79] Findling RL, Aman MG, Eerdekens M, et al, Risperidone Disruptive Behavior Study Group. Long-term, open-label study of risperidone in children with severe disruptive behaviors and below-average IQ. Am J Psychiatry 2004;161(4):677–84.

[80] Masi G, Cosenza A, Mucci M. Prolactin levels in young children with pervasive developmental disorders during risperidone treatment. J Child Adolesc Psychopharmacol 2001;11(4):389–94.

[81] Aman MG, De Smedt G, Derivan A, et al, Risperidone Disruptive Behavior Study Group. Double-blind, placebo-controlled study of risperidone for the treatment of disruptive behaviors in children with subaverage intelligence. Am J Psychiatry 2002;159(8):1337–46.

[82] Snyder R, Turgay A, Aman M, et al, The Risperidone Conduct Study Group. Effects of risperidone on conduct and disruptive behavior disorders in children with subaverage IQs. J Am Acad Child Adolesc Psychiatry 2002;41:1026–36.

[83] Sallee FR, Kurlan R, Goetz CG, et al. Ziprasidone treatment of children and adolescents with Tourette's syndrome: a pilot study. J Am Acad Child Adolesc Psychiatry 2000;39(3):292–9.

[84] Shaw JA, Lewis JE, Pascal S, et al. A study of quetiapine: efficacy and tolerability in psychotic adolescents. J Child Adolesc Psychopharmacol 2001;11(4):415–24.

[85] Marder SR, Essock SM, Miller AL, et al. Physical health monitoring of patients with schizophrenia. Am J Psychiatry 2004;161(8):1334–49.

[86] Croonenberghs J, Fegert JM, Findling RL, et al, Risperidone Disruptive Behavior Study Group. Risperidone in children with disruptive behavior disorders and subaverage intelligence: a 1-year, open-label study of 504 patients. J Am Acad Child Adolesc Psychiatry 2005;44(1): 64–72.

[87] Turgay A, Binder C, Snyder R, et al. Long-term safety and efficacy of risperidone for the treatment of disruptive behavior disorders in children with subaverage IQs. Pediatrics 2002; 110(3):e34.

[88] Dunbar F, Kusumakar V, Daneman D, et al. Growth and sexual maturation during long-term treatment with risperidone. Am J Psychiatry 2004;161(5):918–20.

[89] Lewis R. Typical and atypical antipsychotics in adolescent schizophrenia: efficacy, tolerability, and differential sensitivity to extrapyramidal symptoms. Can J Psychiatry 1998;43(6):596–604.

[90] Toren P, Ratner S, Laor N, et al. Benefit-risk assessment of atypical antipsychotics in the

treatment of schizophrenia and comorbid disorders in children and adolescents. Drug Saf 2004;27(14):1135–56.

[91] Sathpathy S, Winsberg B. Extrapyramidal symptoms in children on atypical antipsychotic drugs. J Clin Psychopharmacol 2003;23(6):675–7.

[92] Demb HB, Nguyen KT. Movement disorders in children with developmental disabilities taking risperidone. J Am Acad Child Adolesc Psychiatry 1999;38(1):5–6.

[93] Grcevich SJ, Findling RL, Rowane WA, et al. Risperidone in the treatment of children and adolescents with schizophrenia: a retrospective study. J Child Adolesc Psychopharmacol 1996; 6(4):251–7.

[94] Mandoki M. Risperidone treatment of children and adolescents: increased risk for extrapyramidal side effects? J Child Adolesc Psychopharmacol 1995;5(1):49–67.

[95] McDougle CJ, Holmes JP, Bronson MR, et al. Risperidone treatment of children and adolescents with pervasive developmental disorders: a prospective open-label study. J Am Acad Child Adolesc Psychiatry 1997;36(5):685–93.

[96] Perry R, Pataki C, Munoz-Silva DM, et al. Risperidone in children and adolescents with pervasive developmental disorder: pilot trial and follow-up. J Child Adolesc Psychopharmacol 1997;7(3):167–79.

[97] Schonberger RB, Douglas L, Baum CR. Severe extrapyramidal symptoms in a 3-year-old boy after accidental ingestion of the new antipsychotic drug aripiprazole. Pediatrics 2004;114(6):1743.

[98] Lindsey RL, Kaplan D, Koliatsos V, et al. Aripiprazole and extrapyramidal symptoms. J Am Acad Child Adolesc Psychiatry 2003;42(11):1268–9.

[99] Addonizio G, Roth SD, Stokes PE, et al. Increased extrapyramidal symptoms with addition of lithium to neuroleptics. J Nerv Ment Dis 1988;176(11):682–5.

[100] Kumra S, Jacobsen LK, Lenane M, et al. Case series: spectrum of neuroleptic-induced movement disorders and extrapyramidal side effects in childhood-onset schizophrenia. J Am Acad Child Adolesc Psychiatry 1998;37(2):221–7.

[101] Campbell M, Armenteros JL, Malone RP, et al. Neuroleptic-related dyskinesias in autistic children: a prospective, longitudinal study. J Am Acad Child Adolesc Psychiatry 1997;36(6): 835–43.

[102] Connor DF, Fletcher KE, Wood JS. Neuroleptic-related dyskinesias in children and adolescents. J Clin Psychiatry 2001;62(12):967–74.

[103] Malone RP, Maislin G, Choudhury MS, et al. Risperidone treatment in children and adolescents with autism: short- and long-term safety and effectiveness. J Am Acad Child Adolesc Psychiatry 2002;41(2):140–7.

[104] Feeney DJ, Klykylo W. Risperidone and tardive dyskinesia. J Am Acad Child Adolesc Psychiatry 1996;35(11):1421–2.

[105] Carroll NB, Boehm KE, Strickland RT. Chorea and tardive dyskinesia in a patient taking risperidone. J Clin Psychiatry 1999;60(7):485–7.

[106] Kwon H. Tardive dyskinesia in an autistic patient treated with risperidone. Am J Psychiatry 2004;161(4):757–8.

[107] Corson AH, Barkenbus JE, Posey DJ, et al. A retrospective analysis of quetiapine in the treatment of pervasive developmental disorders. J Clin Psychiatry 2004;65(11):1531–6.

[108] Ross RG, Novins D, Farley GK, et al. A 1-year open-label trial of olanzapine in school-age children with schizophrenia. J Child Adolesc Psychopharmacol 2003;13(3):301–9.

[109] Blair J, Taggart B, Martin A. Electrocardiographic safety profile and monitoring guidelines in pediatric psychopharmacology. J Neural Transm 2004;111(7):791–815.

[110] Glassman AH, Bigger Jr JT. Antipsychotic drugs: prolonged QTc interval, torsade de pointes, and sudden death. Am J Psychiatry 2001;158(11):1774–82.

[111] Varley CK. Sudden death related to selected tricyclic antidepressants in children: epidemiology, mechanisms and clinical implications. Paediatr Drugs 2001;3(8):613–27.

[112] Bazett H. An analysis of the time-relations of electrocardiograms. Heart 1918;7:353–70.

[113] Wernicke JF, Faries D, Breitung R, et al. QT correction methods in children and adolescents. J Cardiovasc Electrophysiol 2005;16(1):76–81.

[114] Taylor DM. Antipsychotics and QT prolongation. Acta Psychiatr Scand 2003;107(2):85–95.

[115] Ziprasidone [package insert]. New York (NY): Pfizer; 2002.

[116] Goodnick PJ. Ziprasidone: profile on safety. Expert Opin Pharmacother 2001;2(10): 1655–62 [review].

[117] Blair J, Scahill L, State M, et al. Electrocardiographic changes in children and adolescents treated with ziprasidone: a prospective study. J Am Acad Child Adolesc Psychiatry 2005;44(1): 73–9.

[118] Scahill L, Blair J, Leckman JF, et al. Sudden death in a patient with Tourette syndrome during a clinical trial of ziprasidone. J Psychopharmacol 2005;19(2):205–6.

[119] Minov C. [Risk of QTc prolongation due to combination of ziprasidone and quetiapine]. Psychiatr Prax 2004;31(Suppl 1):S142–4 [in German].

[120] Beelen AP, Yeo KT, Lewis LD. Asymptomatic QTc prolongation associated with quetiapine fumarate overdose in a patient being treated with risperidone. Hum Exp Toxicol 2001;20(4): 215–9.

[121] Sala M, Vicentini A, Brambilla P, et al. QT interval prolongation related to psychoactive drug treatment: a comparison of monotherapy versus polytherapy. Ann Gen Psychiatry 2005;4(1):1.

[122] Wehmeier PM, Heiser P, Remschmidt H. Myocarditis, pericarditis and cardiomyopathy in patients treated with clozapine. J Clin Pharm Ther 2005;30(1):91–6.

[123] Trenton A, Currier G, Zwemer F. Fatalities associated with therapeutic use and overdose of atypical antipsychotics. CNS Drugs 2003;17(5):307–24.

[124] Branik E, Nitschke M. Pericarditis and polyserositis as a side effect of clozapine in an adolescent girl. J Child Adolesc Psychopharmacol 2004;14(2):311–4.

[125] Wehmeier PM, Heiser P, Remschmidt H. Pancreatitis followed by pericardial effusion in an adolescent treated with clozapine. J Clin Psychopharmacol 2003;23(1):102–3.

[126] Wehmeier PM, Schuler-Springorum M, Heiser P, et al. Chart review for potential features of myocarditis, pericarditis, and cardiomyopathy in children and adolescents treated with clozapine. J Child Adolesc Psychopharmacol 2004;14(2):267–71.

[127] Physicians' desk reference. Montvale (NJ): Medical Economics Production Company; 2004.

[128] McQuade RD, Stock E, Marcus R, et al. A comparison of weight change during treatment with olanzapine or aripiprazole: results from a randomized, double-blind study. J Clin Psychiatry 2004;65(Suppl 18):47–56.

[129] Addington DE, Pantelis C, Dineen M, et al. Efficacy and tolerability of ziprasidone versus risperidone in patients with acute exacerbation of schizophrenia or schizoaffective disorder: an 8-week, double-blind, multicenter trial. J Clin Psychiatry 2004;65(12):1624–33.

[130] Conley RR, Mahmoud R. A randomized double-blind study of risperidone and olanzapine in the treatment of schizophrenia or schizoaffective disorder. Am J Psychiatry 2001;158(5): 765–74 [erratum: Am J Psychiatry 2001;158(10):1759].

[131] Azorin JM, Spiegel R, Remington G, et al. A double-blind comparative study of clozapine and risperidone in the management of severe chronic schizophrenia. Am J Psychiatry 2001; 158(8):1305–13.

[132] Meltzer HY, Alphs L, Green AI, et al, International Suicide Prevention Trial Study Group. Clozapine treatment for suicidality in schizophrenia: International Suicide Prevention Trial (InterSePT). Arch Gen Psychiatry 2003;60(1):82–91.

[133] Yatham LN, Paulsson B, Mullen J, et al. Quetiapine versus placebo in combination with lithium or divalproex for the treatment of bipolar mania. J Clin Psychopharmacol 2004;24(6): 599–606.

[134] Vieta E, Parramon G, Padrell E, et al. Quetiapine in the treatment of rapid cycling bipolar disorder. Bipolar Disord 2002;4(5):335–40.

[135] Barzman DH, DelBello MP, Kowatch RA, et al. The effectiveness and tolerability of aripiprazole for pediatric bipolar disorders: a retrospective chart review. J Child Adolesc Psychopharmacol 2004;14(4):593–600.

[136] Biederman J, McDonnell MA, Wozniak J, et al. Aripiprazole in the treatment of pediatric bipolar disorder: a systematic chart review. CNS Spectr 2005;10(2):141–8.

[137] McDougle CJ, Kem DL, Posey DJ. Case series: use of ziprasidone for maladaptive symptoms in youths with autism. J Am Acad Child Adolesc Psychiatry 2002;41(8):921–7.

[138] Mukaddes NM, Abali O. Quetiapine treatment of children and adolescents with Tourette's disorder. J Child Adolesc Psychopharmacol 2003;13(3):295–9.

[139] Delbello MP, Schwiers ML, Rosenberg HL, et al. A double-blind, randomized, placebo-controlled study of quetiapine as adjunctive treatment for adolescent mania. J Am Acad Child Adolesc Psychiatry 2002;41(10):1216–23.

[140] McConville B, Carrero L, Sweitzer D, et al. Long term safety, tolerability, and clinical efficacy of quetiapine in adolescents: an open-label extension trial. J Child Adolesc Psychopharmacol 2003;13(1):75–82.

[141] Aman MG, Gharabawi GM. Special Topic Advisory Panel on Transitioning to Risperidone Therapy in Patients With Mental Retardation and Developmental Disabilities. Treatment of behavior disorders in mental retardation: report on transitioning to atypical antipsychotics, with an emphasis on risperidone. J Clin Psychiatry 2004;65(9):1197–210.

[142] Shea S, Turgay A, Carroll A, et al. Risperidone in the treatment of disruptive behavioral symptoms in children with autistic and other pervasive developmental disorders. Pediatrics 2004;114(5):e634–41.

[143] Frazier JA, Biederman J, Tohen M, et al. A prospective open-label treatment trial of olanzapine monotherapy in children and adolescents with bipolar disorder. J Child Adolesc Psychopharmacol 2001;11(3):239–50.

[144] Kant R, Chalansani R, Chengappa KN, et al. The off-label use of clozapine in adolescents with bipolar disorder, intermittent explosive disorder, or posttraumatic stress disorder. J Child Adolesc Psychopharmacol 2004;14(1):57–63.

[145] Masi G, Mucci M, Millepiedi S. Clozapine in adolescent inpatients with acute mania. J Child Adolesc Psychopharmacol 2002;12(2):93–9.

[146] Kumra S, Frazier JA, Jacobsen LK, et al. Childhood-onset schizophrenia. A double-blind clozapine-haloperidol comparison. Arch Gen Psychiatry 1996;53(12):1090–7.

[147] Kumra S, Herion D, Jacobsen LK, et al. Case study: risperidone-induced hepatotoxicity in pediatric patients. J Am Acad Child Adolesc Psychiatry 1997;36(5):701–5.

[148] Szigethy E, Wiznitzer M, Branicky LA, et al. Risperidone-induced hepatotoxicity in children and adolescents? A chart review study. J Child Adolesc Psychopharmacol 1999;9(2):93–8.

[149] Gonzalez-Heydrich J, Raches D, Wilens TE, et al. Retrospective study of hepatic enzyme elevations in children treated with olanzapine, divalproex, and their combination. J Am Acad Child Adolesc Psychiatry 2003;42(10):1227–33.

[150] Stubner S, Grohmann R, Engel R, et al. Blood dyscrasias induced by psychotropic drugs. Pharmacopsychiatry 2004;37(Suppl 1):S70–8.

[151] Alvir JM, Lieberman JA. Agranulocytosis: incidence and risk factors. J Clin Psychiatry 1994; 55(Suppl B):137–8.

[152] Alvir JM, Lieberman JA, Safferman AZ, et al. Clozapine-induced agranulocytosis. Incidence and risk factors in the United States. N Engl J Med 1993;329(3):162–7.

[153] Usiskin SI, Nicolson R, Lenane M, et al. Retreatment with clozapine after erythromycin-induced neutropenia. Am J Psychiatry 2000;157(6):1021.

[154] Miller DD. Review and management of clozapine side effects. J Clin Psychiatry 2000; 61(Suppl 8):14–7 [discussion: 18–9].

[155] Sporn A, Gogtay N, Ortiz-Aguayo R, et al. Clozapine-induced neutropenia in children: management with lithium carbonate. J Child Adolesc Psychopharmacol 2003;13(3):401–4.

[156] McConville BJ, Arvanitis LA, Thyrum PT, et al. Pharmacokinetics, tolerability, and clinical effectiveness of quetiapine fumarate: an open-label trial in adolescents with psychotic disorders. J Clin Psychiatry 2000;61(4):252–60.

[157] Dobbs RL, Brahm NC, Fast G, et al. Thyroid function alterations following quetiapine initiation in a developmentally disabled adolescent. Ann Pharmacother 2004;38(9):1541–2.

[158] Kelly DL, Conley RR. Thyroid function in treatment-resistant schizophrenia patients treated with quetiapine, risperidone, or fluphenazine. J Clin Psychiatry 2005;66(1):80–4.

[159] Hedges D, Jeppson K, Whitehead P. Antipsychotic medication and seizures: a review. Drugs Today (Barc) 2003;39(7):551–7.

[160] Gonzalez-Heydrich J, Pandina GJ, Fleisher CA, et al. No seizure exacerbation from risperidone in youth with comorbid epilepsy and psychiatric disorders: a case series. J Child Adolesc Psychopharmacol 2004;14(2):295–310.

[161] Hedges DW, Jeppson KG. New-onset seizure associated with quetiapine and olanzapine. Ann Pharmacother 2002;36(3):437–9.

[162] Caroff SN, Mann SC, Campbell EC, et al. Movement disorders associated with atypical antipsychotic drugs. J Clin Psychiatry 2002;63(Suppl 4):12–9.

[163] Ananth J, Parameswaran S, Gunatilake S. Side effects of atypical antipsychotic drugs. Curr Pharm Des 2004;10(18):2219–29.

[164] Silva RR, Munoz DM, Alpert M, et al. Neuroleptic malignant syndrome in children and adolescents. J Am Acad Child Adolesc Psychiatry 1999;38(2):187–94.

[165] Hanft A, Eggleston CF, Bourgeois JA. Neuroleptic malignant syndrome in an adolescent after brief exposure to olanzapine. J Child Adolesc Psychopharmacol 2004;14(3):481–7.

[166] Spalding S, Alessi NE, Radwan K. Aripiprazole and atypical neuroleptic malignant syndrome. J Am Acad Child Adolesc Psychiatry 2004;43(12):1457–8.

[167] Abu-Kishk I, Toledano M, Reis A, et al. Neuroleptic malignant syndrome in a child treated with an atypical antipsychotic. J Toxicol Clin Toxicol 2004;42(6):921–5.

[168] Leibold J, Patel V, Hasan RA. Neuroleptic malignant syndrome associated with ziprasidone in an adolescent. Clin Ther 2004;26(7):1105–8.

[169] Zalsman G, Lewis R, Konas S, et al. Atypical neuroleptic malignant syndrome associated with risperidone treatment in two adolescents. Int J Adolesc Med Health 2004;16(2):179–82.

[170] Robb AS, Chang W, Lee HK, et al. Case study. Risperidone-induced neuroleptic malignant syndrome in an adolescent. J Child Adolesc Psychopharmacol 2000;10(4):327–30.

[171] Sharma R, Trappler B, Ng YK, et al. Risperidone-induced neuroleptic malignant syndrome. Ann Pharmacother 1996;30(7–8):775–8.

[172] Elliott SS, Keim NL, Stern JS, et al. Fructose, weight gain, and the insulin resistance syndrome. Am J Clin Nutr 2002;76(5):911–22.

[173] Ludwig DS, Peterson KE, Gortmaker SL. Relation between consumption of sugar-sweetened drinks and childhood obesity: a prospective, observational analysis. Lancet 2001;357(9255): 505–8.

[174] Howarth NC, Saltzman E, Roberts SB. Dietary fiber and weight regulation. Nutr Rev 2001; 59(5):129–39.

[175] Boule NG, Weisnagel SJ, Lakka TA, et al. Effects of exercise training on glucose homeostasis: the HERITAGE Family Study. Diabetes Care 2005;28(1):108–14.

[176] Berkel LA, Carlos Poston WS, Reeves RS, et al. Behavioral interventions for obesity. J Am Diet Assoc 2005;105(5 Pt 2):35–43.

[177] Simpson GM, Angus JW. A rating scale for extrapyramidal side effects. Acta Psychiatr Scand Suppl 1970;212:11–9.

[178] Chouinard G, Ross-Chouinard A, Annabel L, et al. The Extrapyramidal Symptom Rating Scale. Can J Neurol Sci 1980;7:233.

[179] Barnes TR. A rating scale for drug-induced akathisia. Br J Psychiatry 1989;154:672–6.

[180] Guy W, editor. ECDEU assessment manual for psychopharmacology. Publication #ABM 76–338. Washington (DC): US Department of Health, Education, and Welfare; 1976.

[181] Vitiello B, Riddle MA, Greenhill LL, et al. How can we improve the assessment of safety in child and adolescent psychopharmacology? J Am Acad Child Adolesc Psychiatry 2003;42(6): 634–41.

[182] Greenhill LL, Vitiello B, Abikoff H, et al. Developing methodologies for monitoring long-term safety of psychotropic medications in children: report on the NIMH conference, September 25, 2000. J Am Acad Child Adolesc Psychiatry 2003;42(6):651–5.

[183] Greenhill LL, Vitiello B, Fisher P, et al. Comparison of increasingly detailed elicitation methods for the assessment of adverse events in pediatric psychopharmacology. J Am Acad Child Adolesc Psychiatry 2004;43(12):1488–96.

[184] Committee on Nutrition. Prevention of pediatric overweight and obesity. Pediatrics 2003;112: 424–30.

[185] Williams CL, Hayman LL, Daniels SR, et al. Cardiovascular health in childhood: a statement for health professionals from the Committee on Atherosclerosis, Hypertension, and Obesity in the Young (AHOY) of the Council on Cardiovascular Disease in the Young, American Heart Association. Circulation 2002;106(1):143–60.

[186] Kane JM, Woerner M, Lieberman J. Tardive dyskinesia: prevalence, incidence, and risk factors. J Clin Psychopharmacol 1988;8(4 Suppl):52S–6S.

[187] Findling RL, McNamara NK, Youngstrom EA, et al. A prospective, open-label trial of olanzapine in adolescents with schizophrenia. J Am Acad Child Adolesc Psychiatry 2003; 42(2):170–5.

[188] Kumra S, Jacobsen LK, Lenane M, et al. Childhood-onset schizophrenia: an open-label study of olanzapine in adolescents. J Am Acad Child Adolesc Psychiatry 1998;37(4):377–85.

[189] Gerbino-Rosen G, Roofeh D, Tompkins DA, et al. Hematological adverse events in clozapine-treated children and adolescents. J Am Acad Child Adolesc Psychiatry 2005;44(10):1024–31.

ELSEVIER
SAUNDERS

Child Adolesc Psychiatric Clin N Am
15 (2006) 207–220

CHILD AND
ADOLESCENT
PSYCHIATRIC CLINICS
OF NORTH AMERICA

Female Puberty: Clinical Implications for the Use of Prolactin-Modulating Psychotropics

Amy L. Becker, MD[a],*, C. Neill Epperson, MD[b]

[a]*Yale University School of Medicine, Child Study Center, 230 South Frontage Road,
New Haven, CT 06520, USA*
[b]*Yale Behavioral Gynecology Program, Yale University School of Medicine,
100 York Street, New Haven, CT 06511, USA*

Puberty is a complex time in human development. As neuroendocrine functioning awakens, the capacity for reproduction develops, and skeletal mass and bone mineral density (BMD) increase. In the context of this dynamic process, girls may present with psychiatric illness necessitating treatment with psychotropic medications. Pubertal girls are especially vulnerable to medication-associated adverse events. Atypical antipsychotic (AAP) medications and antidepressants have the potential to elevate serum prolactin (PRL) levels, and hyperprolactinemia has the potential to alter the tempo of the pubertal progression and to inhibit the achievement of important developmental milestones. Clinicians must incorporate existing knowledge of normal pubertal development and evidence from clinical trials and case reports to optimize treatment outcomes. Selection of PRL-sparing AAP medications is recommended, as is treatment with the lowest effective dose of selective serotonin reuptake inhibitors (SSRIs). In addition, because many pubertal girls lack the capacity to express outward signs of hypothalamic-pituitary-gonadal (HPG) dysfunction such as galactorrhea or menstrual irregularities, monitoring of serum PRL levels may be necessary to rule out chronic hyperprolactinemia and to prevent the loss of developmentally critical bone mineral deposit.

Dr. Epperson is part of the Speakers' Bureau for Pfizer and GlaxoSmithKline, has received research grant support from Pfizer and Ely Lilly, and serves as a consultant to GlaxoSmithKline.
* Corresponding author.
E-mail address: alb1655@aol.com (A.L. Becker).

doi:10.1016/j.chc.2005.08.006
childpsych.theclinics.com

Rates of psychiatric illness and trends in psychotropic use in pubertal girls

Puberty is the multifaceted period of development between childhood and the attainment of adult reproductive capacity. In girls, it is not only a time for critical somatic growth but also one which heralds the onset of psychiatric illness. Pubertal girls are affected across diagnostic categories and are more commonly afflicted than their male counterparts with anxiety disorders, depression, and eating disorders. The lifetime prevalence of generalized anxiety disorder is estimated to be 5.1%, with a 2:1 female-to-male ratio, and studies of panic disorder in youth reflect an increased frequency of the diagnosis in female subjects [1,2]. Rates of depression in pubertal girls double when compared with males, and adolescent girls are affected approximately 10 times more often than males by anorexia nervosa and bulimia nervosa [3–7].

Illness-associated morbidity and mortality require clinicians to be familiar with substantial treatment options, including potential impacts of psychopharmacology during puberty. Few psychotropic medications have been approved by the Food and Drug Administration for specific indications in children and adolescents (Table 1). However, off-label use of medications is estimated to constitute approximately 75% of pediatric use [8]. Pharmacoepidemiologic studies show that SSRI antidepressants are the second most commonly prescribed psychotropic medications to children and adolescents, and antipsychotic medications seem to be among the seven most commonly prescribed classes of psychotropic medications [9,10]. Studies conducted in the United States, the United Kingdom, and Australia additionally demonstrate that prescription rates for antipsychotic medications have increased dramatically during the past decade, in some settings more than twofold, and recent research found the prevalence of AAP use in girls to peak during puberty [11,12]. SSRIs and AAP medications

Table 1
Medications, indications, and prolactin effects

Medication	Food and Drug Administration indication in children and adolescents/age (years)	Prolactin effect
Fluoxetine	Depression (7–17)	↑
	Obsessive-compulsive disorder (7–17)	
Paroxetine	None	↑
Sertraline	Obsessive-compulsive disorder (6–17)	↑
Citalopram	None	↑
Fluvoxamine	Obsessive-compulsive disorder (8–17)	↑
Venlafaxine	None	↑
Mirtazapine	None	↔
Clozapine	None	↔
Quetiapine	None	↔
Olanzapine	None	↑
Ziprasidone	None	↑
Risperidone	None	↑
Aripiprazole	None	↔

have the capacity to alter pubertal development in girls, so appreciating the interface between pubertal development and psychopharmacology is essential.

Hallmarks of female pubertal progression

Hypothalamic-pituitary-gonadal axis

Puberty begins as the gonadotropin-releasing hormone (GnRH) pulse generator of the hypothalamus becomes active. GnRH signals the anterior pituitary gland to release pulsatile bursts of the gonadotropic hormones, lutenizing hormone (LH), and follicle-stimulating hormone (FSH), and gonadotropin levels increase exponentially throughout the perimenarchal period [13,14]. LH stimulates the theca cells of the ovarian follicles to synthesize androgens from cholesterol. FSH acts on the granulosa cells of the ovarian follicles to convert the androgens to estrogens through activation of the cytochrome P-450 aromatase. The ovaries are the primary source of estrogen synthesis in pubertal girls, and estrogen levels rise as follicular production is stimulated by the gonadotropins. Estrogens exert an autocrine function on ovarian follicles, stimulating the growth and development of granulosa cells.

In addition, estrogens act peripherally in the female body on the vagina, uterus, and mammary glands to promote their maturation. Estrogen receptors are located on peripheral adipocytes, where estrogens probably act to signal the characteristic pattern of fat deposition seen in women, and estrogen receptors are found in dermal papilla cells where they seem to increase the production of androgen receptors and promote hair growth [15,16]. Furthermore, estrogens act centrally in the nervous system where they foster structural and functional brain development, and estrogens continually provide feedback to the HPG axis as the cyclic feedback loop of the menstrual cycle is established [17].

Staging

The staging of this pubertal progression was characterized by Tanner [17a] in his seminal paper from 1969 and includes stages I through V in girls (Table 2). These stages span the time from prepuberty to menarche, the onset of the menstrual cycle. The progression from Tanner stages I to V takes an average of 3 to 4 years [18,19]. Although there is individual variation, and a decline in the age of onset has been noted during the past decade, girls typically begin to develop secondary sex characteristics at age 10 years. Most often girls begin with breast development, thelarche, and then advance to pubic and axillary hair growth and genital development. Menarche typically occurs around age 12 years, a milestone whose timing has not changed in the United States and Europe in approximately 50 years, and regular ovulatory menstrual cycles are attained approximately 2 to 3 years after menarche [20–22].

Table 2
Chronology of female adolescent development

Tanner stage	Clinical signs of development	Developmental features	Approximate age (years)
I	Prepuberty		
II	Breast budding		10
	Minimal pubic hair		
III	Elevation of breast contour	Growth spurt	
	Areolae enlarge	Peak height velocity	
	Course, dark pubic hair spreads over mons pubis		
	Axillary hair develops		
IV	Areola forms secondary mound on breast	Menarche	12
	Pubic hair of adult quality		
V	Adult breast contour	Regular menses	15
	Adult distribution of pubic hair	Whole-body bone mineral density plateaus	16

Somatic growth and skeletal development

Along with developing secondary sexual characteristics, pubertal girls undergo rapid physical growth and skeletal maturation. The timing of the pubertal growth spurt in girls typically occurs during Tanner stage III, approximately 1 year before the age it occurs in boys, and 90% of adult stature is attained as peak height velocity is reached [23,24]. The estimated duration of the growth spurt in girls is 3 years, compared with 4 years in males, and girls average a total stature gain of approximately 25 cm [22].

Linear growth of the bones in the appendicular skeleton precedes the growth of those in the axial skeleton, and skeletal mass is estimated to double between puberty and young adulthood. Metabolic markers of bone turnover in puberty are four times the levels measured in adults, including bone-specific alkaline phosphatase, which seems to peak in girls during Tanner stage III and decline to adult levels during Tanner stage V [25]. These changes reflect an active modeling and remodeling process, and bone mineral content and BMD increase as skeletal size and volume increase [26]. Whole-body BMD seems to plateau in females at approximately age 16 years, which precedes the plateau seen in males by 1 year. The convergence of these dynamic metabolic processes in the first 2 decades of life culminates in the attainment of approximately 90% of peak bone mass (PBM), and optimal accumulation of PBM is important in determining eventual bone strength and in preventing the later development of osteoporosis [23,27].

Determinants of peak bone mass

Multiple factors, including gender and hormones, influence the accrual of PBM. Because girls begin to mature earlier than boys, they have less prepubertal growth of the appendicular skeleton. Moreover, the duration of the pubertal growth spurt is shorter than in boys, and the combination of these factors theoretically leads women to have less overall bone mass.

Adequate circulating levels of functioning hormones are critical in skeletal growth and maturation. Estrogens, growth hormone (GH) and insulin-like growth factor (IGF) seem to serve both independent and interrelated functions in the maturational process [28]. Estrogen stimulates the pulsatile release of GH, whose skeletal effects seem to be mediated by IGF. The GH/IGF combination promotes the proliferation and differentiation of osteoblasts, which are the cells responsible for bone formation. In addition, GH/IGF fosters the retention and production of elements essential for bone mineralization, including renal phosphate, vitamin D, and gastrointestinal calcium [26,29,30]. GH/IGF reciprocally stimulates the ovarian release of estrogen and potentiates its effects on bone. Estrogen functions in a capacity similar to that of the GH/IGF combination. It mediates calcium flux and vitamin D production; in addition, estrogen receptors are located on osteoblasts and chondrocytes, the cartilage-producing cells of the skeleton [31–33]. Estrogen seems to influence the balance between bone formation and resorption, with estrogen deficiency favoring resorption, and high levels of estrogen are necessary for the fusion of epiphyseal growth plates, a phenomenon seen during the latter stages of puberty as growth velocity plateaus [34]. The importance of estrogen in normal skeletal development and maturation is further demonstrated in cases where aberrant estrogen production or function is associated with skeletal abnormalities, including the presumed HPG axis dysfunction associated with psychotropic-induced hyperprolactinemia.

Prolactin

Structure, function, and regulation

PRL is a protein produced in the anterior pituitary gland. The majority of circulating hormone is a 23-kd molecule, but additional polypeptide structures with biologic activity have been described, possibly products of posttranslational modification or dimerization [35]. The specific functions and potential clinical significance of the different PRL species in females has yet to be determined. Serum PRL levels in childhood remain low, but sleep-related increases are noted throughout the pubertal progression. In sexually mature females, PRL is released from the anterior pituitary gland in a pulsatile fashion, and circulating levels are found to be higher than those in sexually mature males [19].

PRL works synergistically with estrogen and progesterone to promote mammary gland development and milk protein production, or lactogenesis. In the postpartum period, PRL also couples with oxytocin to maintain the production and release of milk. PRL also seems to have a role in ovarian follicular maturation and steroid production, and in sexually mature females PRL functions to sustain the corpus luteum, which is essential for the production of progesterone and the maintenance of normal reproductive functioning [36].

PRL secretion is governed by a number of factors, both inhibitory and stimulatory. The main factor inhibiting PRL release is dopamine produced in the tuberoinfundibular tract of the hypothalamus. Dopamine is released from the hypothalamus into the portal circulation, which subsequently binds to the dopamine (D2) receptors on the lactotrophic cells of the anterior pituitary. Stimulation of the D2 receptors activates a complex cascade of intracellular events and second-messenger systems that lead to inhibition of the production and release of PRL.

Conversely, PRL secretion is stimulated by estrogens at the levels of the hypo-thalamus and the pituitary. Estrogens modulate the release of dopamine from the hypothalamus, and they stimulate the expression of the *PRL* gene, the multipli-cation of lactotrophic cells, and the decreased production of D2 receptors on the lactotrophic cell surface [37].

Serotonin (5HT) also seems to affect the release of PRL through a com-bination of direct and indirect mechanisms. Studies examining serotonergic ago-nists such as DL-fenfluramine demonstrate an increase in PRL levels after acute administration of 5HT. Blockade of various 5HT receptor subtypes leads to a blunting of PRL response; the receptor subtypes that seem to mediate the inter-action between 5HT and PRL include 5HT1, 5HT2, and 5HT3 [38,39]. Animal and human studies also have demonstrated that 5HT impairs the production and function of dopamine, the main inhibitory factor regulating PRL release [40].

Effects of elevated prolactin levels

Elevated PRL alters HPG axis functioning in females. It seems to inhibit the release of GnRH from the hypothalamus, which subsequently disrupts the normal pulsatile secretion of FSH and LH from the anterior pituitary gland. Results of longitudinal and cross-sectional studies of lactational amenorrhea and hyper-prolactinemia further suggest that PRL may have a direct role in blocking gonadotropin actions on the ovary [36]. Aberrant follicular development has also been visualized by ultrasound in sexually mature women with elevated PRL levels, and hyperprolactinemia seems to impair the selection of a domi-nant ovarian follicle, leading to the production of an inadequately primed corpus luteum or anovulatory menstrual cycles. In addition, in vitro studies have dem-onstrated inhibition of sex steroid synthesis, so that elevated PRL levels antago-nize LH-directed androgen production and block FSH-induced aromatization of androgens to estrogens [41].

The clinical manifestations of hyperprolactinemia in females have been well documented in reports describing prolactinomas, hormone-secreting tumors of the pituitary gland. Symptoms of prolactinomas include galactorrhea, menstrual irregularities, infertility, and osteopenia. The incidence of galactorrhea in normal sexually mature women subjects is estimated to be as high as 45%. Galactorrhea becomes a better predictor of elevated PRL when combined with menstrual irregularities [42]. Reliance on these indicators in pubertal girls is not always possible, however. Mammary glands may be inadequately primed by sex steroids, preventing the development of galactorrhea, or the menstrual cycle regularity may not be established. Delayed pubertal development, including primary amenorrhea, has been observed in females, and osteopenia has been confirmed in case reports of children and adolescents with prolactinomas [43–45]. Clinical findings are associated with a wide range of serum PRL levels, and although pubertal development and reproductive functioning are frequently restored with dopamine agonist therapy, findings with regard to bone mass are less encouraging. Treatment seems to lead to improvement but not restoration of bone mass, even after normalization of PRL levels for up to 24 months. The duration of hyperprolactinemia may play a role in the development of osteopenia, with longer duration conferring a greater risk, and BMD that is one SD below mean age-population values is thought to double the risk for fractures [46]. Hormonal measures included in studies of prolactinomas vary, and although many studies report gonadotropin and PRL levels, few studies include measures of estrogen. This frequent omission makes it difficult to substantiate the association between hyperprolactinemia and decreased levels of sex steroids in pubertal girls; however, decreased estrogen production is generally believed to be a central factor mediating the development of osteopenia.

Impact of psychotropic medications on prolactin

Antipsychotic medications

AAP medications have been shown to elevate basal PRL levels in females. Studies have included women of reproductive and postmenopausal age and pubertal girls. Youth demonstrate greater PRL elevations in response to AAP medications than do adults, a finding presumably related to a higher density of D2 receptors in the developing striatum or to differential D2 receptor sensitivity in the tuberoinfundibular tract [47,48]. Females demonstrate an increased PRL response to antipsychotic administration when compared with males with equivalent dosing [37,49].

It is estimated that D2 receptor occupancy of greater than 50% results in elevated PRL levels [50]. AAP medications possess unique receptor profiles, and agents vary in their propensity to cause PRL elevation. Clozapine and quetiapine have relatively low affinity for D2 receptors, and results of numerous trials support their description as PRL-sparing agents [49,51–54]. Olanzapine has a receptor profile similar to that of clozapine, and ziprasidone is noted to have a high 5HT2a/D2 affinity ratio. Olanzapine and ziprasidone are generally believed to cause moderate but transient effects on PRL levels, although data on ziprasidone are limited to a single study including few female subjects with Tourette's syndrome [55]. Additionally, a pediatric olanzapine trial conducted at the National Institute of Mental Health found PRL levels elevated above baseline at 6 weeks, and one open-label study in adult men receiving high-dose olanzapine demonstrated sustained PRL elevation at 40 weeks [49,56–59]. Risperidone has a high affinity for D2 receptors and is a potent D2 antagonist. PRL elevation from baseline has been established in controlled trials with risperidone in children and adolescents, and significant elevation has been found to be sustained in adults for up to 60 weeks [56,57,60,61]. Aripiprazole is a novel antipsychotic that acts as a partial D2 agonist. Although studies of aripiprazole in children and adolescents do not include measures of serum PRL, adult subjects in controlled studies demonstrate a decrease in PRL levels from baseline through 6 weeks of drug administration [62,63].

Clinical symptoms associated with AAP-induced hyperprolactinemia include galactorrhea and menstrual irregularities. Young women seem to be more susceptible to these adverse events than adult females [48,60]. The degree of PRL elevation has not consistently been correlated with AAP dose, and results of one study that measured serum drug concentrations suggest that serum levels may be a better correlate than actual dose [47]. Switching from a PRL-elevating to a PRL-sparing agent may lead to a reduction in serum PRL, although the development of galactorrhea and menstrual irregularities has not been associated consistently with extent of hyperprolactinemia [54,56,61]. PRL elevation beyond baseline occurs in up to 100% of subjects, depending on the agent studied, and adverse clinical events appear in up to 12% of subjects, most often in those taking risperidone [48,60]. Studies of AAP use in pubertal girls do not include measures of estrogen or BMD; however, adult women receiving chronic typical antipsychotic therapy demonstrate a significant reduction in BMD. Moreover, an inverse relationship between PRL and BMD has been reported in sexually mature women taking risperidone, with elevated serum PRL levels associated with greater decreases in BMD [37,64,65].

Antidepressant medications

Acute and long-term administration of SSRIs also increases basal PRL levels in females [66,67]. Increased PRL levels have been detected after administration of fluoxetine, sertraline, paroxetine, fluvoxamine, and citalopram with variable dosing and routes of administration. Female subjects included in these studies have been of reproductive age as well as postmenopausal [68]. Investigations that have demonstrated an SSRI-induced increase in serum PRL have included healthy women and those diagnosed with unipolar and bipolar depression [69–73].

Numerous case reports also detail clinical symptoms associated with SSRI use, including galactorrhea and amenorrhea. Serum PRL was not measured in all cases, but those that did found elevated levels, generally around twice the upper limit of normal. Case reports of SSRIs associated with galactorrhea and menstrual irregularities so far include fluoxetine, sertraline, fluvoxamine, and paroxetine, and all subjects demonstrated remission of symptoms after a decrease in medication dosage or discontinuation of its use [74–81].

Methodologies have not been uniform across studies examining the association between SSRIs and hyperprolactinemia. Only one case to date has reported symptoms in an adolescent girl, and, in addition, many studies do not control for variables that potentially complicate outcomes [77]. These factors challenge the ability to draw meaningful conclusions from existing evidence and to apply that knowledge to clinical practice with pubertal girls. For example, there is evidence to suggest that psychiatric illness and the associated biologic underpinnings may impact PRL response to 5HT stimulation, making it difficult to pool data from studies that combine healthy subjects and subjects with a diagnosis of unipolar or bipolar depression [82]. In addition, many SSRI studies permitted female subjects to take concurrent estrogen replacement therapy or benzodiazepines, both of which have been shown to modulate PRL release [83].

Despite the mixed methodologies and a lack of controlled studies in pubertal girls, a number of findings appear consistently in SSRI research. First, females demonstrate a greater sensitivity to the PRL-elevating effects of 5HT than males, potentially related to the stimulatory effects of estrogen. Second, the degree of PRL elevation seems to be positively correlated with increased medication dose, and route of administration may play a role in modulating PRL response to 5HT, at least theoretically, with intravenous administration of SSRIs showing the most robust PRL elevation [67,84]. Finally, although the understanding of the neurodevelopment of the serotonergic system in children and adolescents remains limited, existing data support the theory that youth demonstrate therapeutic responsivity to SSRIs equal to that seen in adults (unlike the case with tricyclic antidepressants, for example), suggesting that children and adolescents may be as susceptible as adults to SSRI-induced adverse events such as elevated PRL levels [85].

Through their serotonergic or dopaminergic mechanisms of action, nefazadone, buproprion, venlafaxine, and mirtazapine theoretically also have the capacity to modulate the release of PRL. Although less is known about the effects of nefazadone and buproprion, cases of galactorrhea have been reported in adult women taking venlafaxine [86,87]. Controlled studies of mirtazapine in adult men showed a decrease in serum PRL after drug administration. This interesting finding is probably related to mirtazapine's atypical mode of action. Although mirtazapine is an indirect 5HT1 agonist, it also acts to block 5HT2 and 5HT3 receptors, and this blocking is believed to be the property responsible for the observed endocrinologic effects [88–90].

Implications for the assessment and treatment of pubertal girls

Once the determination is made to recommend treatment with a PRL-modulating psychotropic medication, informed consent should include the potential for hyperprolactinemia-induced HPG axis dysfunction and the resultant sequelae, such as delayed pubertal development or loss of bone mineral deposit. In addition, premedication screening should include specific questions that determine pubertal stage, and collaboration with pediatricians is essential to monitor the pubertal progression closely and to watch for clinical signs of elevated PRL levels, such as menstrual irregularities or galactorrhea detected on physical examination. Girls initially treated with an AAP or antidepressant may be early in their pubertal development and may not possess the capacity to develop outward signs of elevated PRL levels. Instead, HPG axis function may be less obviously disrupted by antidepressant- or AAP-induced PRL elevation, leading to delayed development and impaired skeletal maturation. The challenge for clinicians becomes identifying these adverse events in a timely fashion. One study of adolescent girls demonstrated that 6 months of HPG axis dysfunction can lead to reduction in BMD to two SD below the population mean [91]. This finding highlights the importance of early intervention during this critical time in skeletal development and BMD accrual. The normal progression from thelarche to menarche can take up to 3 years, and delayed pubertal maturation frequently is not identified in girls until they are 16 years old [92]. Individual variation in the tempo of this progression further complicates the timely identification of delayed maturation.

The difficulty inherent in making a clinical diagnosis of PRL-induced HPG dysfunction in early-pubescent girls requires clinicians to consider alternate preventative and early-intervention strategies. When feasible, selection of a PRL- sparing agent is recommended, as is treatment with the lowest therapeutic dose of SSRIs. If these options do not prove efficacious, and treatment with an alternate AAP or high-dose SSRI is deemed necessary, consideration should be given to monitoring serum PRL levels. The absolute PRL level does not seem to be useful in guiding treatment, because it is not consistently correlated with adverse events. Perhaps the more relevant measure should be the degree of change of serum levels over time or from baseline. Case reports of prolactinomas in children demonstrate that an elevation in PRL level of as little as twice the upper limit of normal can lead to osteopenia [45]. This finding suggests that PRL measures that are twice the upper limit of normal or twice the baseline value may be of concern and justify an AAP switch or SSRI dosage adjustment. In addition, although not presently the standard of care, monitoring serum PRL levels in pubertal girls taking PRL-modulating agents every 6 months may be a reasonable indirect measure of HPG axis function. Until sexual maturity and menstrual cycle regularity are achieved, this practice would probably identify abnormalities early and allow clinical interventions that could minimize irreversible BMD loss.

Future directions

For all psychotropic agents, controlled and longitudinal psychopharmacology studies are needed that include measures of pubertal development, serum levels of hormones, and determinants of BMD and turnover. In addition, because absolute levels of hormones do not consistently correlate with clinical observations, new study paradigms need to be developed to offer explanations for apparent discrepancies. Future considerations may include fractioning PRL of varying molecular weights to correlate with clinical findings or examining the estrogen-to-PRL ratio in HPG axis dysfunction as it relates to loss in BMD.

References

[1] Masi G, Millepiedi S, Mucci M, et al. Generalized anxiety disorder in referred children and adolescents. J Am Acad Child Adolesc Psychiatry 2004;43(6):752–60.

[2] Diler RS, Birmaher B, Brent D, et al. Phenomenology of panic disorder in youth. Depress Anxiety 2004;20:39–43.

[3] Angold A, Worthman C. Puberty onset of gender differences in rates of depression: a developmental, epidemiologic and neuroendocrine perspective. J Affect Disord 1993;29:145–58.

[4] Born L, Shea A, Steiner M. The roots of depression in adolescent girls: is menarche the key. Curr Psychiatry Rep 2002;4(6):449–60.

[5] Ebeling H, Tapanainen P, Joutsenoja A, et al. A practice guideline for treatment of eating disorders in children and adolescents. Ann Med 2003;35:488–501.

[6] Gowers S, Bryant-Waugh R. Management of child and adolescent eating disorders: the current evidence base and future directions. J Child Psychol Psychiatry 2004;45(1):63–83.

[7] Kotler LA, Walsh BT. Eating disorders in children and adolescents: pharmacological therapies. Eur Child Adolesc Psychiatry 2000;9(Suppl 1):I108–16.

[8] Unapproved uses of approved drugs: the physician, the package insert and the Food and Drug Administration: subject review. American Academy of Pediatrics Committee on Drugs. Pediatrics 1996;98(1):143–5.

[9] Jensen P, Bhatara V, Vitiello B, et al. Psychoactive medication prescribing practices for US children: gaps between research and clinical practice. J Am Acad Child Adolesc Psychiatry 1999;38(5):557–65.

[10] Martin A, Van Hoof T, Stubbe D, et al. Multiple psychotropic pharmacotherapy among child and adolescent enrollees in Connecticut Medicaid managed care. Psychiatr Serv 2003;54(1):72–7.

[11] Kaye J, Bradbury B, Jick H. Changes in antipsychotic drug prescribing by general practitioners in the United Kingdom from 1991 to 2000: a population-based observational study. Br J Clin Pharmacol 2003;56:569–75.

[12] Curtis L, Masselink L, Ostbye T, et al. Prevalence of atypical antipsychotic drug use among commercially insured youths in the United States. Arch Pediatr Adolesc Med 2005;159:362–6.

[13] Legro R, Mo Lin H, Demers L, et al. Rapid maturation of the reproductive axis during perimenarche independent of body composition. J Clin Endocrinol Metab 2000;85:1021–5.

[14] Demir A, Dunkel L, Stenman U, et al. Age-related course of urinary gonadotropins in children. J Clin Endocrinol Metab 1995;80:1457–60.

[15] Penny R, Goldstein I, Frasiet D. Gonadotropin excretion and body composition. Pediatrics 1978;61(2):294–300.

[16] Garnett S, Hogler W, Blades B, et al. Relation between hormones and body composition, including bone, in prepubertal children. Am J Clin Nutr 2004;80:966–72.

[17] Alonso L, Rosenfield R. Oestrogens and puberty. Best Pract Res Clin Endocrinol Metab 2002;16(1):13–30.

[17a] Marshall WA, Tanner JM. Variations in the pattern of pubertal changes in girls. Arch Dis Child 1969;44:291–303.

[18] Ducharme JR, Forest MG. Normal pubertal development. In: Bertrand J, Rappaport R, Sizonenko P, editors. Pediatric endocrinology: physiology, pathophysiology and clinical aspects. 2nd edition. Baltimore (MD): Williams and Wilkins; 1993. p. 372–7.

[19] Schwartz ID, Bercu BB. Normal growth and development. In: Hung W, editor. Clinical pediatric endocrinology. St. Louis (MO): Mosby Year Book; 1992. p. 30–3.

[20] Apter D, Hermanson E. Update on female pubertal development. Curr Opin Obstet Gyn 2002; 14(5):475–81.

[21] Legro R, Mo Lin H, Demers L, et al. Rapid maturation of the reproductive axis during perimenarche independent of body composition. J Clin Endocrinol Metab 2000;85:1021–5.

[22] Rogol AD, Roemmich JN, Clark PA. Growth at puberty. J Adolesc Health 2002;31:192–200.

[23] Mora S, Gilsanz V. Establishment of peak bone mass. Endocrinol Metab Clin North Am 2003;32:39–63.

[24] Braillon PM. Annual changes in bone mineral content and body composition during growth. Horm Res 2003;60:284–90.

[25] Fares JE, Choncair M, Nabulsi M, et al. Effect of gender, puberty and vitamin D status on biochemical markers of bone remodeling. Bone 2003;33:242–7.

[26] Saggese G, Baroncelli G, Bertelloni S. Puberty and bone development. Best Pract Res Clin Endocrinol Metab 2002;16(1):53–64.

[27] Javaid MK, Cooper C. Prenatal and childhood influences on osteoporosis. Best Pract Res Clin Endocrinol Metab 2002;16(2):349–67.

[28] Holmes SJ, Shalet SM. Role of growth hormone and sex steroids in achieving and maintaining normal bone mass. Horm Res 1996;45:86–93.

[29] Ho KY, Evans WS, Blizzard RM, et al. Effects of sex and age on the 24-hour profile of growth hormone secretion in man: importance of endogenous estradiol concentrations. J Clin Endocrinol Metab 1987;64(1):51–8.

[30] Libanati C, Baylink DJ, Lois-Wenzel E, et al. Studies on the potential mediators of skeletal changes occurring during puberty in girls. J Clin Endocrinol Metab 1999;84(8):2807–14.

[31] Van Coeverden S, Netelenbos JC, de Ridder CM, et al. Bone metabolism markers and bone mass in healthy pubertal boys and girls. Clin Endocrinol (Oxf) 2002;57:107–16.

[32] Saggese G, Bertelloni S, Baroncelli GI. Sex steroids and the acquisition of bone mass. Horm Res 1997;48(Suppl 5):65–71.

[33] Marcus R. New perspectives on the skeletal role of estrogen [editorial]. J Clin Endocrinol Metab 1998;83(7):2236–7.

[34] Lee PA, Witchel SF. The influence of estrogen on growth. Curr Opin Pediatr 1997;9:431–6.

[35] Duntas LH. Prolactinomas in children and adolescents—consequences in adult life. J Pediatr Endocrinol Metab 2001;14:1227–32.

[36] McNeilly AS, Glasier A, Swanston I, et al. Prolactin and the human ovary. In: Tolis G, Stefanis C, Mountokalakis T, et al, editors. Prolactin and prolactinomas. New York: Raven Press; 1982. p. 173–7.

[37] Wieck A, Haddad PM. Antipsychotic-induced hyperprolactinemia in women: pathophysiology, severity and consequences. Br J Psychiatry 2003;182:199–204.

[38] Laakmann G, Chuang I, Gugath M, et al. Prolactin and antidepressants. In: Tolis G, Stefanis C, Mountokalakis T, et al, editors. Prolactin and prolactinomas. New York: Raven Press; 1982. p. 151–61.

[39] Spigset O, Mjorndal T. The effect of fluvoxamine on serum prolactin and serum sodium concentrations: related to platelet 5–ht2a receptor status. J Clin Psychopharmacol 1997;17:292–7.

[40] Arya DK. Extrapyramidal symptoms with selective serotonin reuptake inhibitors. Br J Psychiatry 1994;165:728–33.

[41] Malarkey W. Effects of hyperprolactinemia on other endocrine systems. In: Olefsky J, Robbins R, editors. Contemporary issues in endocrinology and metabolism, vol. 2: prolactinomas. New York: Churchill Livingstone; 1986. p. 21–33.

[42] Molitch M. Manifestations, epidemiology, and pathogenesis of prolactinomas in women. In: Olefsky J, Robbins R, editors. Contemporary Issues in endocrinology and metabolism, vol. 2: prolactinomas. New York: Churchill Livingstone; 1986. p. 67–89.

[43] Fideleff H, Boquete H, Sequera A, et al. Peripubertal prolactinomas: clinical presentation and long-term outcome with different therapeutic approaches. J Pediatr Endocrinol Metab 2000;13:261–7.

[44] Colao A, Loche S, Cappa M, et al. Prolactinomas in children and adolescents. Clinical presentation and long-term follow-up. J Clin Endocrinol Metab 1998;83(8):2777–80.

[45] Galli-Tsinopoulou A, Nousia-Arvanitakis S, Mitsiakos G, et al. Osteopenia in children and adolescents with hyperprolactinemia. J Pediatr Endocrinol Metab 2000;13:439–41.

[46] Colao A, Di Somma C, Loche S, et al. Prolactinomas in adolescents: persistent bone loss after two years of prolactin normalization. Clin Endocrinol (Oxf) 2000;52:319–27.

[47] Alfaro C, Wudarsky M, Nicolson R, et al. Correlation of antipsychotic and prolactin concentrations in children and adolescents acutely treated with haloperidol, clozapine, or olanzapine. J Child Adolesc Psychopharmacol 2002;12(2):83–91.

[48] Woods S, Martin A, Spector S, et al. Effects of development on olanzapine-associated adverse events. J Am Acad Child Adolesc Psychiatry 2002;41(12):1439–46.

[49] Wudarsky M, Nicolson R, Hamburger S, et al. elevated prolactin in pediatric patients on typical and atypical antipsychotics. J Child Adolesc Psychopharmacol 1999;9(4):239–45.

[50] Naidoo U, Goff DC, Klibanski A. Hyperprolactinemia and bone mineral density: the potential impact of antipsychotic agents. Psychoneuroendocrinology 2003;28:97–108.

[51] Borison R, Arvantis L, Miller B. ICI 204,636, an atypical antipsychotic: efficacy and safety in a multicenter, placebo-controlled trial in patients with schizophrenia. J Clin Psychopharmacol 1996;16:158–69.

[52] Shaw J, Lewis J, Pascal S, et al. A Study of quetiapine: efficacy and tolerability in psychotic adolescents. J Child Adolesc Psychopharmacol 2001;11(4):415–24.

[53] Small J, Hirsch S, Arvanitis L, et al. Quetiapine in patients with schizophrenia. Arch Gen Psychiatry 1997;54:549–57.

[54] Breier A, Malhotra A, Su TP, et al. Clozapine and risperidone in chronic schizophrenia: effects on symptoms, parkinsonian side effects, and neuroendocrine response. Am J Psychiatry 1999; 156(2):294–8.

[55] Sallee F, Kurlan R, Goetz C, et al. Ziprasidone treatment of children and adolescents with Tourette's syndrome: a pilot study. J Am Acad Child Adolesc Psychiatry 2000;39(3):292–9.

[56] Kinon B, Gilmore J, Liu H, et al. Hyperprolactinemia in response to antipsychotic drugs: characterization across comparative clinical trials. Psychoneuroendocrinology 2003;28:69–82.

[57] David S, Taylor C, Kinon B, et al. The effects of olanzapine, risperidone, and haloperidol on plasma prolactin levels in patients with schizophrenia. Clin Ther 2000;22(9):1085–96.

[58] Bronson B, Lindenmayer JP. Adverse effects of high-dose olanzapine in treatment-refractory schizophrenia. J Clin Psychopharmacol 2000;20(3):382–4.

[59] Stigler K, Potenza M, McDougle C. Tolerability profile of atypical antipsychotics in children and adolescents. Paediatr Drugs 2001;3(12):927–42.

[60] Findling R, Kusumakar V, Daneman D, et al. Prolactin levels during long-term risperidone treatment in children and adolescents. J Clin Psychiatry 2003;64(11):1362–9.

[61] Kleinberg D, Davis J, De Coster R, et al. Prolactin levels and adverse events in patients treated with risperidone. J Clin Psychopharmacol 1999;19:57–61.

[62] Marder S, McQuade R, Stock E, et al. Aripiprazole in the treatment of schizophrenia: safety and tolerability in short-term, placebo-controlled trials. Schizophr Res 2003;61:123–36.

[63] Mallikaarjun S, Salazar D, Bramer S. Pharmacokinetics, tolerability, and safety of aripiprazole following multiple oral dosing in normal healthy volunteers. J Clin Pharmacol 2004; 44:179–87.

[64] Abraham G, Friedman R, Verghese C. Osteoporosis demonstrated by dual energy X-ray absorptiometry in chronic schizophrenic patients. Biol Psychiatry 1996;40:430–1.

[65] Abraham G, Halbreich U, Friedman R, et al. Bone mineral density and prolactin associations in patients with chronic schizophrenia. Schizophr Res 2002;59:17–8.

[66] Sagud M, Pivac N, Muck-Seler D, et al. Effects of sertraline treatment on plasma cortisol, prolactin and thyroid hormones in female depressed patients. Neuropsychobiology 2002;45: 139–43.

[67] Attenburrow MJ, Mitter PR, Whale R, et al. Low-dose citalopram as a 5-HT neuroendocrine probe. Psychopharmacology (Berl) 2001;155:323–6.

[68] Urban R, Veldhuis J. A selective serotonin reuptake inhibitor, fluoxetine hydrochloride, modu-

lates the pulsatile release of prolactin in postmenopausal women. Am J Obstet Gynecol 1991; 164:147–52.

[69] Amsterdam J, Garcia-Espana F, Goodman D, et al. Breast enlargement during chronic antidepressant therapy. J Affect Disord 1997;46:151–6.

[70] Dulchin M, Oquendo M, Malone K, et al. Prolactin response to DL-fenfluramine challenge before and after treatment with paroxetine. Neuropsychopharmacology 2001;25:395–401.

[71] Cowen PJ, Sargent PA. Changes in plasma prolactin during SSRI treatment: evidence for a delayed increase in 5-HT neurotransmission. J Psychopharmacol 1997;11(4):345–8.

[72] Laine K, Anttila M, Heinonen E, et al. Lack of adverse interactions between concomitantly administered selegiline and citalopram. Clin Neuropharmacol 1997;20(5):419–33.

[73] Spigset O, Mjorndal T. The effect of fluvoxamine on serum prolactin and serum sodium concentrations: relation to platelet 5–HT2A receptor status. J Clin Psychopharmacol 1997;17(4): 292–7.

[74] Morrison J, Remick R, Leung M, et al. Galactorrhea induced by paroxetine. Can J Psychiatry 2001;46(1):88–9.

[75] Jeffries J, Bezchlibnyk-Bulter K, Remington G. Amenorrhea and galactorrhea associated with fluvoxamine in a loxapine-treated patient. J Clin Psychopharmacol 1992;12(4):296–7.

[76] Peterson M. Reversible galactorrhea and prolactin elevation related to fluoxetine use. Mayo Clin Proc 2001;76:215–6.

[77] Iancu I, Ratzoni G, Weitzman A, et al. More fluoxetine experience. J Am Acad Child Adolesc Psychiatry 1992;31(4):755–6.

[78] Lesaca T. Sertraline and galactorrhea. J Clin Psychopharmacol 1996;16(4):333–4.

[79] Bronzo M, Stahl S. Galactorrhea induced by sertraline. Am J Psychiatry 1993;150(8):1269–70.

[80] Davenport E. A Case of paroxetine-induced galactorrhea. Can J Psychiatry 2002;47(9):890–1.

[81] Gonzalez E, Minguez L, Sanguino RM. Galactorrhea after paroxetine treatment. Pharmacopsychiatry 2000;33:118.

[82] O'Keane V, Dinan T. Prolactin and cortisol responses to D-fenfluramine in major depression: evidence for diminished responsivity of central serotonergic function. Am J Psychiatry 1991; 148(8):1009–15.

[83] Emiliano A, Fudge J. From galactorrhea to osteopenia: rethinking serotonin-prolactin interactions. Neuropsychopharmacology 2004;29:833–46.

[84] Laakmann G, Chuang I, Gugath M, et al. Prolactin and antidepressants. In: Tolis G, Stefanis C, Mountakalakis T, et al, editors. Prolactin and prolactinomas. New York: Raven Press; 1982. p. 151–61.

[85] Ryan N, Varma D. Child and adolescent mood disorders—experience with serotonin-based therapies. Biol Psychiatry 1998;44:336–40.

[86] Sternbach H. Venlafaxine-induced galactorrhea. J Clin Psychopharmacol 2003;23(1):109–10.

[87] Pae CU, Kim JJ, Lee CU, et al. Very low dose quetiapine-induced galactorrhea in combination with venlafaxine. Hum Psychopharmacol Clin Exp 2004;19:433–4.

[88] Laakmann G, Schule C, Baghai T, et al. Mirtazapine: an inhibitor of cortisol secretion that does not influence growth hormone and prolactin secretion. J Clin Psychopharmacol 2000; 20(1):101–2.

[89] Schule C, Baghai T, Goy J, et al. The influence of mirtazapine on anterior pituitary hormone secretion in health male subjects. Psychopharmacology (Berl) 2002;163:95–101.

[90] Schule C, Baghai T, Bidlingmaier M, et al. Endocrinological effects of mirtazapine in healthy volunteers. Prog Neuropsychopharmacol Biol Psychiatry 2002;26:1253–61.

[91] Csermely T, Halvax L, Schmidt E, et al. Occurrence of osteopenia among adolescent girls with oligo/amenorrhea. Gynecol Endocrinol 2002;16:99–105.

[92] Rosenfield R. Diagnosis and management of delayed puberty. J Clin Endocrinol Metab 1990; 70(3):559–62.

ELSEVIER
SAUNDERS

Child Adolesc Psychiatric Clin N Am
15 (2006) 221–237

CHILD AND
ADOLESCENT
PSYCHIATRIC CLINICS
OF NORTH AMERICA

Selective Serotonin Reuptake Inhibitors and Suicidality in Juveniles: Review of the Evidence and Implications for Clinical Practice

Joseph M. Rey, MBBS, PhD, FRANZCP[a],*,
Andrés Martin, MD, MPH[b]

[a]University of Sydney, 72/71 Victoria Street, Potts Point, NSW 2011, Australia
[b]Yale Child Study Center, Yale University School of Medicine, 230 South Frontage Road,
New Haven, CT 06520-7900, USA

In February 2005, a judge in Charleston, South Carolina, sentenced 15-year-old Christopher Pittman to 30 years in prison. Christopher was 12 years old when, in November 2001, he shot his grandparents as they slept. He then set fire to the house and fled. Christopher had been prescribed sertraline by his family doctor 3 weeks earlier. Some experts testified at the trial that selective serotonin reuptake inhibitors (SSRIs) can cause certain patients to become suicidal or violent [1].

[Interviewer] And what drug are you on now?
[Teenager]: Prozac.
[Interviewer]: How is that?
[Teenager]: Perfect. I have no side effects at all to it. It's a security blanket for me, being on my antidepressants. If I wasn't on them I really don't think I would be here [alive] today [2].

At a meeting of the US Food and Drug Administration (FDA) in February 2004, several parents told compelling personal stories about young people who had killed themselves after starting treatment with SSRIs [3]. On October 15,

Dr. Rey serves on the Australian advisory board for Stratera (Ely Lilly) and Concerta (Janssen Cilag). During the past 5 years, Dr. Martin has received career development support from the National Institute of Mental Health (PHS grant MH 01792), and honoraria, research, or travel support from Alza, Bristol-Myers Squibb, Eli Lilly, and Janssen Pharmaceuticals.

* Corresponding author.
E-mail address: jrey@mail.usyd.edu.au (J.M. Rey).

2004, the FDA issued the latest in a series of advisories (that had begun in June 2003) about suicidal behavior in children and adolescents treated with antidepressants, recommending the strongest labeling warning ("black box") about increased suicide risk ("Antidepressants increased the risk of suicidal thinking and behavior (suicidality) in short-term studies in children and adolescents with major depressive disorder and other psychiatric disorders") but not contraindicating their use. In the United Kingdom, paroxetine had been banned for use in children a year earlier [4]. The original FDA black box warning was altered February 9, 2005, to a more precise statement clarifying that use of SSRIs is associated with an increased risk of suicidal ideation and behaviors but no longer indicating that a causal relationship between SSRI use and suicidality had been established. The FDA also stressed that this conclusion was based on short-term studies. Pending the results of a review currently under way, a further advisory was issued by the FDA on June 30, 2005, warning about the possibility that antidepressants may increase suicidality in adults [5]. A detailed description of the regulatory background can be found in reference [6].

Concurrently, much has been said in the professional and lay media about the use of SSRIs in depressed children and adolescents, including concerns about increased suicide risk and the growing number of prescriptions, revised evidence about effectiveness, and revelations of drug companies withholding data [7]. The discovery of unforeseen risks in other drugs such as cycloocygenase-2 inhibitors heightened the climate of uncertainty and mistrust about drug treatment. These reports have caused anxiety and confusion among parents, clinicians, and regulators. Practicing clinicians became reluctant to prescribe SSRIs, and the number of prescriptions fell [8]. Medical professionals further questioned whether the diagnosis of major depression in children should be reconceptualized, arguing that to diagnose major depression in this age group is to medicalize the unhappiness caused by affluence, permissiveness, and decaying family and society structures [9].

Claims that fluoxetine increased the risk of suicide in adults have been around since the early 1990s [10] but were dismissed [11]. Few case reports of increased suicidal behavior and self-harm in the young associated with SSRI use have been published in the professional literature [12,13]. Possible explanations are that suicidal behavior caused by SSRIs is rare; that clinicians did not notice it, either because they attributed suicidality to the depressive illness or believed this behavior to be something else (eg, activation or mood lability); that practitioners had actually noticed this phenomenon but did not report it because of indifference, fear, or questioning the counterintuitive attribution to the drug as causally linked. Finally, it is conceivable that the phenomenon was underreported because of journal editors' reluctance to publish isolated case reports.

Earlier reviews of SSRIs [14] and child psychiatry textbooks [15,16]) published before the initial reports from the United Kingdom (in June 2003) had not highlighted an increase in suicidal behavior in children as an important side effect of these treatments. The practice parameter for the assessment and treatment of children and adolescents with suicidal behavior of the American Academy of Child and Adolescent Psychiatry states that SSRIs may increase suicidal ideation in a small number of adults not previously suicidal and notes that "it would be prudent to carefully monitor children and adolescents on SSRIs to ensure that new suicidal ideation or akathisia are noted" [17]. A review of adolescent suicide states that on rare instances, ruminative suicidal ideation combined with akathisia can occur during the course of antipsychotic or SSRI treatment [18]. Child psychiatry textbooks recommend SSRIs as the drug treatment of choice for major depression and for suicidal children and adolescents, because of the lower toxicity of SSRIs [19]. It follows that before 2003, most practitioners, including child psychiatrists, were unlikely to be aware that increased suicidal behavior in young people could be a clinically significant risk of SSRIs and hence were not likely to mention this risk to their patients.

This article seeks to shed light on these matters by examining the evidence about whether SSRIs increase suicidal behavior in children and, if so, to ascertain by how much and who is at greater danger. Implications of the findings for clinical practice and research are also explored. Although the focus is on juvenile data, relevant adult evidence is also considered. The term "suicidality" is used to denote thoughts of suicide, planning to kill oneself, or deliberate self-harm behaviors, which may or may not have suicidal intent, which sometimes is difficult to establish. The words "child," "juvenile," and "youth" denote children and adolescents, unless otherwise specified.

Changes in the prescription of antidepressants

Prescription of antidepressants for children has grown dramatically since the introduction of the SSRIs, in the United States and in many other countries [20,21]. Although SSRIs are increasingly prescribed instead of the tricyclic antidepressants (TCAs), geographic differences remain. Prescription rates and types of antidepressant prescribed for all ages vary from county to county in the United States. Overall antidepressant prescription is lower, and the ratio of TCA to non-TCA prescription is higher in less densely populated counties, perhaps because rural areas may be poorer or have less access to psychiatrists [22].

Antidepressants are prescribed for a wide range of conditions in children, not just depression. In 2002 in the United States, only 26% of visits by patients aged 1 to 11 years old that resulted in prescription of antidepressants were for a mood disorder, compared with 30% for anxiety disorders and 18% for attention deficit disorder. The respective rates for 12- to 17-year-olds were 59%, 18%, and 8%, respectively [23]. In spite of the widespread use of antidepressants, youth depression is often ignored, underdiagnosed, and undertreated. For example, an Australian national household survey showed that among depressed adolescents, 11% had seen a family doctor or pediatrician, 17% had used mental health services, and only 3% had been prescribed an antidepressant [24]. There is also evidence that earlier-onset disorders are associated with longer delays in treatment [25].

Toxicity

There is considerable data demonstrating that SSRIs are less toxic, particularly in overdose, than TCAs. A study of deaths associated with antidepressants in England and Wales from 1998 to 2000 showed 2 deaths per million prescriptions of SSRIs, compared with 14 deaths per million prescriptions for TCAs. Of the other antidepressant drugs, venlafaxine also showed higher toxicity: 13 deaths per million [26].

Post-mortem data

If SSRIs increase suicide risk, it would be expected that SSRIs would be found more often than expected in suicide victims. A study comparing 14,857 suicides with 26,422 deaths by accident or natural causes in Sweden from 1992 to 2000 showed overall that SSRIs were detected less often than other antidepressants in suicide victims (odds ratio, 0.83; 99% CI, 0.77–0.90). Among those younger than 15 years of age, three of the four (75%) antidepressants detected in the accident/ natural causes group were SSRIs; among the 52 children who had committed suicide, no SSRIs were found. In the 15 to 19 years age group, three of the five (60%) antidepressants discovered in the accident/natural causes group were SSRIs. Among the 326 cases of suicide, 6 of 13 (46%) were SSRIs [27]. A study of completed suicides by persons younger than 18 years of age in New York City from 1990 to 1998 reported that antidepressants had been detected in 4 (7.3%) of the 55 cases in which toxicology was examined less than 4 days after death (two imipramine and two fluoxetine). The parallel number for 407 accident victims ascertained with the same method was 3 (0.07%) (two amitryptiline and one fluoxetine) [28]. Statistical analysis of these data is not appropriate because of a substantial number of exclusions, because 60% of accident victims were younger than 10 years whereas none of the suicides were younger than 10, and because the numbers taking antidepressants were very small.

In the Utah Adolescent Suicide Psychological Autopsy Study, parents of the 32 suicide victims who had a psychiatric diagnosis that required treatment were asked if their child had a current prescription for psychotropic medication. About half (14 of 32) were reported to have had a current prescription (10 antidepressants; two antidepressant plus mood stabilizer; one antipsychotic; one stimulant). No traces of psychotropic medication were found in any of these cases [29].

Although the data refer to adults, Tardiff and colleagues [30] reviewed the 127 murder-suicides that took place in New York City between 1990 and 1998. Blood from murderers who committed suicide was routinely tested for drugs, including antidepressants. Three of the murderers (2.4%) were positive for anti-depressants, one of which was an SSRI (sertraline).

In summary, post-mortem data are scarce. The limited evidence available is inconsistent with the hypothesis that SSRIs are more likely to be found in victims of suicide. Further, the evidence seems to suggest that young suicide victims do not take or have stopped taking prescribed medications (not only antidepressants) before killing themselves. Their noncompliance with treatment may be an indication of high suicide risk [29]. Alternatively, ceasing to take SSRIs may result in withdrawal or worsening of symptoms which, in turn, may increase suicide risk.

Suicide

Adult data

Large-scale ecologic studies in several countries have suggested that a recent reduction in the rate of suicide is associated with an increase in the prescription of SSRIs [31–34], Iceland and Japan being the exceptions [35,36]. Gibbons and colleagues [22], examining the association across counties in the United States from 1996 to 1998 likewise found no overall relationship between the rates of prescribed antidepressants and suicide. After controlling for a variety of confounders such as age, income, and population density, however, increases in the prescription of TCAs were associated with higher suicide rates, whereas increases in non-TCAs (largely SSRIs) were associated with a decrease in suicide.

A review of published and unpublished placebo-controlled trials of antidepressants in adults reported that 9 of 23,804 participants treated with SSRIs had committed suicide [37]. The authors found no evidence that SSRIs increased the risk of suicide compared with placebo (odds ratio, 0.85; 95% CI, 0.20–3.40). Another meta-analysis of 345 randomized, controlled trials with 36,445 participants testing the effectiveness of SSRIs versus placebo or other treatment for all conditions and all ages found no difference in suicide rates between SSRIs and placebo [38]. The adjusted odds ratio of suicide was 0.57 (95% CI, 0.26–1.25) in patients prescribed SSRIs compared with those prescribed TCAs in an observational study of patients attending selected primary care practices in the United Kingdom [39]. The data available from these and other studies [40] provide no evidence to support the view that treatment with SSRIs in adults increases the risk of suicide. Jick and colleagues [40], however, reported that risk was increased in the 9 days after an antidepressant was first prescribed.

Children and adolescents

The youth suicide rate has been steadily climbing in most countries since World War II. Contrary to this trend, there has been for the first time a fall in suicides in the United States during the 1990s, and a similar decline has been observed in other countries [18]. Some argue that, as in adults, increased prescription of SSRIs has contributed to the decline. Olfson and colleagues [41] examined the association between changes in prescription of antidepressants and suicide among 10- to 19-year-olds in regions across the United States. They reported that regions with increased use of SSRIs showed a greater decrease in the rate of suicide, possibly accounted for by a reduction in suicide in males and older adolescents in those areas.

No suicides were reported among the more than 2000 SSRI-treated participants younger than 19 years in controlled trials [7,42]. Similarly, none of the 3831 people younger than 19 years diagnosed with depression and exposed to SSRIs completed suicide in the study by Martinez and colleagues [39], nor among the 6976 10- to 19-year-olds in a similar population reported by Jick and colleagues [40].

In summary, adolescent data on completed suicides, although limited, are inconsistent with an SSRI-induced increase—similar to findings in adults. These data do not necessarily disprove that SSRIs can cause some adolescents to kill themselves. Suicide results from a complex interplay among individual, psychosocial, and mental health factors. It is possible that the reduction in youth suicide reflects the success of preventive programs rather than a putative medication effect, for in recent years there has been much public-policy emphasis on prevention of suicide in youth [18]. If that were the case, the overall drop in suicides could conceal a small increase caused by SSRIs [32].

Suicide attempts and deliberate self-harm

Adults

A prospective study examined the association of deliberate self-harm (DSH) with antidepressant use [43]. It involved 2776 consecutive cases of DSH seen in the emergency department of the Derbyshire Royal Infirmary during 1995 and 1996. Results showed that significantly more DSH events occurred in patients prescribed SSRIs (16.6 of 10,000 prescriptions) than TCAs (5.6 of 10,000 prescriptions). The duration between antidepressant prescription and DSH events was similar for both TCAs and SSRIs. Sixty-seven percent of those who had been prescribed SSRIs had a history of DSH, compared with 54% of those prescribed TCAs. Also, the average age of those prescribed SSRIs was lower (34 years) than those prescribed TCAs (42 years), and 62% of those prescribed SSRIs were between 17 and 34 years of age, compared with 40% of those prescribed TCAs. Thus, although individuals taking SSRIs were more likely to show DSH events, this finding could be the result not of their taking an SSRI but of their being younger. Alternatively, those with a history of DSH may have been more likely to be prescribed SSRIs because practitioners identified their risk and tried to minimize it by prescribing drugs that are less toxic, especially in overdose. Bateman and colleagues [44] examined all patients admitted to the Edinburgh Royal Infirmary (from January 2000 to December 2002) with an overdose involving an antidepressant and compared this number with prevalent antidepressant prescribing patterns. They found no evidence of an excess of presentation with SSRI overdoses, and the likelihood was actually reduced in those taking sertraline. There was a small excess of both admissions and poison inquiries for mirtazapine and venlafaxine.

Jick and colleagues [40], using a large primary-care sample in the United Kingdom, reported no differences in suicide attempts between four specific antidepressants (two SSRIs and two non-SSRIs). They noted, however, that suicide attempts were more likely during the first 29 days after antidepressant prescription. In another study using a similar population, Martinez and colleagues [39] found that risk of nonfatal self-harm in adults prescribed SSRIs was no greater than in those prescribed TCAs, or that risk varied according to time since starting treatment.

A review [37] of more than 40,000 individuals participating in 477 randomized controlled trials of SSRIs reported no increased risk of suicidal thoughts in those taking SSRIs compared with placebo (odds ratio, 0.77; 95% CI, 0.37–1.55). The authors, however, concluded there was a "suggestion" of an increased risk of nonfatal self-harm (odds ratio, 1.57; 95% CI, 0.99–2.55). Another systematic review by Fergusson and colleagues [38] showed that treatment with SSRIs in all patients with all conditions doubled the probability of suicide attempt compared with placebo. This effect was virtually undetectable, however: it would be necessary to treat 684 patients with SSRIs to identify a suicide attempt attributable to the treatment. There were no differences when SSRIs were compared with TCAs.

Children and adolescents

Few anecdotal reports have been published of suicidality in young people attributed to the SSRIs [12,13]. In their primary-care sample from the United Kingdom, Jick and colleagues [40] reported no increase in suicidality among patients younger than 20 years taking SSRIs when compared with those taking TCAs. Contrary to this result, however, Martinez and colleagues [39] found "weak" evidence (odds ratio, 1.59; 95% CI, 1.01–2.50) of an increased risk of nonfatal self harm for current SSRI use among patients aged 18 years or younger, paroxetine having the highest risk of the five SSRIs considered (citalopram, fluoxetine, fluvoxamine, paroxetine, sertraline).

A review commissioned by the FDA [45] of 26 controlled trials (16 for major depression, the rest for a variety of anxiety disorders and ADHD –not all trials were included in all analyses) comprising more than 4400 children showed a higher incidence of suicidality in those receiving antidepressants (4%), mostly SSRIs, compared with placebo (2%) (risk ratio, 1.95; 95% CI, 1.28–2.98). Risk ratio data for 20 of these trials are presented in Fig. 1. The effect was significant for major depression trials (risk ratio, 1.66; 95% CI, 1.02–2.68). Although nonsignificant, the finding was similar for non–major depression trials (risk ratio, 2.17; 95% CI, 0.72–6.48). There was a nonsignificant trend for the effect to be higher with paroxetine and venlafaxine.

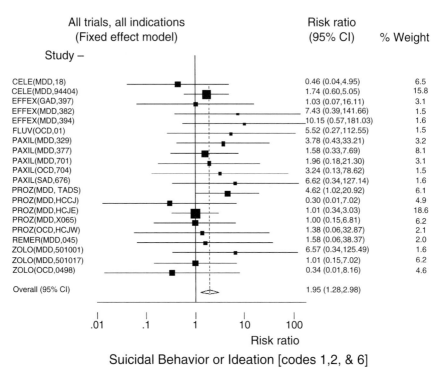

Fig. 1. Risk ratio for suicidality in patients younger than 19 years, comparing antidepressants and placebo from 20 randomized, controlled trials of antidepressants (including TADS), based on adverse-events reports. CELE, Celexa; EFFEX, Effexor; FLUV, fluvoxamine maleate; GAD, generalized anxiety disorder; MDD, major depressive disorder; OCD, obsessive compulsive disorder; PROZ, Prozac; REMER, Remeron; SAD, separation anxiety disorder; ZOLO, Zoloft. (*From* Hammad T. Results of the analysis of suicidality in pediatric trials of newer antidepressants. In: Department of Health and Human Services, Food and Drug Administration Center for Drug Evaluation and Research. Joint Meeting of the CDER Psychopharmacologic Drugs Advisory Committee and the FDA Pediatric Advisory Committee, September 13, 2004. Slide 67. Available at: http://www.fda.gov/ohrms/dockets/ac/04/transcripts/2004-4065T1.pdf and http://www.fda.gov/ohrms/dockets/ac/04/slides/2004-4065S1.htm. Accessed January 6, 2005.)

These analyses were based on adverse-events reports. Adverse-event reports are an unreliable measure: they reflect reports made by the research clinician if, during the regular reviews, patients (or parents) spontaneously, or upon questioning, mentioned thoughts of suicide or described potentially dangerous behavior. In 17 of the trials questionnaire data on suicidal ideation/behavior were completed by patients at each clinical review. Results of this analysis are presented in Fig. 2, which shows that treatment with antidepressants did not worsen suicidality (risk ratio, 0.92; 95% CI, 0.76–1.11). Also, treatment with antidepressants did not increase the risk of developing suicidal behavior in patients who had not reported suicidality at baseline (risk ratio, 0.93; 95% CI, 0.75–1.15).

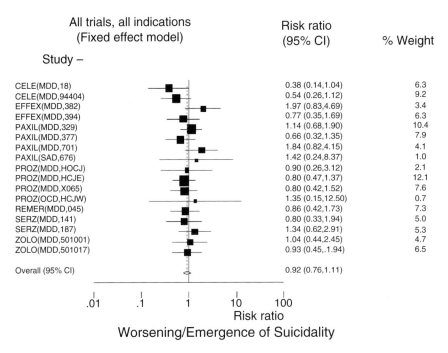

All trials, all indications
(Fixed effect model)

Study –

Risk ratio
(95% CI)   % Weight

Study	Risk ratio (95% CI)	% Weight
CELE(MDD,18)	0.38 (0.14,1.04)	6.3
CELE(MDD,94404)	0.54 (0.26,1.12)	9.2
EFFEX(MDD,382)	1.97 (0.83,4.69)	3.4
EFFEX(MDD,394)	0.77 (0.35,1.69)	6.3
PAXIL(MDD,329)	1.14 (0.68,1.90)	10.4
PAXIL(MDD,377)	0.66 (0.32,1.35)	7.9
PAXIL(MDD,701)	1.84 (0.82,4.15)	4.1
PAXIL(SAD,676)	1.42 (0.24,8.37)	1.0
PROZ(MDD,HOCJ)	0.90 (0.26,3.12)	2.1
PROZ(MDD,HCJE)	0.80 (0.47,1.37)	12.1
PROZ(MDD,X065)	0.80 (0.42,1.52)	7.6
PROZ(OCD,HCJW)	1.35 (0.15,12.50)	0.7
REMER(MDD,045)	0.86 (0.42,1.73)	7.3
SERZ(MDD,141)	0.80 (0.33,1.94)	5.0
SERZ(MDD,187)	1.34 (0.62,2.91)	5.3
ZOLO(MDD,501001)	1.04 (0.44,2.45)	4.7
ZOLO(MDD,501017)	0.93 (0.45,.1.94)	6.5
Overall (95% CI)	0.92 (0.76,1.11)	

.01   .1   1   10   100
Risk ratio
Worsening/Emergence of Suicidality

Fig. 2. Risk ratio for worsening or treatment-emergent suicidality in patients younger than 19 years, comparing antidepressants and placebo from 17 randomized, controlled trials of antidepressants, based on questionnaire reports. CELE, Celexa; EFFEX, Effexor; MDD, major depressive disorder; OCD, obsessive compulsive disorder; PROZ, Prozac; REMER, Remeron; SAD, separation anxiety disorder; SERZ, Serzone; ZOLO, Zoloft. (*From* Hammad T. Results of the analysis of suicidality in pediatric trials of newer antidepressants. In: Department of Health and Human Services, Food and Drug Administration Center for Drug Evaluation and Research. Joint Meeting of the CDER Psychopharmacologic Drugs Advisory Committee and the FDA Pediatric Advisory Committee, September 13, 2004. Slide 39. Available at: http://www.fda.gov/ohrms/dockets/ac/04/transcripts/2004-4065T1.pdf and http://www.fda.gov/ohrms/dockets/ac/04/slides/2004-4065S1.htm. Accessed January 6, 2005.)

The Treatment of Adolescents with Depression Study (TADS) was funded by the National Institute of Mental Health with the aim of examining the effectiveness of four treatments (fluoxetine, cognitive behavioral therapy [CBT], fluoxetine plus CBT, or placebo) among adolescents who had major depressive disorder [42]. Data from this trial deserves more detailed reporting because, unlike most studies, it included a group of patients more akin to those seen in clinical practice: moderate to severe depressive symptoms that were present for more than 6 weeks (mean duration of the major depression, 42 weeks) in at least two of three contexts (home, school, peers). More than half of the participants had comorbid mental disorders. Also,the trial examined suicidal behavior in more detail. Assessment of suicidality was not the primary aim of the study, and statistical power was still limited. The results in relation to suicidal ideation showed that (1) overall, suicidal behavior decreased significantly across all active treatment arms, (2) there were no differences between fluoxetine and placebo, and (3) combined fluoxetine and CBT reduced suicidal ideation compared with placebo. The study also considered a broader category of harm-related events, which comprised suicidal ideation, harm to self (with or without suicidal intent), and harm to others (aggressive thoughts or actual behavior involving harming another person or physical property). Harm-related events were more prevalent among those treated with fluoxetine (alone or in combination with CBT) than in those not taking fluoxetine (odds ratio, 2.19; 95% CI, 1.03–4.62).

Comments

Examination of suicidality in placebo-controlled trials has significant methodological problems, most notably post hoc analyses, trials varying in methodology, limited assessment of suicidality, and suicidal youth being largely excluded from participation [45]. The finding that SSRIs increase the risk of suicidal thoughts and attempts, when based on nonsystematic reports of adverse events, seems robust. When questionnaire data were used, however, no differences were observed.

These findings could have been influenced by methodological shortcomings. For example, suicidal thoughts are common in young people. As many as 25% of females and 14% of males aged 14 to 17 years in the United States endorse the question, "Have you seriously considered suicide in the last 12 months?" Overall suicide attempt rates in the same age group have been relatively consistent at about 8%, with about 2% making attempts serious enough to require medical attention [19]. Rates are much higher among clinically depressed adolescents. The impact of this bias is difficult to foretell but does not seem strong. The TADS showed that suicidal behavior decreased significantly across all active treatment arms. Data from the review of controlled trials showed no difference in emergent suicidal behavior after SSRI treatment between suicidal and non-suicidal children at baseline, although statistical power was limited because of low numbers [45]. The results of nonrandomized studies (eg, [43]) are more difficult to interpret, because suicidality can be confounded by clinicians being more inclined to prescribe SSRIs to younger patients or those with higher suicide risk.

In spite of the very large numbers involved, evidence from adult samples is largely consistent with the youth data. They show no increase in suicidal ideation. SSRIs may elevate the risk of self-harm compared with placebo, but not when compared with TCAs [37–39].

It is noteworthy that most controlled trials report data only for treatment lasting up to 12 or 14 weeks. It is not known what happens to young people in longer-term treatment. Some uncontrolled studies in clinic samples of adults [46] suggest that discontinuation of antidepressant treatment results in an increase in suicidal behavior, but this response could be caused by withdrawal symptoms, among other reasons. The effect of long-term treatment on suicidal behavior requires more research attention.

Possible mechanisms and explanations

Assuming that the finding that SSRI treatment increases suicidal thoughts and attempts in children is accurate, it would be important to ascertain putative mechanisms underlying this outcome, which may help to identify children at particular risk. Several hypotheses have been advanced to explain this phenomenon, including a direct effect on the biochemical pathways controlling suicidal behavior, development of so-called "activation," manic switching, and withdrawal symptoms.

Direct effect on suicidal behavior

It has been suggested that dysfunctions in central serotonergic pathways may be instrumental in patients manifesting suicidal tendencies [47] and that SSRIs may be effective in reducing suicidal behavior. In this line, Verkes and colleagues [48] reported a reduction in suicidal behavior in a subgroup of patients who had attempted suicide more than once but who did not suffer from major depression.

Behavioral activation

SSRIs induce akathisia, agitation, hostility, or irritability in about 10% of patients. This poorly understood phenomenon is often described as "behavioral activation" [12] and may be caused by frontal lobe disinhibition, agitation secondary to akathisia [49], or perhaps related to serotonin syndrome or hypomania. These side effects are typically thought to be dose related [14] and may be particularly common among slow-metabolizers. Data from the review of controlled trials show that activation is more common among children treated with SSRIs than with placebo (relative risk, 1.79; 95% CI, 1.16–2.76), and particularly with paroxetine (relative risk, 7.69; 95% CI, 1.80–32.99). Participants who showed activation were seven times more likely to show treatment-emergent suicidal thoughts or attempts [45].

Manic switching

Like other antidepressants, SSRIs can trigger manic switches, often with unstable mood, which may increase suicide risk (for a recent review, see [50]). Further, differences between activation and mania or hypomania in children may be difficult to detect in clinical practice. Martin and colleagues [51] examined this problem in a sample of 87,920 patients aged 5 to 29 years followed for a median of 41 weeks. They reported that overall 6% of patients became manic during the 5-year period of observation, and that both patient age and antidepressant class contributed to the risk of conversion. The conversion rate among antidepressant-treated patients (7.7%) was threefold that among unexposed patients (2.5%). Risk was highest for TCAs (odds ratio, 3.9) and lowest for SSRIs (odds ratio, 2.1). Risk was highest for 10- to 14-year-olds.

Patients with agitated depression [52] or unrecognized bipolar depression, which often cannot be diagnosed because of unclear symptoms or a lack of a history of manic behaviors, may be particularly at risk of manic switching or suicidality when treated with antidepressants [53].

Withdrawal symptoms

Noncompliance or ceasing medication altogether may trigger withdrawal symptoms, which are common in SSRIs with a shorter half-life (eg, paroxetine). As indicated previously, teenagers who completed suicide often had not adhered to treatment [29]. It is possible the emergence of these symptoms may cause dysphoria, a worsening of the symptoms of the illness being treated, and an increase in suicidal behavior. No systematic data are available on this issue. The review of controlled trials, however, did not find that dropping out of a trial increased the risk of suicidality [45].

Discussion

The evidence available is still inconclusive. Data based on adverse-event reports from controlled trials suggest that SSRIs increase suicidality (thoughts, attempts) in children. When questionnaire-based data are used, however, no comparable increase in suicidality is observed. In the TADS study, SSRIs were associated with higher rates of harm-related events (when aggression and self-cutting without suicidal intent were added to suicidal thoughts and attempts). If an association exists, the effect is small: between 20 and 50 children need to be treated with antidepressants for one to develop suicidality in its widest sense (Table 1). Children who develop activation or a manic switch or who are treated with paroxetine may be at higher risk, although this possibility needs con-firmation. The larger adult data allow similar conclusions.

To demonstrate irrefutably whether SSRIs increase the risk of completed suicide, a rare event, would require very large trials (enrolling up to 2 million individuals according to Gunnell and colleagues [37]. Such trials will not be conducted. Hence, clinicians and regulators must continue to live with the ambiguity and to rely on the accumulation of specks of information from a variety of experimental, epidemiologic, and observational studies to draw conclusions. As a result, experts will probably continue to disagree in their interpretations of the evidence. The data currently available indicate that SSRIs do not increase the risk of completed suicide in either children or adults. Further, the ratio of attempts to completed suicides has been estimated as 6000 to 1 among girls and 400 to 1 among boys in the United States [17]. This finding suggests that, even if SSRIs produce a small increase in suicidal attempts, this increase is unlikely

Table 1
Summary of risk–benefit evidence for suicidality in youths treated with selective serotonin reuptake inhibitors

Treatment effects	Treatment	Response (%)	NNT[a]
TADS (March et al, 2004 [42])	FLU	61	4
	FLU + CBT	71	3
	CBT	43	12
	Placebo	35	—

Suicidal ideation/attempts/self-harm	Treatment	Treatment-emergent suicidality (%)	NNH[a]
FDA reassessment (Hammad, 2004 [45])	Active (SSRI)	4	50
	Placebo	2	—
TADS (March et al, 2004 [42])	FLU + CBT	6	50
	FLU	8	25
	Placebo	4	—

Summary risk assessment of suicidal ideation	NNT[a]	NNH[a]	LHH[a]
Hammad, 2004 [45]: SSRI	4[b]	50	13
TADS (March et al, 2004 [42]): FLU	4	25	7
TADS (March et al, 2004 [42]): FLU + CBT	3	50	17

Abbreviations: FLU, fluoxetine; LHH, likelihood of being helped to harmed; NNH, number needed to harm; NNT, number needed to treat.

[a] LHH, NNH, and NNT point estimate calculations are based on the numbers shown and the formulae derived from Sackett DL, Straus SE, Richardson WS, et al. Evidence-based medicine: how to practice and teach EBM. Edinburgh (UK): Churchill Livingston; 2000. All results are rounded to the higher next integer.

[b] With TADS, FLU used as NNT referent.

to have substantial effect on the number of completed suicides, particularly if such attempts are managed appropriately.

Adult data show that SSRI treatment does not increase suicidal ideation, although it may increase nonlethal suicide attempts. In youth, a significant minority of those who self-harmed in the TADS trial showed self-cutting without suicidal thoughts. This finding seems inconsistent with the widely held view that there is continuity in suicidal behavior, from ideation to attempts to completed suicide. SSRIs may specifically increase deliberate self-harm events (eg, self-cutting to relieve distress). This possibility requires further investigation, which will need better instruments to assess suicidality and behavioral side effects in controlled trials and in postmarketing surveillance.

Implications for clinical practice

In this rapidly evolving field new data are becoming available all the time, and clinicians need to change their practice accordingly, considering that the balance between benefit and harm, although paramount, is neither simple nor static. For example, conclusions derived from clinical trials may not apply to individual patients for methodological, genetic, physiologic, psychosocial, and cultural reasons. Also, the weight given to the evidence may vary in line with changes in personal and social values. Hence, clinical practice should be guided by a careful appraisal of benefit and risk (including whether risks can be managed successfully, as is the case with clozapine) based on best evidence, clinical experience, and the needs, circumstances, and wishes of individual patients.

It is essential that clinicians and patients have access to a range of interventions, pharmacologic and psychosocial, that alone or in combination can best meet the needs and circumstances of individual children and families. SSRIs have been widely and increasingly used in children from the early 1990s. Nevertheless, data about benefit in a variety of conditions, including depression, are limited. More evidence showing whether SSRIs are effective for particular disorders and in certain types of patients is a pressing need to inform treatment decisions. Until that information is available, the balance of the evidence for the use of fluoxetine in moderate to severe depression is favorable. According to TADS, four children will need to be treated for one to show much or very much improvement, compared with the need to treat 25 children for 1 to display a harm-related event (see Table 1), yielding a favorable likelihood of being helped to harmed (LHH) of 7. The numbers are even more compelling when using fluoxetine combined with CBT (3 and 50, respectively, for an LHH of 17) or when using the number needed to harm (NNH) estimate derived from the FDA reassessment study (4% versus 2%, for an NNH of 50) [45]. When balanced against the fact that depression in the young is a serious, recurring condition that produces much personal suffering and can lead to professional and social problems, poor physical health, and suicide, the overall weight of the evidence clearly supports treatment with the SSRIs over nontreatment.

During the evaluation phase, particular care must be taken to ascertain a family or individual history of manic symptoms and suicidal behaviors. When treatment is initiated, patients and family must be informed of the risk of increased suicidality and the side effects that may emerge, so that they can detect symptoms of activation, manic switch, or increase in suicidality. This information would be accompanied by a discussion of practical ways of dealing with these unwanted effects and of enhancing the patient's safety. Particularly, immediate contact with the clinician should be encouraged should any comments or behaviors indicative of self-harm or suicidality arise, especially during early treatment with an antidepressant. Leaflets that provide useful information on these issues for patients and parents and provide assistance to clinicians in this endeavor are available at:

- http://www.parentsmedguide.org/parentsmedguide.htm (information for patients and families concerning the use of medication in treating childhood and adolescent depression; accessed March 28, 2005).
- http://www.parentsmedguide.org/physiciansmedguide.htm (information for physicians concerning the use of medication in treating childhood and adolescent depression; accessed March 28, 2005).

Dose reduction or antidepressant discontinuation may become warranted at times, always balancing the decision against the risks of having the underlying depressive disorder go untreated or undertreated.

It is imperative to monitor side effects closely and to review patient outcomes often, particularly during the first few weeks of treatment. In the case of depression, psychiatrists have known for a long time that suicide risk is higher during the first weeks of treatment. During that time physical symptoms and energy levels may improve, but psychologic well-being usually lags, thus creating a window of increased vulnerability and potential risk. Frequent visits, based on the clinical needs of each individual patient, during the early stages of treatment are also likely to facilitate the development of trust and improve adherence. Noncompliance with treatment may reflect increased suicide risk and needs to be kept in mind and monitored during all follow-up visits. These cautions and the generally good advice for close monitoring need to be balanced against the challenge of securing weekly follow-up, even on a time-limited basis, especially in under-served areas, and the possibility that setting an unrealistic expectation of monitoring may paradoxically lead to undertreatment of this critical, sometimes deadly condition.

References

[1] Springer J. Jurors find teenager guilty of murdering his grandparents. February 16, 2005. Available at: http://www.cnn.com/2005/LAW/02/15/zoloft.trial/. Accessed July 11, 2005.

[2] Teenage depression. SBS Insight November 9, 2004. Available at http://news.sbs.com.au/insight/archive.php?daysum=2004-11-09#. Accessed July 11, 2005.

[3] Moynihan R. FDA advisory panel calls for suicide warnings over new antidepressants. BMJ 2004;328(7435):303.

[4] Medicines CoSo. Use of selective serotonin reuptake inhibitors (SSRIs) in children and adolescents with major depressive disorder (MDD). Available at: http://www.mhra.gov.uk. Accessed February 9, 2004.

[5] Food and Drug Administration. Suicidality in adults being treated with antidepressant medications. FDA Public Health Advisory, June 30, 2005. Available at: http://www.fda.gov/cder/drug/advisory/SSRI200507.htm. Accessed July 11, 2005.

[6] Leslie LK, Newman TB, Chesney PJ, et al. The Food and Drug Administration's deliberations on antidepressant use in pediatric patients. Pediatrics 2005;116:195–204.

[7] Whittington CJ, Kendall T, Fonagy P, et al. Selective serotonin reuptake inhibitors in childhood depression: systematic review of published versus unpublished data. Lancet 2004;363(9418):1341–5.

[8] Valuck RJ, Libby AM, Sills MR, et al. Antidepressant treatment and risk of suicide attempt by adolescents with major depressive disorder: a propensity-adjusted retrospective cohort study. CNS Drugs 2004;18(15):1119–32.

[9] Timimi S. Rethinking childhood depression. BMJ 2004;329(7479):1394–6.

[10] Teicher MH, Glod C, Cole JO. Emergence of intense suicidal preoccupation during fluoxetine treatment. Am J Psychiatry 1990;147(2):207–10.

[11] Beasley Jr CM, Dornseif BE, Bosomworth JC, et al. Fluoxetine and suicide: a meta-analysis of controlled trials of treatment for depression. BMJ 1991;303(6804):685–92.

[12] King RA, Riddle MA, Chappell PB, et al. Emergence of self-destructive phenomena in children

and adolescents during fluoxetine treatment. J Am Acad Child Adolesc Psychiatry 1991; 30(2):179–86.

[13] Vorstman J, Lahuis B, Buitelaar JK. SSRIs associated with behavioral activation and suicidal ideation. J Am Acad Child Adolesc Psychiatry 2001;40(12):1364–5.

[14] Leonard HL, March J, Rickler KC, et al. Pharmacology of the selective serotonin reuptake inhibitors in children and adolescents. J Am Acad Child Adolesc Psychiatry 1997;36(6):725–36.

[15] Rutter M, Taylor E, editors. Child and adolescent psychiatry. 4th edition. Oxford (UK): Blackwell Science; 2002.

[16] Martin A, Scahill L, Charney DS, et al, editors. pediatric psychopharmacology: principles and practice. New York: Oxford University Press; 2003.

[17] American Academy of Child and Adolescent Psychiatry. Practice parameter for the assessment and treatment of children and adolescents with suicidal behavior. J Am Acad Child Adolesc Psychiatry 2001;40(7 Suppl):24S–51S.

[18] Gould MS, Greenberg T, Velting DM, et al. Youth suicide risk and preventive interventions: a review of the past 10 years. J Am Acad Child Adolesc Psychiatry 2003;42(4):386–405.

[19] Shaffer D, Gutstein J. Suicide and attempted suicide. In: Rutter MT, Taylor E, editors. Child and adolescent psychiatry. 4th edition. Oxford (UK): Blackwell Science; 2002. p. 529–54.

[20] Zito JM, Safer DJ, DosReis S, et al. Rising prevalence of antidepressants among US youths. Pediatrics 2002;109(5):721–7.

[21] Martin A, Leslie D. Psychiatric inpatient, outpatient, and medication utilization and costs among privately insured youths, 1997–2000. Am J Psychiatry 2003;160(4):757–64.

[22] Gibbons RD, Hur K, Bhaumik DK, et al. The relationship between antidepressant medication use and rate of suicide. Arch Gen Psychiatry 2005;62(2):165–72.

[23] Rigoni GC. Drug utilization for selected antidepressants among children and adolescents. US Food and Drug Administration. Psychopharmacologic Drugs Advisory Committee and Pediatric Subcommittee of the Anti-Infective Drugs Advisory Committee. February 2, 2004. Available at: http://www.fda.gov/ohrms/dockets/ac/04/slides/4006s1.htm. Accessed March 16, 2005.

[24] Rey JM, Sawyer MG, Clark JJ, et al. Depression among Australian adolescents. Med J Aust 2001;175(1):19–23.

[25] Wang PS, Berglund P, Olfson M, et al. Failure and delay in initial treatment contact after first onset of mental disorders in the National Comorbidity Survey Replication. Arch Gen Psychiatry 2005;62:603–13.

[26] Cheeta S, Schifano F, Oyefeso A, et al. Antidepressant-related deaths and antidepressant prescriptions in England and Wales, 1998–2000. Br J Psychiatry 2004;184:41–7.

[27] Isacsson G, Holmgren P, Ahlner J. Selective serotonin reuptake inhibitor antidepressants and the risk of suicide: a controlled forensic database study of 14,857 suicides. Acta Psychiatr Scand 2005;111:286–90.

[28] Leon AC, Marzuk PM, Tardiff K, et al. Paroxetine, other antidepressants, and youth suicide in New York City: 1993 through 1998. J Clin Psychiatry 2004;65(7):915–8.

[29] Moskos M, Olson L, Frazier S, et al. Utah Adolescent Suicide Psychological Autopsy Study. Suicide Life Threat Behav, in press.

[30] Tardiff K, Marzuk PM, Leon AC. Role of antidepressants in murder and suicide. Am J Psychiatry 2002;159(7):1248–9.

[31] Isacsson G. Suicide prevention—a medical breakthrough? Acta Psychiatr Scand 2000;102(2): 113–7.

[32] Gunnell D, Ashby D. Antidepressants and suicide: what is the balance of benefit and harm. BMJ 2004;329(7456):34–8.

[33] Barbui C, Campomori A, D'Avanzo B, et al. Antidepressant drug use in Italy since the introduction of SSRIs: national trends, regional differences and impact on suicide rates. Soc Psychiatry Psychiatr Epidemiol 1999;34(3):152–6.

[34] Hall WD, Mant A, Mitchell PB, et al. Association between antidepressant prescribing and suicide in Australia, 1991–2000: trend analysis. BMJ 2003;326(7397):1008.

[35] Helgason T, Tomasson H, Zoega T. Antidepressants and public health in Iceland. Time series analysis of national data. Br J Psychiatry 2004;184:157–62.

[36] Desapriya EBR, Iwase N. New trends in suicide in Japan. Inj Prev 2003;9:284.

[37] Gunnell D, Saperia J, Ashby D. Selective serotonin reuptake inhibitors (SSRIs) and suicide in adults: meta-analysis of drug company data from placebo controlled, randomised controlled trials submitted to the MHRA's safety review. BMJ 2005;330(7488):385.

[38] Fergusson D, Doucette S, Glass KC, et al. Association between suicide attempts and selective serotonin reuptake inhibitors: systematic review of randomised controlled trials. BMJ 2005; 330(7488):396.

[39] Martinez C, Rietbrock S, Wise L, et al. Antidepressant treatment and the risk of fatal and non-fatal self harm in first episode depression: nested case-control study. BMJ 2005;330(7488):389.

[40] Jick H, Kaye JA, Jick SS. Antidepressants and the risk of suicidal behaviors. JAMA 2004;292(3):338–43.

[41] Olfson M, Shaffer D, Marcus SC, et al. Relationship between antidepressant medication treatment and suicide in adolescents. Arch Gen Psychiatry 2003;60(10):978–82.

[42] March J, Silva S, Petrycki S, et al. Fluoxetine, cognitive-behavioral therapy, and their combination for adolescents with depression: Treatment for Adolescents with Depression Study (TADS) randomized controlled trial. JAMA 2004;292(7):807–20.

[43] Donovan S, Clayton A, Beeharry M, et al. Deliberate self-harm and antidepressant drugs. Investigation of a possible link. Br J Psychiatry 2000;177:551–6.

[44] Bateman DN, Chick J, Good AM, et al. Are selective serotonin re-uptake inhibitors associated with an increased risk of self-harm by antidepressant overdose? Eur J Clin Pharmacol 2004;60(3):221–4.

[45] Hammad T. Results of the analysis of suicidality in pediatric trials of newer antidepressants. In: Department of Health and Human Services, Food and Drug Administration Center for Drug Evaluation and Research. Joint Meeting of the CDER Psychopharmacologic Drugs Advisory Committee and the FDA Pediatric Advisory Committee, September 13, 2004. p. 152–200. Available at: http://www.fda.gov/ohrms/dockets/ac/04/transcripts/2004-4065T1.pdf. and http://www.fda.gov/ohrms/dockets/ac/04/slides/2004-4065S1.htm. Accessed January 6, 2005.

[46] Yerevanian BI, Koek RJ, Feusner JD, et al. Antidepressants and suicidal behaviour in unipolar depression. Acta Psychiatr Scand 2004;110(6):452–8.

[47] Van Praag HM. Serotonergic dysfunction and aggression control. Psychol Med 1991;21(1): 15–9.

[48] Verkes RJ, Van der Mast RC, Hengeveld MW, et al. Reduction by paroxetine of suicidal behavior in patients with repeated suicide attempts but not major depression. Am J Psychiatry 1998;155(4):543–7.

[49] Walkup J, Labellarte M. Complications of SSRI treatment. J Child Adolesc Psychopharmacol 2001;11(1):1–4.

[50] Lim C, Leckman JF, Young CM, et al. Antidepressant-induced manic conversion: a developmentally-informed synthesis of the literature. International Review of Biology 2005; 65:25–52.

[51] Martin A, Young C, Leckman JF, et al. Age effects on antidepressant-induced manic conversion. Arch Pediatr Adolesc Med 2004;158(8):773–80.

[52] Akiskal HS, Benazzi F, Perugi G, et al. Agitated "unipolar" depression re-conceptualized as a depressive mixed state: implications for the antidepressant-suicide controversy. J Affect Disord 2005;85(3):245–58.

[53] Shi LZ, Thiebaud P, McCombs JS. The impact of unrecognized bipolar disorders for patients treated for depression with antidepressants in the fee-for-services California Medicaid (Medi-Cal) program. J Affect Disord 2004;82(3):373–83.

ELSEVIER
SAUNDERS

Child Adolesc Psychiatric Clin N Am
15 (2006) 239–262

CHILD AND
ADOLESCENT
PSYCHIATRIC CLINICS
OF NORTH AMERICA

Teamwork: The Therapeutic Alliance in Pediatric Pharmacotherapy

Shashank V. Joshi, MD

Stanford University School of Medicine, 401 Quarry Road, Stanford, CA 94305, USA

"Medicating a child" is full of potential implications regarding patient autonomy and confidentiality, parental rights, and physician beneficence. This task must be approached thoughtfully. The prescriber (pharmacotherapist) is often the person with ultimate diagnostic and treatment authority, despite sometimes meager contact with the patient. This situation is aggravated by the time constraints of modern pharmacotherapy encounters. The therapeutic bond between patient and physician is vulnerable and may be neglected in contemporary practice [1]. Because the "offer" of any treatment to patients is much more than a neutral act [2], prescribing medications for children and adolescents requires that special attention be paid to communication styles and messages [3]. Does the clinician's language and affect convey a hope and confidence in things to come [4]? Does the prescription signal the end of the interview or the beginning of an alliance [5]? (Among the very first pediatrician-psychiatrists, DW Winnicott [4] reminds us that the term "prescription" is really a misnomer: one is never written in a vacuum, devoid of relational and diagnostic context.)

Moreover, in pediatric work, a *dual alliance* is required. The parents/guardians must play an important role, while not impeding the therapeutic activity between doctor and patient. All aspects of psychiatric encounters with patients and families convey important meanings [6], including, at times, inflated expectations regarding the prescription itself. Psychiatrists may share the same "magic-cure" fantasies of the perfect potion or combination of medications that their patients and families entertain [4].

E-mail address: svjoshi@stanford.edu

Although the fields of psychotherapy and sociotherapy directly acknowledge these principles and are prepared to examine the potential implications, pharmacotherapy too often has ignored them [2]. There is, in fact, an established literature to support the empiric basis of the therapeutic alliance (the working alliance) in psychotherapeutic work [1,7–12]. This literature addresses ways of establishing the doctor–patient relationship itself and for maximizing clinical outcomes and maintaining these gains. (In this article, the terms "doctor," "pharmacotherapist," and "clinician" refer to any medical provider who may be prescribing medications, including nurse practitioners and physician assistants.) Recent investigators have demonstrated that the strength of the alliance may independently predict the clinical outcome of pharmacotherapy and psychotherapy [11,13].

This article addresses the role of the "pharmacotherapeutic alliance" in child and adolescent psychiatry, the psychologic implications of administering medications, specific developmental issues important when working with children and adolescents of varying ages, the role of the dual alliance (with both patients and parents) for practitioners in both specialty and primary care settings, and, finally, recommendations for clinical practice and further research.

The role of the therapeutic alliance in child and adolescent pharmacotherapy

The *psychology of psychopharmacology* has become a subfield within psychiatry. Although some thought-provoking material has been written regarding the psychologic aspects of pharmacotherapy with adult patients [3,5,11,14–21], and formal empiric studies have been done [13], aspects of this field germane to children and adolescents are, at best, early in their development. Some scientific journals and standard texts on psychiatric drug treatment in children have devoted specific sections to the topic [2,4,8,22–25]. Other authors have written about the myriad factors involved in children's and adolescents' adherence or nonadherence to medication [25–27]. The term "pharmacotherapy" includes all medication interactions with children, adolescents, and families and includes more than just medication management. Pharmaco*therapy* implies all of the inherent mindfulness that characterizes a thorough work-up for children and adolescents referred for consideration of medication treatments. The term "psychopharmacotherapy" has been described previously [4,22] and may be defined as the combined use of psychoactive medication and psychotherapy (by the same person). This construct may also be referred to as "integrated treatment" or "combined treatment." Unfortunately, it may be a rare entity in current psychiatric practice.

Gabbard and Kay [28] have outlined some of the distinct advantages of the one-person treatment model in general (adult) psychiatry, in which a psychiatrist conducts the psychotherapy while prescribing medication. Given the many providers and caregivers in a pediatric patient's life, similar arguments could be made for integrated treatment in work with children and adolescents.

The concepts discussed in this article may be applied to either integrated treatment or split treatment.

Joshi and colleagues [2] have described how psychologic aspects of pharmacotherapy observed in children and adolescents are derived from the characteristics of the pediatric patient, the characteristics of the important adults in that patient's life, and the characteristics of their social environment.

Pediatric patients and their internal working models of receiving support, help, nurturance, and treatment are based on previous experiences with caregivers, both within and outside of the family. These experiences may include past relationships with physicians, teachers, and counselors, for example. Sometimes referred to as "transference," this working model influences the patient's capacity to form a helping alliance with the clinician who administers the medication. Attachment status, age of the child, and past outcomes of interacting with caregivers in times of hurt and need also influence the formation of the helping alliance. Clinicians who understand these influences are best positioned to maximize adherence and optimize clinical outcomes.

In considering the characteristics of the important adults (caregivers/family and school staff) in the youth's life, the most salient factor is that children are context-dependent upon these adults, especially at young ages. The way that family members or school personnel handle the supervision and administration of medication may have profound influences on how this process will unfold, and whether it will support or hinder the child's taking medication under optimal conditions. Adherence is promoted when teachers and parents echo support for the child's striving toward self-care, rather than giving backhanded compliments such as, "You're doing really well today—you must have taken your meds." Children and adolescents are likely to attribute success more to their inherent abilities, rather than to medication, when the adults in their lives are attentive to the specific language they use.

Patients may be more likely to accept taking medication when there is a connection to a peer or famous person with a similar problem. Media influences may include internet information (or misinformation), music video depictions of adolescents with mental health problems, and mental illness themes in television, film, and printed media. Thus, it is especially important to elicit the child's or adolescent's *self-perception of what it means* to be taking psychotropic medication.

All these factors guide cultivation of a *working alliance*. A strong working alliance has at its core the concept of *mutual collaboration against* the common foe of the patient's presenting problems. It integrates the relational and technical aspects of treatment [29]. Somewhat distinct from a "helping alliance," the "working alliance" identifies the patient's own efforts as bringing about changes, with an emphasis on shared responsibility for working out the treatment goals and on the patient's ability to do what the therapist does [12]. In actual pediatric practice, clinicians may skillfully employ aspects of both a warm, nurturing helping alliance and a shared, collaborative working alliance so that the interaction is, at its core, therapeutic. Formation of the therapeutic alliance becomes a critical first step to any successful intervention, be it psychotherapy or pharmacotherapy.

A strong alliance includes a mutual understanding and agreement about goals for change and about the necessary tasks to achieve these goals [30,31]. The collaboration between therapist and client involves three essential components: tasks, goals, and bonds. *Tasks* are the in-therapy behaviors and cognitions that form the basis of the therapeutic process. Bordin [30,31], Horvath and Greenberg [32], and Beitman and colleagues [18] have emphasized that, if the relationship is strong, both therapist and client perceive the tasks in therapy as relevant and potentially effective, and each party accepts responsibility to take part in these tasks. A strong working alliance involves the therapist and patient mutually endorsing and valuing the *goals* (outcomes) that are the targets of an intervention. The term *"bonds"* acknowledges patient–therapist attachment status and includes mutual trust, acceptance, and confidence [18,32]. The following case exemplifies the need for this responsibility to be shared.

A 15- year-old boy with debilitating anxiety and bipolar traits was enrolled in weekly cognitive-behavioral therapy (CBT), integrated with pharmacotherapy by the same psychiatrist. Although initially enthusiastic, after the third session the patient regularly forgot to bring his CBT manual or to do the homework. He promised to complete intersession tasks, but his nonadherence to the CBT continued. Although he consistently took his prescribed medications, his symptoms continued to worsen. Understanding some of the factors related to CBT nonadherence (shame, embarrassment, a family unable to set limits) became crucial in understanding his resistance to progress. Ultimately, a supportive residential treatment setting that was mindful of these factors and that reinforced them throughout the day allowed him to complete the work in class (his milieu group setting). The lack of progress in CBT had as much to do with context and setting (family messages undermining treatment) as with the disorder itself. Within 1 year the patient's symptoms improved substantially. A strong working alliance allowed the doctor to prescribe medication while patiently processing the resistance to full participation with the team.

A body of research has addressed the alliance in psychotherapy in children and adolescents. Most of this work focuses on interpersonal process, such as therapeutic engagement with children and adolescents [33–35]. Newer research investigates factors related to the dual alliance with caregivers as well [35–37]. Recent work has also begun to focus on the mediators and moderators of the alliance, such as client and parent variables, in-therapy process variables, and therapist contributions to the alliance [38]. The overall theme from the body of work conducted during the last 30 years (in both pediatric and adult patients) indicates the quality of the alliance is an important element in all forms of effective therapies [38]. Horvath's [38] comprehensive review indicates effect sizes of about 0.21 to 0.25. Although this effect may be considered modest, other research on psychotherapy effectiveness indicates that the therapeutic alliance and specific therapist variables contribute significantly to outcomes in psychotherapy [39]. Variables associated with improvement include interpersonal skills (expressed responsiveness and the ability to generate a sense of hope), open and clear communication style, emoted empathy, and minimal negative therapist behaviors (eg, a take-charge attitude that fosters patient dependency in the early phases, an attitude the client experiences as cold, the premature offering of insight or interpretation, and irritability or impatience with patient efforts) [38,40–43]. Although the alliance in adult psychotherapy is often established early, by the third to fifth session [29,44,45], a meta-analysis of outcomes in child and adolescent psychotherapy found that relationship measures obtained later in therapy were more strongly associated with outcome than measures taken early [46]. The authors postulate that relationship formation may evolve more slowly with younger patients [46]. As of this writing, the session at which the alliance is usually established in pediatric pharmacotherapy is unclear, but one might assume that an early alliance may be important for the *work with the adults* (eg, parents and teachers) in the patient's life.

The alliance in pharmacotherapy has been examined in adults who have depression. Weiss and colleagues [13] examined the role of the therapeutic alliance on the efficacy of pharmacotherapy in 31 outpatients treated with antidepressants over 2 years. The alliance in pharmacotherapy was highly and directly correlated with clinical outcomes. Although previous research in the psychotherapy process indicates that the *patient's* perception of the alliance best predicts outcome [47], in this study the *pharmacotherapist's* perception of the alliance was the more reliable predictor.

Psychologic implications of prescribing medications

Physicians treat people with illness ("a girl who has ADHD"), not simply the illness itself ("an ADHD patient"). Havens [48] cautions that, to many patients, the doctor's trustworthiness and decency are not givens, and that mental illness in particular is often a delicate subject. He describes three "psychological analgesics" that may facilitate the approach to painful topics in therapy. For the pharmacotherapist, these psychologic analgesics might be "prescribed" for difficult matters, such as the need to take psychotropic medication. These measures can be modified to approach parents as well [48]:

1. *Protect self-esteem:* The patient has been potentially affected by having to come to a psychiatrist, and the parent may feel guilty for having caused the illness through bad parenting, poor gene contribution, or both.
2. *Emote a measure of understanding and acceptance:* When this measure is successful, the patient's problem is grasped intellectually, and the patient's and family's predicament is understood from *their* point of view.
3. *Provide a sense of future:* Many families have experienced frustration and failure in attempting to find solutions and may have lost hope. Discussion about expectations for treatment that still acknowledges fears or even

hopelessness may still preserve opportunities for change: "It seems hope-less to you *now*."

Sabo and Rand [21] emphasize the importance of spending adequate time with the patient (and family) in the initial evaluation. Patients too often feel as though they are merely "the next appointment" unless the doctor listens to the personal and unique elements of their story. Active empathic listening is necessary to create a special, common language between the patient and therapist. If a full work-up cannot be completed in the first session, follow-up sessions (preferably within a week) may be necessary to sustain the developing alliance. Pruett and Martin [4] caution against prescribing for patients who are difficult for the pharmacotherapist to remember, whether because of excess patient volume or some other reason. They advise those practicing pharmacotherapy to examine carefully those circumstances in which neither doctor nor patient seems sufficiently invested in a relationship to make it worth remembering [21]. Prescribing clinicians who have a large patient volume may need to record and review information collected during the initial assessment to remind them of the patient *as a person*, beyond the necessary streamlined medical data. Sabo and Rand [21] suggest these reminders might be something anecdotal but significant (or even interesting to the clinician), such as the patient's best friend's or pet's name, favorite sports figure, or best subject in school. Such specifics help physicians quickly re-establish the relationship and demonstrate interest in this patient and this family as they detail emotionally laden and other personal information. Asking parents about, and then documenting, the patient's strengths similarly helps highlight distinguishing characteristics. It also aids in recognizing each patient as an individual, while contributing to the formation of a relationship not focused entirely on pathology or inadequacies. This process may strengthen the doctor–patient relationship and encourage parents to recall their child's strengths, granting them permission to enjoy and acknowledge their role in fostering those strengths, rather than dwelling solely on what necessitated the visit to the psychiatrist. In subsequent patient visits, the treatment provider can address symptom complaints within a more person-centered (and less disease-centered) approach.

How and when to present the idea of prescribing medication

Patients and their patients often wonder why a clinician would consider the use of psychoactive medication. For example, questions (sometimes directly expressed) such as "Why now? Am I such a failure as a patient (or parent)?" can interfere with treatment adherence and undermine the best-conceived interventions. Further, these questions may arise whether treatment is integrated or divided. Discussing the possibility of a medication intervention at the time of initial assessment and treatment plan can be quite useful. It allows an open and frank discussion regarding potential benefits and side effects, making the family and patient aware of medication options early in treatment and of the use of medication as one option to begin considering as the assessment proceeds. This introduction eases the task of "bringing up the subject of meds" as an intervention later in the course of therapy. Also, discussing medication options with the primary therapist enhances collaboration and helps convey a unified message to the patient and family.

A full discussion of medication options

When feasible, the acts of writing and handing a prescription should be allocated sufficient time to evaluate benefits and risks for the particular patient, to monitor patient and family reactions to the proposal of medication, and to answer questions of both patient and parent. In many cases, multiple visits are required before medication can be proposed to, and accepted by, patients and their families. Accordingly, early attention to pharmacotherapy as an option may be needed so patients and their families can consider, investigate, and concur on this modality.

The meaning of the medication itself, and on the self

Children and adolescents alike may have preconceived notions about medication, based partly on direct-to-consumer marketing campaigns encouraging them to "ask your doctor about the purple pill." Potential barriers to adherence include feeling different from or damaged compared with friends who do not take medication, experiencing new feelings when the medicine takes effect, feeling like a different person when medicated (and likeable only in this altered state), and seeing the prescriber more as an agent of the parent and less as an ally of the adolescent. If the *intended therapeutic effect* of a medication (decrease in symptoms) conflicts with *its meaning to the patient* (feeling changed or controlled in some way), the medicine may be less effective (higher risk of nonadherence, greater subjective perception of side effects) [49]. As Schowalter [22] has noted, "All too often it is unclear whether a medication heals directly or mainly removes obstacles to self-healing ... [A] balance should be strived for, as some clinicians try to snuff out all discomfort pharmacologically, while others overvalue anxiety and discomfort as necessary motivation for psychotherapy."

The name of the medicine can influence attitudes and thus, adherence. A patient of this author was reluctant to take a certain medication (Abilify), fearing it could make him feel "vilified," whereas another patient felt it could "abilify" him (give him ability) to control his mood swings. A third patient in the author's clinic eventually chose to try Geodon because the name resembled a Pokemon character (Geodude), and this familiarity made the medication seem more acceptable.

Do children and adolescents feel changed as people?

Some patients and families fear a change in personality or worry about a "zombie effect." Anticipating and pre-emptively addressing such topics or fears directly in the initial assessment phase allows the prescribing clinician to diminish this resistance, while cultivating the alliance, by emphasizing that these effects are unnecessary and unacceptable.

Other patients worry that medication will alter their perceptions of themselves: "I love my symptoms, Doc, they make me myself!" [4]. This attitude may be especially true for patients with a psychotic thought process, as illustrated in early writings after the introduction of the phenothiazines in the 1950s. As Havens [50] wrote, "If the illness is serving a positive function for the patient, he may resist efforts to be cured of it ... for example, [when] hallucinatory figures restore the lost parents."

Winer and Andriukaitis [3] reiterate that if the patients' clinical symptoms are, in part, "the armor by which they protect themselves ... then any move to eradicate these may be threatening to their defensive system ... thus, being medicated could be experienced by patients as a swift housecleaning during which vital and treasured items are discarded." Psychotic patients in particular, require an unambiguous, esteem-preserving communication style from the doctor:

> It is precisely because of the impairment in his/her mental processes caused by the psychosis that the patient is most in need of deliberate and careful consideration of his or her capacity to participate in decisions about medication. The psychotic patient can be acutely aware of attitudes and beliefs of others that are communicated via the *slightest gesture or word* [emphasis added]. In the course of adjusting or initiating medication, your irritation or amusement at symptoms can be easily interpreted as irritation or amusement at the patient. A patient with poor reality testing may not realize that your attempt to control the illness is not an attempt to control himself/herself.

Praise by adults

Even well-meaning parents, teachers, and other adults must be reminded about the use of appropriate language when praising or checking for adherence. One approach is for parents to keep track (discreetly) of the number of pills in the prescription bottle, then subtly but regularly to give appropriate praise for good decision making, good behavior, and adherence to family requests and doctor's instructions.

Transitions in treatment providers and institutional transference

Effective medication regimens too often collapse when a resident on a 6-month "psychopharmacology rotation" leaves at the end of the clinical assignment. A patient's feelings of loss and abandonment in such a case may be just as important to acknowledge as those of a patient whose psychotherapist leaves for the next assignment. In a study examining patient outcomes during transfer to a new pharmacotherapist, Mischoulon and colleagues [7] surveyed 38 psychiatric residents and found that nearly one third of their patients were negatively affected by treatment transfer or termination. These patients required medication changes or deteriorated clinically. The authors concluded that the relationship with the prescribing physician was very important to patients, such that forced termination had negative effects similar to those of transfers to a new psychotherapist [7]. The authors recommend that enough notice be given to help patients deal with the forthcoming loss/change and describe specific suggestions and scripts to aid in processing this transition with patients. In this writer's clinic, trainees are encouraged to inform families and patients of these transfers at the halfway point in a given clinical rotation to allow subsequent processing as needed.

The context and setting of the medication prescription

An observant patient once told about the irony in getting a prescription for Prozac, written by the doctor with a Wellbutrin-logo pen, and with titration instructions written on a Depakote notepad. In keeping with the theme that all of a doctor's actions have potential meaning to the patient and family, mindful pharmacotherapists should be aware of the subliminal messages they are broadcasting through their nonverbal acts. At Stanford, all staff members are encouraged to keep the waiting room and their offices free of drug company advertising by avoiding the use of pens, pads, coffee cups, and clipboards with medication logos. Many medical schools and training programs in psychiatry now include didactic seminars on managing interactions with pharmaceutical industry representatives. These contacts often lead to opportunities for convenient lunches, expensive dinners, and other perks. Pruett and Martin [4] have provided an insightful summary of the commercial pressures in modern medical practice: "The parallel process begs description; drug rep caters to future doc in a setting that encourages docs to prescribe ("cater") reps' drugs to patients—now and, it is hoped, long into the future."

Although some industry representatives have written about marketing's "real and proven value" for patient care [51], other authors encourage an increased vigilance regarding the "pharmaceutical-academic complex" [52] that characterizes the "easy traffic" between residents, drug representatives, teaching hospitals, their research funding base, and the pharmaceutical industry [53–56]. Regardless of how prescribing doctors see themselves, patients may see clinicians as influenced and potentially tainted [4,57] and may wonder about the appropriateness of a medicine for them specifically. Thoughtful discussion of medication recommendations, alternatives, and even inquiries into patient familiarity with psychotropic agents (family members who have taken the drugs, or media exposures) can reveal patient concerns and enhance alliance formation.

Important developmental issues

Children are brought to doctors by their caregivers and thus, are more dependent on the alliance constructs (goals, tasks, bonds) for themselves and also for their parents. The prescribing physician should never assume a child's advance willingness to participate [58]. There are, however, numerous ways in which the warmth, acceptance, attentiveness, and credibility of the doctor can promote a true therapeutic alliance.

In adolescence, patients usually assume more responsibility for their own care. Helping parents to avoid intrusive, controlling styles and attitudes around medication, while still maintaining a proper monitoring and supervisory relationship, is a crucial task for successful pharmacotherapy. Pruett and Martin [4] stress the importance of the *new developmental terrain* of adolescence that must be negotiated by both adolescent patient and prescribing physician [4]. This important time may lead patients to ascribe new meanings to medication itself as well as to the act of accepting a medication [20]. Any agent that in the prepubescent past may have affected appetite (resultant weight gain or loss), endocrine function (galactorrhea, amenorrhea), skin appearance (acne), sexual function (genital arousal or dysfunction), mood, alertness, or sleep may now be viewed or experienced quite differently. Adolescents may manifest simple and overt nonadherence arising from ignorance of the importance of medication, general nonadherence because of familial factors (parental ambivalence regarding need for medication, family history of poor response or of drug addiction), covert nonadherence caused by oppositionality, or intermittent nonadherence because of preoccupation with other activities [2,4].

Dosing itself may become a relevant issue for parents, children, and adolescents (Box 1). For example, patients may have erroneous perceptions about medications that require hundreds of milligrams for effectiveness, compared with medications that require only a few milligrams [4].

Great care must be taken to ensure that there is appropriate, regular, and delineated supervision of medication administration. Specific directions are often required: "Your mom will put the medicine out with your cereal every morning. You can take it right after you finish your cereal, before you put your dishes in the sink. How does that sound to you?" Physicians should also be prepared to engage with adolescents who may become confused or upset by the changing objectives of pharmacotherapy (eg, no longer used for impulsivity, but now for sustaining focus) and interpret them as an indication that he or she is irreparably deficient or damaged in some way. Other issues may include fear of being controlled or impeded by the medication, or of becoming permanently dependent upon an external substance to function ("a happy pill") or upon the adults who administer it.

Parents'/caregivers' guilt about their child's problems, worries about cost of pharmacotherapy, and concerns regarding long-term, possibly unknown, side effects complicate their alliance with the doctor. In addition, parents sometimes feel they do not have an option of refusing medication if they are being pressured by school personnel. If pharmacotherapy is advocated by the physician, they may feel even more uncomfortable discussing the situation, fearing that others hold them responsible for their child's disorder and view them as incapable of implementing behavioral or other nonpharmacologic interventions.

Box 1. Children's concepts about medication

<u>Physical properties of the medication itself</u>

Name: The name of a medication may help enhance or decrease adherence, depending on association (eg, the medicine's name may sound like a superhero or cartoon character (Geodon/"Geodude") or evoke a particular word (Abilify/ability or Abilify/vilify).

Form: Liquid, tablet, capsule, or injectable forms may carry specific and different meanings (eg, liquid formulations may be associated with infants; bad-tasting or injectable medications may be considered punishments).

Special caution must be taken in using injectable medications for children and adolescents with a history of trauma.

Size: A patient may interpret a large pill or dosage as indicating a more severe or more important problem.

Labeling and printing: The patient may have personal associations with imprinted numbers or letters (eg, some children have reported their belief that the numbers on their pills are coded to destroy the monsters inside them or that the shape of or initials on the pills have special meaning to them).

<u>The need to take medicine</u>

The patient may believe that only children who are "sick" or "bad" have to take medicine.

<u>Timing of the dose</u>

Frequency: Greater frequency may be perceived as causing more trouble or, conversely, as offering more help.

Morning or evening dosing: Patients may perceive morning dosing as preparation for school and neglect such dosing (with or without the prescriber's agreement) on weekends. Evening dosing may be perceived as addressing sleeping or dreaming troubles.

During school: The patient's or the parents' concerns about stigma may impede adherence.

Administration: Self-administration suggests trust in the patient; teacher/parent administration may be perceived by the patient as distrust or an adult conspiracy.

(*Adapted from* Pruett KD, Martin A. Thinking about prescribing: the psychology of psychopharmacology. In: Martin A, Scahill L, Charney DS, et al, editors. Pediatric psychopharmacology: principles and practices. New York: Oxford University Press; 2003. p. 419; with permission.)

It is critical to gauge the developmental level of the patient, regardless of chronologic age, and to tailor an explanation to that level to facilitate a working alliance. For most adolescents aged 14 years and older, the doctor can address comments directly to the patient and hand the prescription directly to her/him rather than to the parents. This procedure sends an empowering message. Efforts to include the adolescent in appropriate medication decisions (when/where to take the pill, preferences for specific agents or regimens, mechanisms for reporting side effects) can increase these patients' investment in treatment. These measures can also help clinicians avoid what Krener and Mancina [59] have described as direct or indirect coercion of the child/teen patient under the guise of "informed consent."

Still, separation and individuation tasks may lead to arguments about independence between adolescents and their parents, and medication adherence can become the battlefield upon which control issues are fought. Moreover, the defense mechanisms typically used by adolescents (denial and acting out) often intrude upon the doctor–patient alliance [27].

In addition to developmental variables, varying cultural beliefs regarding the youth's role in the family, ultimate parental authority in all decision making, and the meaning bestowed on the pill itself are often important considerations in pharmacotherapy.

Youth adherence to pharmacotherapy

Adherence to pharmacotherapy significantly influences the effectiveness of any treatment [60]. Adolescents may be especially vulnerable to poor adherence [61]. Factors affecting adherence in child and adolescent psychopharmacology include (1) caregivers' attitudes and their roles; (2) medication side effects; (3) treatment accessibility, acceptability, and satisfaction; and (4) the therapeutic relationship [1,16].

Adherence to pharmacotherapy hinges on the working relationship, the transference and countertransference relationships with the prescribing clinician, the therapeutic interventions being used, and the "relationship" that the patient forms with the pills themselves [16,62]. These relationships may be especially important for adolescents. To promote the working alliance, prescribing clinicians can identify the patient's expectations and wishes for the treatment, and restate them to ensure that they are correctly understood. Because the psychotherapist is in a powerful position to strengthen medication adherence (or to undermine it), *a collaboration between prescribing clinician and psychotherapist can be critically important* [63]. Sharing sufficient information about diagnosis, treatment options, rationale for the choices made, and plans for treatment follow-up and session frequency positions the psychotherapist to support pharmacotherapy [16], and also helps the pharmacotherapist support the psychotherapeutic interventions.

Research in adults indicates that there may be a positive direct effect on better clinical outcomes from the alliance itself (independent of adherence per se)

[11]. Frank and colleagues [64] presented the treatment experience as an experiment in which clinician and patient are co-investigators, with active engagement of the family as well. The clinician became the expert on the disorder and its treatment in general, and the patient became the expert on his/her own symptoms and experience of the treatment [64]. Sabo and Rand [21], however, found that some patients expect the doctor to play a more traditional role. Patients from cultures in which doctors have very high status may fare better, for example, if the doctor assumes a more directive (but still beneficent) stance [21]. Finally, pediatric pharmacotherapists often find themselves in the role of adjunctive therapist. Although other members of the treatment team have greater contact with the child, some parents still defer to the prescribing physician for supervisory management of the child's treatment. Although they seek to focus on the pharmacotherapy, prescribers may still be consulted about psychotherapy or behavioral interventions provided by others. Whenever feasible, collaboration and consistent messages from all team members are preferable to disagreements playing out between the treaters (akin to parental conflicts). Thus, ongoing communication among team members is crucial.

Although there is emerging evidence for the predictive role of the alliance in clinical outcomes during pharmacotherapy with adult patients [11,13], literature about children and the therapeutic alliance in pharmacotherapy is limited, with most peer-reviewed articles specifically reporting on adherence or compliance within pediatric psychopharmacology [25]. Most studies have looked at stimulant compliance among children with ADHD and report average adherence rates of 40% to 70%. Thiruchelvam and colleagues [65] described impacts of adherence on outcomes among children who had ADHD. In their 3-year prospective, placebo-controlled study of 71 children, ages 6 to 12 years who had ADHD, response to treatment at 12 months was not associated with adherence per se, because some patients got better even with suboptimal adherence. Adherence declined over time, from 81% in year one to 67% in year two, and 52% in year three. Adherence and outcomes were best in the first year of the study, possibly because of the frequency of contacts and perceived quality of support from the research team [11,65], suggesting a possible role for the alliance in treatment success.

Lewis [26] describes the parent–child dynamic in ADHD as often involving a battle for control. The disruptive behavior that may accompany the condition leads parents to exert their authority. The medication may become a symbol or agent of this control and is thus rejected by the child. Attitude toward medication may mirror feelings toward parents. When the child–parent relationship is harmonious, medicine may be taken readily. When there is tension, it may be refused [26].

The role of the dual alliance

When discussing medications for the first time, one must always consider the different levels of parent/teacher understanding, as well as feelings and receptiveness about psychiatric drug treatment. Although not useful in every situation, some patients and families experience a sense of relief if they are led to understand mental illness as a neurotransmitter (or chemical) imbalance rather than as the result of parenting defects. With depressive illness, for example, adolescents may be relieved when the pharmacotherapist links self-criticism, low energy, depressed mood, and irritability, to a biologic illness beyond the willful control of the patient [21]. In other cases, however, a self-attribution may lead to more sustainable adherence. For example, Lewis [26] cites the usefulness of a soccer metaphor for a 10-year-old child who "wanted to feel that (she), and not the pill, got the goal." She was able to accept the medication when she came to see it as help, similar to a pass that allowed her to score.

Parents invest more helpfully when seen as partners by the therapeutic team [45]. Alexander and Dore [45] examined the negative beliefs about parents often held by therapists from varying disciplines. Occasionally, clinicians get locked into viewing parents as prime contributors to the child's pathology (and therefore as obstacles to the child's therapeutic success rather than as resources who support a positive outcome). Child and adolescent mental health treatment is sometimes too exclusively child-focused, in effect excluding parents in treatment [67]. Alexander and Dore [45] found that, although all therapists are susceptible, psychiatrists were more likely than psychologists or social workers to hold the belief that parents contributed mightily to their child's disorder. In pharmacotherapy, it must be remembered that if parents do not endorse the medication intervention, they may consciously or unconsciously undo the treatment (through failing to fill prescriptions or not adhering to the treatment plan, constant lateness, or missed/cancelled sessions). Prescribing doctors therefore must pay careful attention to the way they include or exclude parents in treatment. DeChillo and colleagues [68] have written how effective partnership practice normalizes the reality that families have variable responses to stressors in their lives. Some will need the physician to take a more proactive stance in decision making, particularly in stressful situations [68]. Thus, partnerships with difficult, hard-to-reach, or vulnerable families can be just as important as those with less impaired families. Accordingly, the type and severity of family problems should not pose insurmountable barriers to effective partnerships, as long as the clinician is truly committed to the process and possesses the skills to engage these families [68].

To evaluate clinical outcomes related to this dual alliance, Hawley and Weisz [37] examined both youth–therapist and parent–therapist alliances in psychotherapy. They found that the parent (but not youth) alliance was significantly related to more frequent family participation, less frequent cancellations and no-shows, and greater therapist concurrence with the decision to end treatment. In contrast, the youth (but not parent) alliance was significantly related to both youth and parent reports of symptom improvement. Thus, the findings indicate that both alliance relationships are crucial, even if they differ in important ways [37]. Kazdin and colleagues [69] found that a poor alliance was one of the factors predictive of treatment dropout within families of children with externalizing symptoms on the oppositional-defiant-antisocial continuum [69]. Nevas and Farber [36] found that parents who experience primarily positive attitudes and feelings about their child's therapist feel hopeful, understood, and grateful [36]. Alexander and Dore [45] noted that outcomes associated with a positive therapeutic alliance include reduced symptom severity, improved global functioning and service satisfaction, increased treatment participation, and avoidance of premature termination, as well as increased medication adherence [45].

In preadolescent children, the doctor–caregiver alliance seems especially key [45]. Horvath and Greenberg [29] suggest that although a strong working alliance does not have to occur immediately, a "good enough alliance" (with both patient and parent/caregiver) is crucial for the therapy to proceed:

> [A]lliance development is a series of windows of opportunity, decreasing in size with each session ... [T]he foundation for collaborative work entails adjustments in both the client's and therapist's procedural expectations and goals. The longer the participants find themselves apart on these issues, the more difficult it becomes to develop a collaborative framework.

Difficult families

Despite the clinician's understanding gained from research and clinical wisdom, certain parents and families remain difficult to work with. Some are afflicted with mental health problems of their own. Others are sufficiently unfamiliar with psychiatric disorders and their treatment so that they vacillate between ambivalence about treatments and unreasonable expectations. This vacillation can impede alliance formation and make any intervention difficult. Groves [66] identified the insatiable dependence of "hateful patients" leading to behaviors that suggested four different groups (which may be applied to work with difficult parents): "dependent clingers," "entitled demanders," "manipulative help-rejecters," and "self-destructive deniers." The physician's negative reactions to each difficult family constitute important clinical data that should facilitate better understanding and lead to more appropriate psychologic management for these situations [66].

Other alliance partners

Teachers and other school staff can be important sources in the alliance relationship [2], sometimes having initiated the medication consultation. The physician may need direct contact with specific personnel. It may be necessary, for example, to correct the school staff's "delusion of precision" [14,15] that pharmacotherapy might have the power to eliminate symptoms with magical precision—if only the physician would prescribe the correct agents. Parents may fear that the school seeks to medicate their children into docility and behavioral compliance, more for reasons of understaffing and overcrowding than for the best interests of the child [4]. The doctor is at his or her best when seen as part of a team on the patient's behalf. There is always at least a four-way relationship involving the patient, parent, teacher, and prescribing physician. The doctor who works with the teacher or school nurse to find ways for the student to take medication (eg, coming up with a signal or giving the student an errand to run at just the right time) optimizes adherence. Once-daily preparations have further improved adherence while diminishing risks of patient embarrassment or humiliation at being publicly "reminded" to take medication.

The alliance in primary care settings

Because primary care providers (PCPs) have a crucial role in pharmacotherapy, their psychotherapeutic role must also be appreciated. What Milton Senn, the Cornell University pediatrician, wrote in 1948 remains relevant in 2006 [69a]:

> From the fields of psychology, psychiatry, education, and that less easily classified area which is called "growth and development", the pediatrician is advised how to make pediatric practice more effective through the use of techniques which have been found useful in each of these disciplines. For example, the pediatrician is urged to become acquainted with the facts of growth and development so that as a "developmental pediatrician" he may predict and interpret behavior of children to their parents; and, along with proper understanding of the parents, may relieve their hopes, fears, and mental conflicts...Actually to help the patient it is neither necessary nor desirable in every instance to offer anything more than *opportunity for the establishment of a relationship* [emphasis added].

Because the PCP interacts directly with both child and parent, a dual alliance is present, as in the practice of psychiatry. Beresin [70] describes the most important elements of a sound PCP–family–patient relationship in pediatrics: a quiet setting that is comfortable and amenable for interviewing, an atmosphere embodied with both a sense of timelessness and a time limit, and a PCP

- Who is comfortable with interviewing (and who always greets each family member cordially, asking how each wishes to be called)
- Who pays attention to both verbal and nonverbal cues during the interview (remembering that patients are also observing the doctor)
- Who is aware of his/her own feelings toward the patient and family
- Who practices culturally informed and developmentally relevant care
- Who can skillfully do psychosocial screening (using the HEADSS mnemonic for teens that includes Home, Education, Activities, Drugs, Sex, Suicide [71])
- Who can employ some basic therapeutic skills essential to the doctor–patient–family relationship

Special populations

Patients with developmental disabilities, including pervasive developmental disorders and mental retardation, fall into a special category. The physician's role often extends to becoming an advocate for this vulnerable group of patients who too often "fall through the cracks" in the regular medical care system. These patients seem especially prone to being kept on the same medication regimen for long periods of time, despite being at higher risk for certain side effects [72]. Their care is sometimes neglected, because systemic resistances may impede "changes" for their home and school behavior. A separate alliance must be established with the guardian (often the director of a group home) and special education classroom staff, in addition to the parents. Although rational pharmacotherapy can be quite helpful, clinicians must guard against pressures to medicate these clients unnecessarily, striving instead to maximize educational and vocational potential and attending to healthy functioning in peer relationships. These patients often have very little cognitive reserve, making them especially susceptible to the dulling effects of mood stabilizers, alpha-agonists, and antipsychotic medicines.

Other groups of special patients that society deems particularly important (the "VIP") may find themselves at risk of being either under- or overtreated. Their status in society may present real and unique barriers to the usual standard of care, and physicians must be aware of the potential countertransference issues when caring for this group of patients [73].

Future directions

The importance of the therapeutic alliance in pediatric pharmacotherapy has led to the creation of instruments to measure this construct more precisely. For example, the Therapeutic Alliance in Pediatric Pharmacotherapy Scale (TAPPS) includes patient, parent, teacher, prescriber, and observer perceptions of the therapeutic relationship in pharmacotherapy treatment. The TAPPS is a relatively short scale that can be used in both outpatient and inpatient settings to measure the alliance more objectively, and is adapted from the California Pharmacotherapy Alliance Scale [13,79], Helping Alliance Questionnaire, revised [74], Helping Alliance Questionnaire for children [75], and Therapeutic Alliance Scale for Children, revised [58]. The TAPPS contains content and face validity, and as of this writing is being piloted in two academic psychiatry clinics for further psychometric validation so that it can be administered in community-based settings as well. Clinical use of the TAPPS may allow the prescribing physician to assess systematically the alliance with patients, parents, and teachers, as well as to assess attitudes toward medication and toward the physician. Finally, instruments such as these may help in teaching the therapeutic alliance in pharmacotherapy as a measurable skill during residency training [76]. Box 2 contains sample questions in the TAPPS versions for parents, children, and therapists.

Box 2. Therapeutic Alliance in Pediatric Pharmacotherapy Scale

Scoring

0 not at all
1 a little/somewhat
2 moderately
3 very much

Parent version sample questions

1. I believe the doctor is trying to help my child get better 0 1 2 3
2. I understand why my child is taking this medication 0 1 2 3
3. It is **not** easy to trust my child's doctor 0 1 2 3
4. I consider the doctor to be an ally of mine 0 1 2 3
5. I feel that the doctor really listens to me 0 1 2 3
6. I think the medicine is helping my child 0 1 2 3
7. I felt that the doctor "pushed" us to start medication for my child 0 1 2 3

IF YOUR CHILD'S TEACHER IS AWARE THAT HE IS TAKING MEDICA-
TION THEN PLEASE COMPLETE THE FOLLOWING:

8. The doctor has done a good job of explaining medication to the teacher 0 1 2 3
9. The doctor should have had more contact with the school 0 1 2 3
10. The doctor helped the teacher manage my child's feelings and behaviors in ways other than using medication 0 1 2 3

Child version sample questions

1. I believe the doctor is trying to help me get better 0 1 2 3
2. I understand why I am taking this medication 0 1 2 3
3. It is **not** easy to trust my doctor 0 1 2 3
4. I consider the doctor to be on my side 0 1 2 3
5. I feel that the doctor really listens to me 0 1 2 3
6. I think the medicine is helping me 0 1 2 3
7. My doctor talked about the medication in a way I could understand 0 1 2 3

Therapist version sample questions

1. The child believes you are trying to help him/her get better 0 1 2 3
2. The child understands why s/he is taking this medication 0 1 2 3
3. The child feels that it is **not** easy to trust you 0 1 2 3
4. Both parent and child consider you to be an ally 0 1 2 3
5. The child feels that you really listen to him/her 0 1 2 3
6. The child thinks the medicine is helping him/her 0 1 2 3
7. The child feels that you talked about the medication in a way he/she could understand 0 1 2 3

(Courtesy of S.V. Joshi, MD, and M. Weiss, MD, PhD, San Francisco, CA.)

Recommendations for practitioners

The recommendations in Box 3 are based on work done thus far in the specialty area of the alliance in pediatric pharmacotherapy [2–4,22–24, 56,64].

Box 3. Recommendations for establishing an effective working alliance in pediatric pharmacotherapy

The pharmacotherapist should strive to:

- Ensure that case formulation always precedes the prescription
- Emote a real sense of understanding in all communications with patients and families
- Involve the patient in the decision-making process, especially in the case of adolescents
- Assess the understanding of the mental illness and the meaning of medication for the patient and family
- Nurture all professional relationships necessary to sustain the child's health (parents, family members, other therapists, teachers, PCPs)
- Visit consumer websites often and help families connect to appropriate support groups
- Identify references and books to help patients obtain useful, accurate understanding about mental health disorders
- When the subject of pharmacotherapy emerges, pause and listen to the patient's and parents' associations and responses to the word "medication"
- Provide a small number of choices of medications whenever possible, so that past associations with a particular product do not derail treatment; remain mindful that any change, including improvement, may be threatening to the patient and family
- Respect the patient's and family's right to informed consent and need to know about common side effects, without burdening them with so much information that they become overwhelmed
- Practice the three C's of good pharmacotherapy:
  1. Collaboration (with therapists, families, other providers)
  2. Conscientiousness (of the evidence base, the standard of practice, the specific sociocultural needs of the patient and family)
  3. Communication (return telephone calls and e-mails promptly, be available between sessions for quick questions, document so that others can follow the pharmacotherapy reasoning if they participate in this patient's care)
- Remember that all actions have potential meanings for patients and families, from the pens used to write prescriptions, to the language employed to explain about mental illness, to the way the pharmacotherapist provides realistic hope for the future

---

Summary

Psychopharmacologic practice is part of child psychiatric practice, and it requires expertise with a variety of therapeutic techniques. Skilled physicians must first promote an alliance, then identify and treat symptoms, and finally enhance adherence on the road to the best possible clinical outcomes. In fact, unless the psychologic aspects of care are attended to carefully, pharmacologic aspects may be only suboptimal at best [77].

A strong therapeutic alliance lays the foundation upon which positive outcomes in mental health treatment are built. Effective pharmacotherapists should be mindful of both the target symptoms and the context and settings in which they occur.

These principles apply in the psychiatrist's office and in other treatment settings such as that of the PCP, where psychotropic medicines are often prescribed for children and adolescents.

In pediatric psychopharmacology specifically, there is always *at least* a dual alliance that must be acknowledged and nurtured. Prescribing clinicians should strive to include both patient and parent/guardian into the working-alliance paradigms of goal identification, task consolidation, and therapeutic bond establishment. Research thus far shows that knowledge of the psychologic factors and developmental implications present when medicines are prescribed will improve therapeutic outcomes.

Finally, physicians should never underestimate their role in helping families and patients *really learn about* mental health and illness. Kandel [78] predicted the enlightened relationship that could develop between psychiatry and neurobiology and how it applies to patient care:

> As a result, when I speak to someone and he or she listens to me, we not only make eye contact and voice contact, but the action of the neuronal machinery in my brain is having a direct and, I hope, long-lasting effect on the neuronal machinery in his/her brain (and vice versa). Indeed, I would argue that it is only insofar as words produce changes in each others' brains that psychotherapeutic intervention produces changes in patients' minds. From this perspective, the biologic and psychologic processes are joined.

Acknowledgments

The author gives special thanks to Drs. Jeff Bostic, Carl Feinstein, and Andrés Martin for their thoughtful editorial suggestions.

References

[1] Metzl JA. Forming an effective therapeutic alliance. In: Tasman A, Riba MB, Silk KR, editors. The doctor-patient relationship in pharmacotherapy: improving treatment effectiveness. New York: Guilford Press; 2000. p. 25–47.

[2] Joshi S, Khanzode L, Steiner H. Psychological aspects of pediatric medication management. In: Steiner H, editor. Handbook of mental health interventions in children & adolescents: an integrated developmental approach. San Francisco (CA): Jossey-Bass; 2004. p. 465–81.

[3] Winer J, Andriukaitis S. Interpersonal aspects of initiating pharmacotherapy: how to avoid becoming the patient's feared negative other. Psychiatr Ann 1989;19(6):318–23.

[4] Pruett KD, Martin A. Thinking about prescribing: the psychology of psychopharmacology. In: Martin A, Scahill L, Charney DS, et al, editors. Principles and practice of pediatric psychopharmacology. New York: Oxford University Press; 2003. p. 417–25.

[5] Blackwell B. Drug therapy: patient compliance. N Engl J Med 1973;289:249–52.

[6] Tasman A, Riba MB, Silk KR. Using the interview to establish collaboration. In: Tasman A, Riba MB, Silk KR, editors. The doctor-patient relationship in pharmacotherapy: improving treatment effectiveness. New York: Guilford Press; 2000. p. 49–69.

[7] Mischoulon D, Rosenbaum J, Messner E. Transfer to a new psychopharmacologist: its effect on patients. Acad Psychiatry 2000;24(3):156–63.

[8] Rappaport N, Chubinsky P. The meaning of psychotropic medications for children, adolescents, and their families. J Am Acad Child Adolesc Psychiatry 2000;39:1198–200.

[9] Luborsky L. Therapeutic alliances as predictors of psychotherapy outcomes: factors explaining the predictive success. In: Horvath A, Greenberg L, editors. The working alliance: theory, research, and practice. New York: John Wiley & Sons; 1994. p. 314.

[10] Luborsky L, McLellan AT, Woody GE, et al. Therapist success and its determinates. Arch Gen Psychiatry 1985;42:602–11.

[11] Krupnick J, Sotsky S, Simmens S, et al. The role of the therapeutic alliance in psychotherapy pharmacotherapy outcome: findings in the National Institute of Mental Health Treatment of Depression Collaborative Research Program. J Consult Clin Psychol 1996;64(3):532–9.

[12] Morgan R, Luborsky L, Crits-Cristoph P, et al. Predicting the outcomes of psychotherapy by the Penn Helping Alliance Rating Method. Arch Gen Psychiatry 1982;39:397–402.

[13] Weiss M, Gaston L, Propst A, et al. The role of the alliance in the pharmacologic treatment of depression. J Clin Psychiatry 1997;58(5):196–204.

[14] Gutheil TG. The psychology of psychopharmacology. Bull Menninger Clin 1982;46:321–30.

[15] Gutheil TG. Improving patient compliance: psychodynamics in drug prescribing. Drug Ther (NY) 1977;7:82–95.

[16] Ellison JM. Enhancing adherence in the pharmacotherapy treatment relationship. In: Tasman A, Riba MB, Silk KR, editors. The doctor-patient relationship in pharmacotherapy: improving treatment effectiveness. New York: Guilford Press; 2000. p. 71–94.

[17] Carli T. The psychologically informed psychopharmacologist. In: Riba MB, Balon R, editors. Psychopharmacology and psychotherapy: a collaborative approach. Washington (DC): American Psychiatric Press; 1999. p. 179–96.

[18] Beitman BD, Blinder BJ, Thase ME, et al. Psychotherapy during pharmacotherapy. Integrating psychotherapy and pharmacotherapy: dissolving the mind-brain barrier. New York: WW Norton; 2003. p. 35–71.

[19] Adelman S. Pills as transitional objects: a dynamic understanding of the use of medication in psychotherapy. Psychiatry 1985;48:246–53.

[20] Tasman A, Riba MB. Psychological management in psychopharmacologic treatment, and combination pharmacologic and psychotherapeutic treatment. In: Lieberman J, Tasman A, editors. Psychiatric drugs. Philadelphia: WB Saunders; 2000. p. 242–9.

[21] Sabo A, Rand B. The relational aspects of psychopharmacology. In: Sabo A, Havens L, editors. The real world guide to psychotherapy practice. Cambridge (MA): Harvard University Press; 2000. p. 34–59.

[22] Schowalter JE. Psychodynamics and medication. J Am Acad Child Adolesc Psychiatry 1989; 28:681–4.

[23] Kutcher SP. Practical clinical issues regarding child and adolescent psychopharmacology. Child Adolesc Psychiatr Clin N Am 2000;9:245–60.

[24] Kutcher SP. Child and adolescent psychopharmacology. 1st edition. Philadelphia: WB Saunders; 1997.

[25] Hack S, Chow B. Pediatric psychotropic medication compliance: a literature review and research-based suggestions for improving treatment compliance. J Child Adolesc Psychopharmacol 2001;11:59–67.

[26] Lewis O. Psychological factors affecting pharmacologic compliance. Child Adolesc Psychiatr Clin N Am 1995;4(1):15–22.

[27] Shaw RJ, Palmer LL. Consultation in the medical setting: a model to enhance treatment adherence. In: Steiner H, editor. Handbook of mental health interventions in children and adolescents: an integrated developmental approach. San Francisco (CA): Jossey-Bass; 2004. p. 917–41.

[28] Gabbard G, Kay J. The fate of integrated treatment: whatever happened to the biopsychosocial psychiatrist? Am J Psychiatry 2001;158:1956–63.

[29] Horvath A, Greenberg L. Introduction. In: Horvath A, Greenberg L, editors. The working alliance: theory, research, and practice. New York: John Wiley & Sons; 1994. p. 304.

[30] Bordin E. The generalizability of the psychoanalytic concept of the working alliance. Psychotherapy Theory, Research, and Practice 1979;16:252–60.

[31] Bordin E. Theory and research on the therapeutic working alliance: new directions. In: Horvath A, Greenberg L, editors. The working alliance: theory, research, and practice. New York C: John Wiley & Sons; 1994. p. 304.

[32] Horvath A, Greenberg L. Development of the working alliance inventory. In: Greenberg L, Pinsof W, editors. The psychotherapeutic process: a research handbook. New York: Guilford Press; 1987.

[33] Oetzel K, Scere D. Therapeutic engagement with adolescents in psychotherapy. Psychotherapy Theory, Research, and Practice 2003;40(3):215–25.

[34] Castonguay L, Constantino M. Engagement in psychotherapy: factors contributing to the facilitation, demise, and restoration of the working alliance In: Castro-Blanco D, editor. Treatment engagement with adolescents. Washington (DC): American Psychological Association; in press.

[35] Morrisey-Kane E, Prinz R. Engagement in child and adolescent treatment: the role of parental cognitions and attributions. Clin Child Fam Psychol Rev 1999;2(3):183–97.

[36] Nevas D, Farber B. Parents' attitudes toward their child's therapist and therapy. Prof Psychol Res Pr 2001;32(2):165–70.

[37] Hawley KM, Weisz JR. Youth versus parent working alliance in usual clinical care: distinctive associations with retention, satisfaction, and treatment outcome. J Clin Child Adolesc Psychol 2005;34(1):117–28.

[38] Horvath A, Bedi R. The alliance. In: Norcross JC, editor. Psychotherapy relationships that work. New York: Oxford University Press; 2002. p. 37–69.

[39] Wampold B. The great psychotherapy debate: models, methods, and findings. Mahwah (NJ): Erlbaum; 2001.

[40] Sexton H. Process, life events, and symptomatic change in brief, eclectic psychotherapy. J Consult Clin Psychol 1996;64:1358–65.

[41] Lichenberg J, Wettersten K, Mull H, et al. Relationship and control as correlates of psychotherapy quality and outcome. J Consult Clin Psychol 1988;45:322–37.

[42] Hersoug A, Monsen J, Havik O, et al. Prediction of early working alliance: diagnoses, relationship, and intrapsychic variables as predictors. Presented at the Society for Psychotherapy Research. Chicago, June 21–25, 2000.

[43] Henry W, Strupp H. The therapeutic alliance as interpersonal process. In: Horvath A, Greenberg L, editors. The working alliance: theory, research and practice. New York: Wiley; 1994. p. 51–84.

[44] Horvath A. Research on the alliance. In: Horvath A, Greenberg L, editors. The working alliance: theory, research, and practice. New York: John Wiley & Sons; 1994. p. 259–86.

[45] Alexander L, Dore M. Making the Parents as Partners principle a reality: the role of the alliance. J Child Fam Stud 1999;8(3):255–70.

[46] Shirk S, Karver M. Prediction of treatment outcome from relationship variables in child and adolescent therapy: a meta-analytic review. J Consult Clin Psychol 2003;71(3):452–64.

[47] Horvath A, Symonds B. Relation between working alliance and outcome in psychotherapy: a meta-analysis. J Couns Psychology 1991;38:139–49.

[48] Havens L. Forming effective relationships. In: Havens L, Sabo A, editors. The real world guide to psychotherapy practice. Cambridge (MA): Harvard University Press; 2000. p. 17–33.

[49] Mintz D. Meaning and medication in the care of treatment-resistant patients. Am J Psychother 2002;56(3):322–38.

[50] Havens L. Problems with the use of drugs in the psychotherapy of psychotic patients. Psychiatry 1963;26:289–96.

[51] Beary J. Pharmaceutical marketing has real and proven value. J Gen Intern Med 1996;11(10): 635–6.

[52] Angell M. Is academic medicine for sale? N Engl J Med 2000;342(20):1516–8.

[53] Wolfe S. Why do American drug companies spend more than $12 billion a year pushing drugs? Is it education or promotion? J Gen Intern Med 1996;11(10):637–9.

[54] Stryer D, Bero L. Characteristics of materials distributed by drug companies: an evaluation of appropriateness. J Gen Intern Med 1996;11(10):575–83.

[55] Temple R, O'Brien R. Why would anyone have expected anything else? J Gen Intern Med 1996;11(10):640–1.

[56] Landefeld C, Chren M-M. Drug companies and information abut drugs: recommendations for doctors. J Gen Intern Med 1996;11(10):642–5.

[57] Mainous III A, Houeston W, Rich E. Patient perceptions of physician acceptance of gifts from the pharmaceutical industry. Arch Fam Med 1995;4:335–9.

[58] Shirk S, Saiz C. Clinical, empirical, and developmental perspectives on the therapeutic relationship in child psychotherapy. Dev Psychopathol 1992;4:713–28.

[59] Krener PK, Mancina RA. Informed consent or informed coercion? Decision-making in pediatric psychopharmacology. J Child Adolesc Psychopharmacol 1994;4:183–200.

[60] Brown RT, Sammons MT. Pediatric psychopharmacology: a review of new developments and recent research. Prof Psychol Res Pr 2002;33(2):135–47.

[61] Cromer B, Tarnowski K. Noncompliance in adolescents: a review. J Dev Behav Pediatr 1989; 10(4):207–15.

[62] Book H. Some psychodynamics of non-compliance. Can J Psychiatry 1987;32:115–7.

[63] Sederer LI, Ellison JM, Keyes C. Guidelines for prescribing psychiatrists in consultative, collaborative, and supervisory relationships. Psychiatr Serv 1998;49:1197–202.

[64] Frank E, Kupfer D, Siegel L. Alliance not compliance: a philosophy of outpatient care. J Clin Psychiatry 1995;56(Suppl 1):11–6.

[65] Thiruchelvam D, Charach A, Schachar R. Moderators and mediators of long-term adherence to stimulant treatment in children with ADHD. J Am Acad Child Adolesc Psychiatry 2001; 40(8):922–8.

[66] Groves JE. Taking care of the hateful patient. N Engl J Med 1978;298(16):883–7.

[67] Johnson H, Cournoyer D, Fisher G. Worker cognitions about parents of children with emotional and emotional disabilities. Journal of Emotional and Behavioral Disorders 1994;1:99–108.

[68] DeChillo N, Koren P, Schultze K. From paternalism to partnership: family and professional collaboration in children's mental health. Am J Orthopsychiatry 1994;64:564–76.

[69] Kazdin A, Holland L, Crowley M. Family experience of barriers to treatment and premature termination from child therapy. J Consult Clin Psychol 1997;65:453–63.

[69a] Senn MJE. The psychotherapeutic role of the pediatrician. Pediatrics 1948;2(2):147.

[70] Beresin E. The doctor-patient relationship in pediatrics. In: Kaye D, Montgomery M, Munson S, editors. Child and adolescent mental health. Philadelphia: Lippincott, Williams, and Wilkins; 2002. p. 8–17.

[71] Goldenring J, Cohen E. Getting into adolescent heads. Contemp Pediatr 1988;July:75–90.

[72] Madrid A, State M, King B. Pharmacologic management of psychiatric and behavioral symptoms in mental retardation. Child Adolesc Psychiatr Clin N Am 2000;9:1225–39.

[73] Martin A, Bostic J, Pruett KD. The VIP: hazard and promise in treating "special" patients. J Am Acad Child Adolesc Psychiatry 2004;43(3):366–9.

[74] Luborsky L, Barber J, Siqueland L, et al. The revised helping alliance questionnaire (HAq II). J Psychother Pract Res 1996;5:260–71.

[75] Kabuth B, Remy C, Saxena K, et al. The modified therapeutic alliance questionnaire for children & parents (HAq-CP). Scientific Proceedings of the American Academy of Child & Adolescent Psychiatry. Miami (FL), October 14–19, 2003.

[76] Summers R, Barber J. Therapeutic alliance as a measurable psychotherapy skill. Acad Psychiatry 2003;27(3):160–5.

[77] Pillay SS, Ghaemi SN. The psychology of polypharmacy. In: Ghaemi SN, editor. Polypharmacy in psychiatry. New York: Marcel Dekker; 2002. p. 299–310.

[78] Kandel E. Psychotherapy and the single synapse: the impact of psychiatric thought on neurobiologic research. N Engl J Med 1979;301(19):1028–37.

[79] Gaston L, Marmar C. The California Pharmacotherapy Alliance Scale. San Francisco: University of California; 1991.

CHILD AND
ADOLESCENT
PSYCHIATRIC CLINICS
OF NORTH AMERICA

ELSEVIER
SAUNDERS

Child Adolesc Psychiatric Clin N Am
15 (2006) 263–287

Gained in Translation: Evidence-Based Medicine Meets Pediatric Psychopharmacology

Vinod Srihari, MD[a], Andrés Martin, MD, MPH[b],*

[a]Department of Psychiatry, Yale University School of Medicine, New Haven, CT 06508, USA
[b]Yale Child Study Center, Yale University School of Medicine, 230 South Frontage Road,
New Haven, CT 06520-7900, USA

Eschew obfuscation

—Bumper sticker, sighted by Professor Glen Gabbard

Since its inception at McMaster University as an effort to improve clinicians' ability to appraise the scientific literature and its subsequent articulation as an approach to medical practice, evidence-based medicine (EBM) has become a much-used term in the medical literature. Given its explicit approach to clinical uncertainty, the model allows for fruitful critique and refinement. EBM has also entered a longstanding debate about the relative value of clinical experience, clinical research, and physiologic knowledge in medical education. In this context EBM has sometimes been used unfairly as a euphemism for clinically irrelevant randomized controlled trials (RCTs) or for the kind of practitioner who uses a narrow emphasis on quantitative measures to hide from clinical complexity. The practice of moving empirically validated treatments into more widespread practice, although a laudable goal, has also linked EBM with policies that are seen as a straightjacket on clinical judgment.

Dr. Martin has received career-development support from the National Institute of Mental Health (PHS grant MH 01792), and honoraria, research, or travel support from Alza, Bristol-Myers Squibb, Eli Lilly, and Janssen Pharmaceuticals.

An earlier version of this manuscript was presented as a workshop at the American Association of Directors of Psychiatric Residency Training Annual Meeting, Tucson (AZ), March 12, 2005.

* Corresponding author.
E-mail address: andres.martin@yale.edu (A. Martin).

Despite its wide dissemination in general medical practice and teaching, EBM has only recently appeared in the psychiatric literature. The time is right for psychiatry to claim the clinical usefulness of this tool for the primary purpose for which it was designed: to help the busy clinician navigate the burgeoning medical literature to inform decision making with and for individual patients. The authors believe that EBM provides an approach to clinical uncertainty based on a sound emphasis on epistemology: that the best way to guide the search for an answer is first to become aware of just how it is that investigators can know. This guiding epistemology allows clinicians to determine to what extent the information available satisfies the criteria for knowing, that is, to evaluate the quality of the evidence that constitutes the current level of knowledge— or ignorance.

What is evidence-based medicine?

An early proponent defined EBM as "the conscientious, explicit, and judicious use of current best evidence in making decisions about the care of individual patients" [1]. This definition can hardly have generated much comment. This process is, after all, what many clinicians see themselves as doing in their routine care of patients and does not do justice to the specific emphasis of EBM. The decision making in any clinical encounter is a result of a number of considerations: reasoning based on pathophysiology, clinical habit, the values and preferences of the patient, contingencies such as the availability and costs (both temporal and monetary) of interventions, and the 'evidence'—information drawn from carefully conducted clinical studies of groups of similar patients. The EBM approach provides a powerful and systematic way to proceed through such decision making. Perhaps most unique is its explicit attention to the process of finding relevant information, to appraising that information, and then to making careful inferences and applications to individual patients.

How can one find and use information from clinical studies to inform the care of an individual patient? Put another way, how can data from large groups that share some similarities with a patient, and yet are distant and anonymous in many other ways, be used to address questions about fundamental clinical activities such as making a diagnosis or prognosis, considering the etiologic factors in an illness, or planning an intervention [2]? The EBM approach highlights the role of such data drawn from human subjects in supplementing theories of pathophysiology or clinical habit. Although for many clinical questions there is a paucity of good data, and one must extrapolate from knowledge of physiology (when possible) or from accumulated experience with patients (when available), EBM urges the practitioner to search for and evaluate the clinical research data before resorting implicitly or exclusively to such approaches. Although this new emphasis has been described as a paradigm shift in the philosophy of medical practice [3], we prefer to focus on the pragmatic and less polarizing aspects of EBM as a tool for continuing medical education. As we hope this article illustrates, an evidence-based approach to clinical practice does not involve a break from traditional knowledge and skills but rather a sharpening of those skills in identifying gaps in knowledge and an appreciation of the available information in databases with which to fill such gaps.

Clinical uncertainty is ubiquitous, and each practitioner has imperfect knowledge of a growing and often overwhelming clinical literature. Much of this literature is of little relevance to daily clinical practice, is difficult to find, and, when stumbled upon, is often difficult to apply, with its value often concealed within a haze of impenetrable statistical jargon. And then there is the matter of limited time.

In the next section the authors attempt to demonstrate an EBM-style approach to clinical uncertainty. A recent paper in the *Child and Adolescent Psychiatric Clinics of North America* eloquently described the background, rationale, and implications of an EBM approach for continuing education in a pediatric psychiatry program [4]. Here, we apply EBM principles to an individual case, attempting to illustrate how such an approach might make the search for information more efficient and productive. We also attempt to keep close to the clinical realities of the case and hope thereby to illustrate the limitations of the evidence and the vital role for clinical judgment and patient preferences in real-world choices. The purpose here is illustrative, not prescriptive: we have chosen a common clinical problem (the treatment of a depressed adolescent) to arrive at relatively well-accepted therapeutic interventions (selective serotonin reuptake inhibitors [SSRIs] and cognitive behavior therapy [CBT]) and a particularly well-designed study, the Treatment for Adolescents with Depression Study (TADS) RCT with which the reader may be familiar. We aim to illustrate how one can use the literature to arrive at an evidence-informed decision for a given individual patient.

How does one "do" evidence-based medicine?

The practice of EBM involves five broad domains of activity, summarized in the "five A's" (Box 1). The authors attempt to show how EBM offers a way to translate everyday clinical challenges into explicit steps, to approach them systematically, and thereby, one hopes, to respond to clinical uncertainty more productively. The reader who is stimulated by this approach is directed to one of several well-written manuals, the last of which has been prepared specifically with psychiatrists in mind [3,5,6].

Case vignette

SL is a 13-year-old boy who presented for his first psychiatric consultation with a 2-year history of a significant decline in school performance, moderately depressed mood, feelings of low self-esteem, a marked decrease in pleasur-able activities, social withdrawal, and vegetative symptoms that included low energy and appetite. The academic decline was reflective of poor attention and concentration in the classroom. On examination he displayed psychomotor retardation, intermittently hiding his face behind his hands and frequently becoming tearful, although he denied suicidal ideation and had no history of self-harm. This presentation occurred against a background of 4 years of behavioral change, mostly marked by social withdrawal, with the depressive symptoms manifesting more clearly to the family and teachers in the preceding 2 years. Additionally, there was a family history of depression (in the father, treated successfully with sertraline) and of bipolar disorder (in the pater-nal grandmother).

ASK: translating global uncertainty into well-built clinical questions or translating a mystery into a problem

Multiple questions can arise from this encounter. When classified into types, these questions suggest different places in which to look for answers. Did SL ever have manic or mixed symptoms (a question about clinical data)? This question can be answered only with careful and repeated discussions with the patient and use of collateral sources. How does one make a diagnosis of dysthymia? This is a typical 'background' question that is best addressed by referral to a textbook or journal review article that explicates current diagnostic criteria and how one might clinically assess for them. There are also 'foreground' [5] questions that are directly relevant to making decisions in this particular case. For example, what is the accuracy of a structured interview in detecting adolescent depression (a question about a diagnostic test)? What is the risk

---

Box 1. The five steps of evidence-based medicine

1. ASK a well-built clinical question.
2. ACCESS the best available evidence.
3. Critically APPRAISE the evidence: Is it valid? Is the size of the effect clinically important? Is it applicable to the patient?
4. APPLY the evidence: Is it possible to generalize or particu-larize the group data to this individual patient in light of the practitioner's clinical expertise, available resources, and the patient's preferences?
5. ASSESS the outcome in this patient.

(*Adapted from* Del Mar C, Glasziou P, Mayer D. Teaching evidence based medicine. BMJ 2004;329:989; with permission.)

of future manic episodes in this adolescent presenting with a first episode of depression (a question about prognosis)? One might wonder what the best pharmacologic maneuver would be for such a patient, whether psychotherapy should be considered first, or whether there is any basis on which to decide between pharmacology and psychotherapy (a question about treatment). Clinical encounters frequently stir up a variety of information needs, and EBM is most useful in addressing foreground questions that typically arise at the point when the clinician has satisfied himself with the quality of the clinical assessment, has sufficient background knowledge to interpret this information, and is poised to make a clinical decision.

After extended discussions with SL and his parents, a history of mania was excluded. After reviewing the course and severity of depressive symptoms and the relevant Diagnostic and Statistical Manual of Mental Disorders IV *criteria, a diagnosis of major depressive disorder superimposed on dysthymia was made.*

A typical clinical encounter can generate a large number of 'foreground' questions that necessitate information from clinical studies. Given time constraints, one way to decide which questions to look up is suggested by the following considerations [5]:

- Which is most important for the patient's well-being?
- Which is likely to arise frequently in the clinician's practice?
- Which is likely to be feasible to answer within the time available?
- Which is the most interesting?

Given the severity and duration of SL's depressive symptoms and the attendant dysfunction, treatment questions were clearly uppermost in the minds of the family and treatment team. The family expressed considerable concern about recent news reports of SSRIs causing suicidal behavior in children and adolescents. Although the father had experienced a good response to sertraline, he expressed a preference for nonpharmacologic approaches. The psychiatry fellow on the treatment team expressed her belief that antidepressant treatment would be the more effective option in this case, citing SL's severe symptoms and concern that these symptoms might limit his ability to engage effectively in psychotherapy. Other members on the team did not feel as strongly, however, and the fellow decided to search the literature to verify her belief.

A well-built clinical question can be framed in response to this query. It has the advantage of being structured to guide effective searches of medical databases. The question, described by the acronym PICO, includes:

1. P: A definition of the problem or patient
2. I: The intervention being contemplated (a drug or non-pharmacologic treatment)
3. C: A comparison intervention (which can be a placebo)
4. O: The clinical outcome of interest

The PICO question thus translates global uncertainty to focused ignorance, or, as one of our colleagues prefers, changes a mystery into a problem, which suggests the kinds of resources that could inform its solution.

> *The fellow framed the following question: in an adolescent male with major depressive disorder (P), what is the comparative efficacy of antidepressants (I) versus psychotherapy (C) in rates of remission (O), and what are the comparative rates of serious side effects, such as suicidal ideation or attempts (O)?*

ACCESS: translating an unfocused literature search into a selective approach

We prefer the broadest definition of evidence as "any empirical observation about the apparent relation between events" [3]. In treatment questions, evidence is any observation about the relationship between an intervention and an outcome and can be drawn from sources as disparate as the unsystematic clinical observation of clinicians, expert consensus, or clinical trials. In this sense, calling decisions "evidence-based" is redundant, given that some kind of evidence underlies any decision-making process. What is at issue here is the *quality* of the evidence that determines the strength of the inferences drawn from it. EBM asks that investigators explicitly identify the various kinds of information used, that they privilege inferences drawn from studies that are less likely to be biased, and that they remain aware of the degree of unavoidable error in these inferences. Thus, for questions about therapeutic interventions, the double-blind RCT is much less susceptible to various kinds of bias than observational studies or clinicians' recollections of patients they have treated in the past. Furthermore, a collection of such well-conducted studies reduces the influence of chance variation in the measured outcome in individual studies and thereby improves the precision of the estimated effect. A systematically collected group of such studies can be integrated either qualitatively or quantitatively (meta-analyzed) to provide the best estimate of the true treatment effect. Such a systematic review can provide a meaningful way to contextualize different trials and resolve the inevitable variation in their results.

Fundamental to EBM is this hierarchy of evidence sources. The strength of influence that various sources of evidence should have in our decision-making is judged by the extent to which they answer three questions (reviewed in detail in the next section):

- How valid is the information, or how carefully has bias been minimized?
- How sizeable or clinically significant is the estimate of effect and how precise is this estimate?
- How relevant is the information to this patient?

Box 2 provides a hierarchy of study types for questions of treatment.

This is not the hierarchy of a dictatorship (where some voices can be silenced without explicit reason), a theocracy (where some voices are silenced on the basis

---

Box 2. Hierarchy of evidence sources for treatment questions

- N of 1 RCT
- Systematic review of RCTs
- Single RCT
- Systematic review of observational studies
- Single observational study
- Physiologic studies
- Unsystematic clinical observation

(*Adapted from* Guyatt G, Haynes B, Jaeschke R, et al. Introduction: the philosophy of evidence-based medicine. In: Guyatt G, Rennie D, editors. Users' guide to the medical literature. Chicago: AMA Press; 2002. p. 12; with permission.)

---

of indefensible belief), or a bureaucracy (where some voices are silenced on the basis of sometimes explicit, often rigid, and essentially arbitrary rules). While allowing a plurality of information sources, EBM offers a means to weigh their relative merit and then encourages the integration of this information with the investigator's clinical experience and the preferences of the patient. The criteria of minimizing bias or the internal validity of a study are often in conflict with the criteria of its external validity or relevance to the individual patient. As discussed later, these considerations must be weighed in appraising a particular article for a particular patient.

The inclusion of n-of-one trials at the top of the hierarchy reflects a rarely achieved ideal that combines exquisitely specific relevance to an individual patient while retaining many safeguards against bias, such as randomization and blinding [7]. Unfortunately, the relatively long duration required for treatment response makes this design unfeasible for most psychiatric interventions.

Once investigators have established their preferences, this hierarchy allows selective interrogation of the vast medical literature in a more time-efficient manner. In the case of SL, the investigator began by looking for systematic reviews of RCTs comparing individual psychotherapy and antidepressants. Although our informal polls indicate that at this point most clinicians would choose to search their favorite primary database, such as Medline or PsycINFO, it is worth pausing for a moment to consider the available options.

In addition to the attributes of relevance, size of effect, and validity, an ideal source of clinical information also should be easily accessible. Much of the published biomedical literature is of little immediate relevance for clinical decision making and often reflects preliminary findings communicated among investigators. Furthermore, the manner in which this information is indexed in the major databases is not intuitively obvious to clinicians. The equation below, modified from Slawson and Shaugnessy [8], represents the contingencies involved in what could easily become a time-consuming, low-yield expedition through the notoriously red-herring rich literature:

usefulness of medical information
= (relevance)(validity)(size of effect)/work

Fortunately, several secondary sources are available that are oriented toward clinically relevant questions, pay explicit attention to study quality and effect

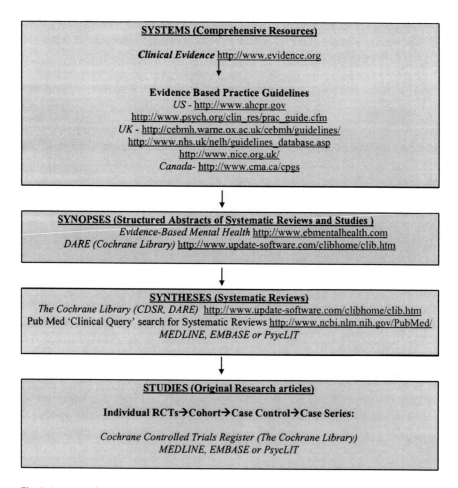

Fig. 1. A systematic approach to identifying the best evidence. (*Adapted from* Geddes J. From science to practice. In: Gelder MG, López-Ibor JJ, Andreasen N, editors. The new Oxford textbook of psychiatry. New York: Oxford University Press; 2000. p. 138; and Haynes RB. Of studies, summaries, synopses, and systems: the "4S" evolution of services for finding current best evidence. Evid Based Ment Health 2001;4:37; with permission.)

size, and synthesize the information in a more easily digestible form. The explicit and comprehensive methods by which these databases are assembled are available on their websites. Examples include The Cochrane Collaboration, which attempts to provide one database for all systematic reviews of various therapies that have been conducted by members of the group (Cochrane Database of Systematic Reviews) or published elsewhere (Database of Abstracts of Reviews of Effectiveness). The quarterly journal *Evidence Based Mental Health* (*EBMH*) screens a wide range of clinical publications for the attributes presented above and publishes single-page summaries structured as responses to clinical questions in a format allowing more rapid appraisal. The biannually updated *Clinical Evidence* is a valuable summary of the best available evidence on an increasingly wide number of clinical questions. *Clinical Evidence* is unique in that its approach begins with clinically relevant questions, which are then followed by systematic searches through the literature. The results are presented in summary form in a condensed paper format; the attached CD-ROM with hyperlinked references allows more detailed reading of the primary sources. Although the range of questions covered by *Clinical Evidence* in the area of child and adolescent psychiatry is limited at present, it can offer a good first stop in the search for relevant systematic reviews or RCTs. The articles are found through an exhaustive search down a hierarchy of resources, which are then appraised and presented according to explicit criteria that address issues of validity, clinical importance, and relevance.

In summary, the task of accessing clinical information that is valid, relevant, and important in size, while minimizing the time and effort involved, can be addressed by attending to two related questions:

- What to look for? Begin with higher quality studies and proceed down the hierarchy.
- Where to look? Begin with pre-appraised secondary sources before proceeding to the primary literature.

One approach that can be used for questions about treatment, combining these two considerations, is presented in Fig. 1.

> *The fellow conducted a quick scan of* Clinical Evidence *(edition 11) under the section on depression in children and adolescents (search date, January 2004). This scan revealed several pieces of useful information that provided her some perspective on treatment approaches. She summarized her findings:*
>
> - *There was insufficient data to support the use of monoamine oxidase inhibitors in adolescents.*
> - *A systematic review of RCTs of tricyclic antidepressants found no clear improvement versus placebo in children, with burdensome side effects. There was some suggestion, however, of possible benefit in adolescents.*
> - *Much of the pharmacotherapy data in the adolescent population was based on studies of SSRIs, with RCT data reported for fluoxetine, sertra-*

line, and paroxetine. Fluoxetine, in particular, had support from more than one RCT, but two of the three trials reported neutral results, and all were brief in duration.

- *There was reference to a Food and Drug Administration advisory against the use of paroxetine in people under the age of 18 years; however, this advisory was based on unpublished data.*
- *In terms of individual psychotherapies, there were no available comparable data for the modalities of psychodynamic, interpersonal, or CBT. The bulk of the controlled data supported the efficacy of CBT.*
- *None of the cited trials addressed the comparison of interest, that is, between pharmacotherapy and psychotherapy.*

She therefore refined her question:

In an adolescent male with major depressive disorder and dysthymia (P), what is the comparative effectiveness of fluoxetine or sertraline (I) versus psychotherapy (any modality) (C) in rates of remission and also in the rates of serious side effects such as suicidal ideation or attempts (O)?

Clinical Evidence had no references to trials comparing SSRIs (or other antidepressants) with psychotherapies. Proceeding down the list of resources arranged in Fig. 1, no recent practice guidelines were available. Had any relevant comparative studies been published since the last edition of *Clinical Evidence 11* (updated in January of 2004)? The journal *EMBH* is ideally suited for such a query. Published quarterly, this secondary journal provides a systematic browsing service, periodically scanning a large selection of clinically relevant publications in psychiatry, psychology, and mental health nursing. Articles are screened for validity, relevance, and clinical importance, and the results are presented as a structured abstract with a commentary. A broad search of *EBMH* titles using the term "depress*" from January 2004 through April 2005 revealed four summaries relevant to the treatment of adolescent depression. One referred to an interesting study of school-based interpersonal therapy, and another summarized a 2003 article about two RCTs comparing sertraline with placebo (already included in *Clinical Evidence 11*). The third summary referred to a maintenance study showing efficacy of fluoxetine in patients who had already responded to this treatment. The fourth reference abstracted an article of direct relevance to the fellow's question: "Fluoxetine, cognitive- behavioral therapy and their combination for adolescents with depression. Treatment for Adolescents with Depression Study (TADS) randomized controlled trial." This order of searching thus averted time-intensive searches of primary databases such as Medline, EMBASE, or PsycINFO.

The one-page *EBMH* structured abstract (reproduced in Appendix 1) provides a summary that facilitates its appraisal. This trial is an RCT with four intervention arms providing comparisons of CBT, fluoxetine, their combination, and placebo. After scanning the descriptors of study methodology and assuring an adequate degree of validity in the study, the investigator

Table 1
Summary results for the Treatment of Adolescent Depression Study: mean score improvement and response to treatment at 12 weeks

Treatment	Mean improvement in Children's Depression Rating Scale–Revised score	Response rate[a] (95% CI)
Fluoxetine plus CBT	27.0	71 (62–80)
Fluoxetine	22.6	61 (51–70)
CBT	17.6	43 (34–52)
Placebo	19.4	35 (26–44)

[a] Response defined as Clinical Global Impression improvement score of 1 or 2.
Data from March J, Silva S, Petrycki S, et al. Fluoxetine, cognitive-behavioral therapy, and their combination for adolescents with depression: Treatment for Adolescents with Depression Study (TADS) randomized controlled trial. JAMA 2004;292:807–20.

could proceed to the outcomes summary statement presented in the *EBMH* abstract [9]:

> At 12 weeks, fluoxetine plus CBT significantly improved symptoms of *depression* compared with placebo in adolescents with major depressive disorder (p = 0.001) Fluoxetine plus CBT was more effective at reducing symptoms of *depression* than fluoxetine alone or CBT alone (fluoxetine plus CBT v fluoxetine, p = 0.02; fluoxetine plus CBT v CBT, p = 0.001). There was no significant difference in reduction of depressive symptoms between fluoxetine alone or CBT alone compared with placebo (fluoxetine v placebo, p = 0.1; CBT v placebo, p = 0.4).[1] Fluoxetine plus CBT significantly improved response rate compared with placebo or CBT alone (p = 0.001), but not compared with fluoxetine alone (p = 0.11). Fluoxetine plus CBT produced the greatest reduction in suicidal thoughts (p = 0.02).

A summary table with clinically relevant results (Table 1) is provided on the *EBMH* website.

The clinician who is familiar with the principles of appraising such an RCT could apply the results presented in this table to inform the decision to be made with SL. The next section, however, discusses in some detail the steps involved in appraising the primary article. The authors hope this discussion will highlight the value of a preappraised resource such as *EBMH*, which can effectively shortcut this next step for the clinician.

APPRAISE: translating the literature into usable evidence

In the early 1990s the *Journal of the American Medical Association* began a series of articles entitled "User's Guide to the Medical Literature" with subtitles

---

[1] In terms of the primary dichotomous outcome of response however, fluoxetine alone was reported by the authors of the study as superior to CBT alone. This claim is examined in the next section on appraisal.

such as "How to Use an Article about Therapy or Prevention. A. Are the results valid?" [10] and "B. What Were the Results and Will They Help Me in Caring for My Patients?" [11]. What began as an attempt by clinicians and epidemiologists to provide pragmatic assistance to clinicians in appraising the literature grew into an articulation of a model of how to approach clinical uncertainty, decision making, and continuing medical education. This process has since come to be known widely as EBM. The concepts behind the series have recently been collected and contextualized in a user-friendly manual [3]. Chapters are organized around the assessment of studies for clinical tasks (therapy, harm, diagnosis, and prognosis.) Also, a CD-ROM with links to a periodically updated interactive website provides several additional features, including worked-through examples of the appraisal and application of evidence from a

---

Box 3. Worksheet for appraising controlled trials of treatments

A. How internally valid are the results? Did experimental and control groups begin with the same prognosis?
  1. Were patients randomly allocated?
  2. Was the random allocation concealed?
  3. Were patients analyzed in the groups to which they were randomly allocated?
  4. Were patients in the treatment and control groups similar with respect to known prognostic factors? Did experimental and control groups retain the same prognosis after the study started?
  5. Were patients blind to group allocation?
  6. Were clinicians blind to group allocation?
  7. Were outcome assessors blind to group allocation?
  8. How complete was follow-up?
B. What were the results?
  1. How large was the treatment effect?
  2. How precise was the estimate of the treatment effect?
C. How can the results be applied to patient care (ie, how externally valid are the results)?
  1. Were the study patients similar to this patient?
  2. Were all clinically important outcomes considered?
  3. Are the likely treatment benefits worth the potential harm and costs?

(*Adapted from* Guyatt G, Cook D, Devereaux PJ, et al. Therapy. In: Guyatt G, Rennie D, editors. Users' guide to the medical literature. Chicago: AMA Press; 2002. p. 86; with permission.)

variety of sources. Worksheets that prompt clinicians to query articles concerning issues of validity, size, and relevance are provided; an adapted sample is shown in Box 3.

The rationale for such a worksheet is discussed briefly before it is completed for this study and this patient. For a detailed discussion of the concepts of bias (systematic error) and chance (random error) on which EBM appraisals are based, the reader is referred to one of the many excellent manuals referred to earlier.

Bias, which can be defined as "a systematic tendency to produce an outcome that differs from the underlying truth" [3] manifests in a clinical trial as the many ways in which the presented outcomes are affected by factors other than the interventions being compared (in this case fluoxetine, CBT, their combination, and placebo). Greenhalgh [12] offers a summary of some common biases, reproduced in Fig. 2.

An appraisal of the Methods section of the TADS study for each of these biases shows that selection bias has been minimized by the random and concealed allocation of subjects to one of the four interventions, thereby minimizing the chance that one group differed from the other in terms of prognosis before receiving the interventions being compared.

Performance bias was limited by keeping the treaters unaware (albeit only for the fluoxetine and placebo pill interventions) of what they were administering,

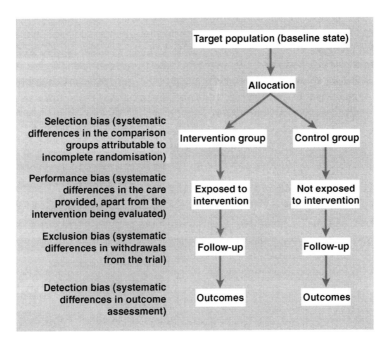

Fig. 2. Sources of bias in a controlled trial. (*From* Greenhalgh T. Assessing the methodological quality of published papers. BMJ 1997;315(7103):306; with permission.)

lest there be some systematic difference in the treatment of patients receiving one or the other intervention. This precaution could not realistically be achieved for the CBT intervention, and although attempts were made to standardize all treatments, the subjects receiving the 15 CBT sessions had more contact with treaters than those who did not, raising the question of whether this additional time (acting as a hidden cointervention), rather than the therapeutic technique itself, was decisive for the outcome.

Exclusion bias was minimized by the careful follow-up and documentation of reasons for which participants dropped out of the trial. The first table in the original study describes the flow of patients with detailed reasons for dropouts in each arm of the study. A quick scan of this table confirms the authors' report that "treatment assignment did not influence the probability of dropping out or premature termination" [13].

Finally, detection bias was minimized by keeping the raters who assessed the outcomes blind to the treatment assignments of the subjects. One wonders, however, if the subjects who received CBT had expectations of this approach that could have skewed their reporting (detection bias) of outcomes.

Are the results valid?

Section A of the worksheet (see Box 3), prompts the reader to appraise the study for these biases before coming to a conclusion about its internal validity.

A brief review of the *EBMH* one-page abstract reveals that much of the information necessary to fill in such a worksheet is summarized here, thus saving clinician time and effort. The various kinds of biases described in the worksheet and the preceding discussion are not meant to be a comprehensive list but rather a set of screening questions to weigh the quality of a study. When such information is not available in an abstract, the clinician must first assess the methods of the study and exclude serious bias before continuing with the next steps in appraisal.

For the TADS, the possible sources of bias discussed in the previous section were judged as not likely to seriously threaten the internal validity of the study.

What were the results?

Two questions address the importance of the results. The first is the size of the effect, and the second is the precision of the estimate of the effect. Instead of reviewing exhaustively all the outcomes presented in the TADS report, we focus on those outcomes relevant to our question.

The investigators used two scales to provide continuous quantitative measures of depressive symptoms, namely the Childhood Depression Rating Scale–Revised and the Reynolds Adolescent Depression Scale. They also defined dichotomous outcomes, with a positive response defined as either a Clinical Global Impression (CGI) score of 1 (very much improved) or 2 (much improved). Using these dichotomous outcomes in the analysis allows the generation of meaningful estimates of the likelihood of response in this particular patient.

How large is the effect?

A review of the raw percentages for the response rates (see Table 1) suggests that the combination approach is more effective than fluoxetine or CBT alone, and in that order. But just how much more effective is the combination approach? There are several ways to express a difference between two rates: as a relative risk (RR), relative risk reduction (RRR), absolute risk reduction (ARR), and the EBM-favored NNT. Each conveys slightly different information, and the translation statements below reflect their unique contributions. These measures can be used to communicate information to the patient and family to enable an informed decision. The reader can assess, by this standard of comprehensibility, each of these different approaches.

By convention, the control event rate (CER) is the proportion of undesirable outcomes in the comparison group. The experimental event rate (EER) similarly refers to the rate of such outcomes in the intervention group. When comparing the outcomes in the combination versus the placebo alone groups the numbers are

$$CER = \% \text{ of nonresponders to placebo} = 1 - 0.35 = 0.65, \text{ or } 65\%$$

$$EER = \% \text{ of nonresponders to combination treatment} = 1 - 0.71$$
$$= 0.29, \text{ or } 29\%$$

The relative risk, calculated as EER/CER, is 0.44; that is, the risk of remaining significantly depressed at the end of 12 weeks of combination treatment is almost half of that of placebo.

The ARR, calculated as CER − EER, is 0.36; that is, over 12 weeks there were 36% fewer cases of significant depression in the subjects treated with the intervention than in those given placebo only.

The RRR, calculated as (CER − EER)/CER, is 0.55; that is, there is a 55% reduction in the risk of remaining significantly depressed at 12 weeks in those subjects given the combination treatment in comparison with those receiving placebo.

The NNT refers to the number of subjects who would need to be treated over the specified period of the study to prevent one bad outcome. It is calculated as the reciprocal of the ARR and in this case equals 1/0.36, or 2.77, which is rounded off to the next higher integer, 3. Thus, for every three subjects treated with the combination intervention rather than placebo over 12 weeks, one additional case of depression will be alleviated.

The values calculated for the various treatment comparisons are presented in Table 2.

How precise is the effect?

Aside from an estimate of the difference in outcomes between two possible interventions, traditional reports of studies usually also present *P* values that reflect the probability that the observed differences occurred purely by chance

Table 2
Evidence-based medicine translation of results from the Treatment of Adolescent Depression Study

Comparisons	CER (%)	EER (%)	RR (%)	RRR (%)	ARR (%)	NNT (95% CI)
Combination versus fluoxetine	39	29	74	26	10	10 (4 to −37)
Combination versus CBT	57	29	51	49	28	4 (3 to 7)
Combination versus placebo	65	29	44	56	36	3 (2 to 4)
Fluoxetine versus placebo	65	29	60	40	26	4 (3 to 8)
Fluoxetine versus CBT	57	39	69	31	17	6 (3 to 27)
CBT versus placebo	65	57	87	13	8	12 (5 to −20)

Data from March J, Silva S, Petrycki S, et al. Fluoxetine, cognitive-behavioral therapy, and their combination for adolescents with depression: Treatment for Adolescents with Depression Study (TADS) randomized controlled trial. JAMA 2004;292:807–20.

or the probability that the null hypothesis of no difference between the experimental and control arms is in fact true. A *P* value of .05 or lower, which reflects a 95% or better probability that this difference did not occur purely by chance, is regarded by convention as a statistically significant difference. Of course, this value has nothing to do with the clinical significance of a finding ("truly improved mood") but rather suggests the likelihood that, if additional patients were to receive this same treatment, one would detect the same (not necessarily beneficial) result. Once the possibility of an accidental effect has been eliminated, one can assess whether the effect is clinically significant. This assessment involves appreciating the size and the precision of the effect. Recognizing that one has only an estimate of the true difference is an acknowledgment of inevitable random error: even well-designed studies that carefully minimize bias can arrive at different estimates of an effect in similar populations. This uncertainty can be expressed in the Confidence Intervals (CIs) around the treatment effect. A 95% CI thus answers the question, "What is the plausible range of values within which the true value of the effect lies, with a 95% probability?" The TADS study exemplifies an emerging trend of providing CIs around NNT estimates for each of the three interventions in comparison with placebo. This presentation greatly aids the interpretation of these studies for the range of possible effect sizes and thereby for clinical rather than mere statistical significance. Also presented in Table 2 are NNTs and CIs calculated for other comparisons. Although CIs may also be calculated from the experimental and control event rates [3], they are often provided in secondary sources such as *EBMH*.

It is now possible to respond to questions A and B for the various comparisons of interest. The initial question concerned the relative effectiveness of fluoxetine and CBT, and the results presented above are compatible with the following statement:

Fluoxetine use in this trial population, over 12 weeks, seems to have proven more effective than CBT, wherein for every six subjects treated with fluoxetine instead of CBT, one would be saved from a significant persistence in depressive symptoms.

The CIs of this estimate are wide, however, and the results are compatible with a difference as strong as an NNT of three or as weak as an NNT of 27. The smaller the NNT, the greater is the difference in efficacy, and therefore fewer additional patients need to be treated to realize this advantage. Another way of expressing this situation would be to state that although the results indicated a point estimate of 17% (ARR) for the comparison of fluoxetine versus CBT, or a difference of 17% in the number remaining significantly depressed at the end of the trial in favor of fluoxetine, the actual estimate could be as little as 14% or as much as 31% (the 95% CIs for the ARR, not shown in the table). This information makes it possible to assess the clinical as opposed to the mere statistical significance of these results. If the NNT of 27 or an ARR of 14% is judged to be clinically meaningful, it would favor the use of one intervention over another (if it was necessary to choose only one). Similarly, for the other comparisons, it would be possible to derive statements about the size and precision of the relative efficacy of the various interventions.

The comparisons between the combination treatment arm and fluoxetine alone and between CBT and placebo include a negative number in the CIs for the NNTs. In the latter case, the effectiveness of CBT could be as high as an NNT of five or as low as -20, and it is not possible to exclude the possibility of no additional benefit or even harm from the use of CBT rather than placebo in this population. The reader is encouraged to contrast this EBM-style interpretation of the results with the more traditional summary containing P values. Would this information help or hinder a discussion of comparative benefits with the family and patient?

What about the risk of suicidal ideation or behavior?

The EBMH summary reports a reassuring reduction in suicidal ideation in all the arms of the study. An examination of the primary study indicates that although 27% of the study entrants reported significant suicidal ideation, only 6% experienced suicide-related adverse events (defined as a worsening of suicidal ideation or an attempted suicide) during the study, with no significant differences between the groups. On a broader measure of harm-related adverse events, which also included nonsuicidal self-harm behaviors, the odds ratios for each of the three interventions in comparison with placebo are presented. The odds ratios (which can be interpreted for this rare outcome as relative risks) are highest for the fluoxetine arm (2.39), lower for the combination (1.62), and lowest for CBT alone (0.83), suggesting some possible protective effect of CBT. The CIs for all these values, however, include an odds ratio of 1 (no difference). This study alone thus cannot give a clear sense of the size or precision of the comparative risk of this rare outcome for the various treatments.

Are the results applicable to the patient?

Section C of the worksheet (see Box 3) first prompts the question whether the subjects in this study were similar enough to the patient for the results to be applicable. The description of the inclusion and exclusion criteria summarized in the *EBMH* abstract and the primary article show that SL would have been admitted as a subject in this study. Of note, the study included patients with moderate to severe symptoms, with average episode durations of 72 weeks, and some with comorbid dysthymia. Therefore the results found in this group of patients could be extrapolated to SL's particular case with some confidence.

Were all clinically important outcomes considered?
    The study defined response as a CGI improvement score of 1 (very much improved) or 2 (much improved). The baseline CGI scores for the patients entering the study averaged 4.77. After a brief discussion about what SL's current CGI score would be (comparable to the study baseline), the team agreed that his achieving the study-defined response would be a clinically meaningful goal. The study investigators also monitored a variety of adverse events. Suicidality, of particular interest to the patient's family and treatment team, was assessed in TADS, with a suicidal ideation questionnaire, and careful follow-up which assured the team that no suicidal events were missed.

Benefits versus risks in a particular patient
    It now is possible to proceed to a more detailed consideration of the results in responding to the final question in the worksheet: will the benefits of the interventions outweigh their risks in this particular patient? The authors consider the beneficial outcome first.
    One cannot easily extrapolate the average benefit of an intervention in a study population to an individual patient, but doing so is part of the task in any informed decision. Once it has been determined that the study is of sufficient validity and relevance to the patient, some inferences can be drawn. Table 2 shows that all three interventions (combination, fluoxetine, and CBT) produce significant RRRs (56%, 40%, and 13%, respectively) in comparison with the placebo arm, with the greatest benefit derived from the combination treatment. Even a high RRR can be misleading, however, if the baseline level of risk is low. For instance, if the risks of remaining depressed without treatment were trivial (eg, 5% instead of the 65% rate of the placebo group), and the risk with combination treatment were similarly trivial (eg, 2% instead of the actual rate of 29%), the RRR would still be 56%, conveying an inflated sense of the value of this intervention. Herein lies the advantage of the NNT: its magnitude includes a measure of the baseline risk and hence the clinical, rather than merely numerical, significance of the treatment effect.
    From Table 2 it can be inferred that for every three adolescents treated with the combination of fluoxetine and CBT over 12 weeks, one would be prevented from remaining significantly depressed. The confidence limits around this NNT can be used to refine this statement to reflect the uncertainty around this estimate: as few as two and as many as four patients might have to be treated

to prevent one such adverse outcome. In the same way, it can be inferred that fluoxetine offers a comparable chance of benefit. The comparison of the combination treatment versus fluoxetine alone can be interpreted as not excluding the possibility that there is no difference between the two options. As discussed earlier, a CI that includes a negative NNT suggest that the available data are too imprecise to exclude the possibility of no benefit or even harm, and more studies would be necessary to arrive at a more precise (ie, a narrower CI) estimate of the true effect. Similarly, it can be concluded that CBT alone failed to separate convincingly from the placebo arm. This conclusion does not mean that CBT is an ineffective treatment; rather, the data from this study were unable to exclude the possibility that CBT was no more effective than placebo.

In the comparison most relevant to the question raised by the family, namely, whether there was any reason to choose fluoxetine over CBT, the data, although favoring fluoxetine (NNT = 6; CI, 3–27), indicate considerable uncertainty about this estimate, which can be translated as the possibility that up to 27 adolescents would have to be treated with fluoxetine rather than with CBT to generate one additional responder.

How significant is an NNT of 27, 6, or even 3? NNTs derived for other medical interventions can provide some perspective. For example, it has been estimated that one would have to treat three adults with severe elevated diastolic blood pressure (115–129 mm Hg) for 1.5 years to prevent one cardiovascular event such as a stroke, myocardial infarction, or death. On the other hand, up to 128 people with less severe elevations (90–109 mm Hg) would have to be treated for 5 years to prevent the same outcomes [5]. The NNT is often interpreted in light of the seriousness of the outcomes for the individual patient. Additionally, while it may be easy for physicians to justify treating many people with hypertension to prevent one catastrophic stroke or myocardial infarction, a careful case for intervention must always be made in the context of the patients' values and preferences. A few NNTs for common psychiatric interventions are provided in Table 3.

What about the other outcome of interest in the initial question: the risk of worsening suicidal ideation or attempts? The results of this trial, although reassuring, illustrate the limitations of individual RCTs in assessing rare outcomes. Larger numbers of subjects, as potentially available by combining the results of several RCTs in a systematic review or through observational studies that can follow more subjects for longer periods of time, can provide valuable information on this outcome.

APPLY: translating the evidence into action

How can one use a seemingly distant metric such as an NNT to communicate risk to an individual patient? After all, few patients would agree to a treatment, even if it had a good chance of reducing the average burden of disease in a population, if it did not offer benefit to them individually. Clinical studies (except

Table 3

Examples of numbers needed to treat for common psychiatric disorders and interventions

Target disorder	Intervention	Outcome measure	Follow-up	NNT (95% CI)
Acute mania[a]	Lithium versus placebo	$\geq 50\%$ improvement in mania score on Schedule for Affective Disorders and Schizophrenia-Change scale	3–4 wk	5 (3–20)
Depressive disorders[b]	Continuing antidepressants in responders	Preventing relapse	6 mo 12 mo 24–36 mo	6 (5–8) 5 (4–6) 4 (3–7)
Schizophrenia[c]	Haldol versus placebo	Psychiatrist rated global improvement	6 wk	3 (2–5)
Obsessive-compulsive disorder (6- to 17-year-olds)[d]	Sertraline versus placebo	25% decrease in the Children's Yale-Brown Obsessive Compulsive Scale score	12 wk	6 (3–47)

[a] *Data from* Poolsup N, Li Wan Po A, de Oliveira IR. Systematic overview of lithium treatment in acute mania. J Clin Pharm Ther 2000;25:139–56.

[b] *Data from* Geddes JG, Carney SM, Davies C, et al. Relapse prevention with antidepressant drug treatment in depressive disorders: a systematic review. Lancet 2003;361:653–61.

[c] *Data from* Joy CB, Adams CE, Lawrie SM. Haloperidol versus placebo for schizophrenia. In: The Cochrane Library, Issue 3. Chichester (UK): John Wiley & Sons, Ltd.; 2004.

[d] *Data from* March JS, Biederman J, Wolkow R, et al. Sertraline in children and adolescents with obsessive-compulsive disorder. A multicenter randomized controlled trial. JAMA 1998;280:1752–6.

for the N of 1 RCT) cannot provide such an individualized certainty. Given that SL matches the profile of the patients in this study, there is a strong probability that he might benefit from the combination or fluoxetine therapy, but it is impossible to predict for certain if he would be the one of three or four patients to benefit from such an intervention over the study period of 12 weeks. Also, the application of the data would involve integrating these probabilistic estimates from the literature with the clinician's own clinical judgment and the patient's (and his family's) preferences.

> In light of the father's preference for nonpharmacologic approaches, the family was advised about the uncertainty regarding the effectiveness of CBT as a lone treatment in a patient such as SL (whose severity of illness matched the study population). A combination of fluoxetine in addition to CBT was recommended instead. To express the likelihood of response, the family was told that for about every three individuals treated with this combination, one would respond over 12 weeks, whereas for CBT alone the comparable number was around 12 but possibly much higher. The family was informed of the placebo response rate of about 35% in the TADS study but also of the team's clinical judgment that SL would not, given his prolonged symptoms and functional decline, want to take the chance of delaying treatment. The fellow stated that although there was

some evidence of an increased risk of self-harm behaviors were SL to be treated with an SSRI, this adverse affect was rare and would be watched for carefully. Regardless of SL and his family's choice or particular response to an intervention, the team also reiterated its commitment to care for him and to continue to try alternatives. The family elected for the combination intervention, but, because of a delay in finding a local therapist proficient in CBT, the family chose to initiate treatment with fluoxetine alone. Given some data indicating that the effects of CBT might be greater in the follow-up rather than the acute treatment phase and might offer some protection against self-harm behaviors, the family was encouraged to continue to pursue this option.

ASSESS: translating reported trial efficacy into a measurement of clinical effectiveness

The final step in the process of evidence-based practice reflects an acknowledgment that although the evidence is a part of any clinical decision, it does not offer certainty about the outcome once this decision is made. Rather, the patient is presented with a probabilistic estimate of efficacy. The NNT is an important tool to estimate the likelihood of a response, and the CIs can indicate the range of this likelihood, but physicians treat individuals whose particular physiology, preferences, and beliefs will influence the outcome in ways that cannot be entirely predicted or statistically modeled. The skill and experience of the physician in monitoring the response, in maintaining compliance and hope, and in following up with alternatives that are less well supported in the literature when the intervention of choice fails are essential parts of evidence-based practice.

Limitations and challenges while eschewing obfuscation

EBM is an effective tool to bring epidemiologic principles to the bedside [5]. Awareness of principles of bias and random error allows clinicians to evaluate claims and make more careful inferences from the literature. EBM stands on an epistemic assumption that tests of hypotheses in carefully conducted clinical experiments provide uniquely valid information that can confirm or correct inferences from unsystematic clinical observation. It allows physicians to know the "error of their ways" [14]. But EBM does not discount evidence from other levels in the hierarchy of sources. Although the hierarchy is a reminder of their degree of susceptibility to bias, a variety of sources are important. For example, observational studies are critical for assessing the frequency of rare events, such as suicidality, which cannot be feasibly addressed by relatively small, short RCTs that are often conducted in carefully selected and therefore rarefied and somewhat unrealistic patient populations.

Practitioners who might use EBM are concerned with much more than the careful appraisal of the literature. Inferences from study populations must be applied to individual patients with unique biology, experiences, and values, and often limited evidence is available on the many clinical questions involved in making a single clinical decision. Some would argue that it is this integration of several levels of imperfect evidence with factors unique to the patient that constitutes clinical expertise or the art of medical practice [14].

The language of EBM has a key role to play in communicating to patients [15] what is more uniquely the expertise of the physician: a working knowledge of population data. The doctor can work strenuously to understand the predicament and values of the individual patient and family without abdicating his role in teaching about risk and benefit derived from studies of groups [16]. It is in this sense that the physician needs to be conversant with the "language of populations and the language of individuals" [17].

The presentation of EBM as a paradigm shift may have elicited an unnecessarily polarized debate with traditional modes of practice. The goals here have been more modest: to illustrate what this approach might look like in an individual case. Can it empower clinicians and their patients to act in the face of clinical uncertainty? Straus and McAlister [18] have carefully addressed a range of limitations and misunderstandings of the EBM model. Several are apparent in this example. First, learning the skills of searching and appraising the literature requires setting aside considerable time and effort in contrast with a more efficient "curbside" consultation with a trusted colleague. The payoff in supplementing traditional modes of continuing medical education with EBM is a growing and more fine-grained knowledge of the literature, especially for questions that arise frequently in one's practice. Second, the reality of publication bias, wherein neutral or negative trials do not reach publication, can subvert even the most careful appraisal of the available data. This so-called "file-drawer bias" has been especially clear with the emerging story of RCTs for SSRIs. A recent systematic review [19] that attempted to gather unpublished data on childhood depression demonstrated how these data would negatively alter the risk–benefit assessment for several antidepressants, excluding fluoxetine (also see commentary in Appendix 1). Although there are encouraging movements to correct this potential bias [20], an awareness of the nonscientific forces that inevitably influence the information available is an important element of the enlightened skepticism advocated here. There is little justification for dogmatic insistence on one or another therapy as evidence-based. Instead, what is called for is awareness of the degree of methodological rigor of the current best evidence and openness to correcting earlier conclusions when previously suppressed, forgotten, or new evidence comes to light.

We find it ironic that EBM is sometimes criticized for not providing resolution of uncertainty, an expectation it is designed to frustrate. This expectation can mistakenly lead to therapeutic nihilism when, for instance, no systematic reviews or RCTs can be found to address a question about an intervention. It can also lead to rigid attachment to a particular set of results as embodying the truth rather than an inevitably flawed, probabilistic estimate that invites revision with further study. Socrates (who might have known something about facing uncertainty in his final hours) warned against this "misology," or loss of confidence that comes from placing "irrational confidence" in the reasoning of others without oneself engaging in the "art of reasoning" [21]. EBM offers one way to begin this engagement.

Finally, the role of EBM in highlighting the value of epidemiologic principles in clinical decision making has perhaps inevitably brought into relief those issues that lie outside their province. Among these are the private, existential questions that require an "empathic witnessing ... [a] commitment to be with the sick person and help build narrative to make sense of and give value to experience" [22]. Indeed, the facing of un-answerable questions is an essential challenge and privilege of clinical work. EBM cannot claim a comprehensive account of the clinical encounter, but, when integrated with an understanding of personal narratives [2], it can enrich medical practice.

Acknowledgments

The authors appreciate the helpful comments of Dr. Christopher Varley on an earlier draft manuscript.

Appendix 1. Structured abstract of Treatment of Adolescent Depression Study

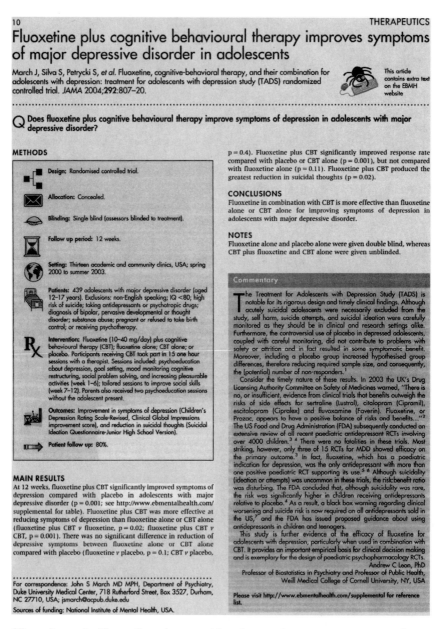

10   THERAPEUTICS

Fluoxetine plus cognitive behavioural therapy improves symptoms of major depressive disorder in adolescents

March J, Silva S, Petrycki S, et al. Fluoxetine, cognitive-behavioral therapy, and their combination for adolescents with depression: treatment for adolescents with depression study (TADS) randomized controlled trial. *JAMA* 2004;**292**:807–20.

This article contains extra text on the EBMH website

Q Does fluoxetine plus cognitive behavioural therapy improve symptoms of depression in adolescents with major depressive disorder?

METHODS

Design: Randomised controlled trial.

Allocation: Concealed.

Blinding: Single blind (assessors blinded to treatment).

Follow up period: 12 weeks.

Setting: Thirteen academic and community clinics, USA; spring 2000 to summer 2003.

Patients: 439 adolescents with major depressive disorder (aged 12–17 years). Exclusions: non-English speaking; IQ <80; high risk of suicide; taking antidepressants or psychotropic drugs; diagnosis of bipolar, pervasive developmental or thought disorder; substance abuse; pregnant or refused to take birth control; or receiving psychotherapy.

Intervention: Fluoxetine (10–40 mg/day) plus cognitive behavioural therapy (CBT); fluoxetine alone; CBT alone; or placebo. Participants receiving CBT took part in 15 one hour sessions with a therapist. Sessions included: psychoeducation about depression, goal setting, mood monitoring cognitive restructuring, social problem solving, and increasing pleasurable activities (week 1–6); tailored sessions to improve social skills (week 7–12). Parents also received two psychoeducation sessions without the adolescent present.

Outcomes: Improvement in symptoms of depression (Children's Depression Rating Scale-Revised, Clinical Global Impressions improvement score), and reduction in suicidal thoughts (Suicidal Ideation Questionnaire-Junior High School Version).

Patient follow up: 80%.

MAIN RESULTS

At 12 weeks, fluoxetine plus CBT significantly improved symptoms of depression compared with placebo in adolescents with major depressive disorder (p = 0.001; see http://www.ebmentalhealth.com/ supplemental for table). Fluoxetine plus CBT was more effective at reducing symptoms of depression than fluoxetine or CBT alone (fluoxetine plus CBT v fluoxetine, p = 0.02; fluoxetine plus CBT v CBT, p = 0.001). There was no significant difference in reduction of depressive symptoms between fluoxetine alone or CBT alone compared with placebo (fluoxetine v placebo, p = 0.1; CBT v placebo,

p = 0.4). Fluoxetine plus CBT significantly improved response rate compared with placebo or CBT alone (p = 0.001), but not compared with fluoxetine alone (p = 0.11). Fluoxetine plus CBT produced the greatest reduction in suicidal thoughts (p = 0.02).

CONCLUSIONS

Fluoxetine in combination with CBT is more effective than fluoxetine alone or CBT alone for improving symptoms of depression in adolescents with major depressive disorder.

NOTES

Fluoxetine alone and placebo alone were given double blind, whereas CBT plus fluoxetine and CBT alone were given unblinded.

Commentary

The Treatment for Adolescents with Depression Study (TADS) is notable for its rigorous design and timely clinical findings. Although acutely suicidal adolescents were necessarily excluded from the study, self harm, suicide attempts, and suicidal ideation were carefully monitored as they should be in clinical and research settings alike. Furthermore, the controversial use of placebo in depressed adolescents, coupled with careful monitoring, did not contribute to problems with safety or attrition and in fact resulted in some symptomatic benefit. Moreover, including a placebo group increased hypothesised group differences, therefore reducing required sample size and, consequently, the (potential) number of non-responders.[1]

Consider the timely nature of these results. In 2003 the UK's Drug Licensing Authority Committee on Safety of Medicines warned, "There is no, or insufficient, evidence from clinical trials that benefits outweigh the risks of side effects for sertraline (Lustral), citalopram (Cipramil), escitalopram (Cipralex) and fluvoxamine (Faverin). Fluoxetine, or Prozac, appears to have a positive balance of risks and benefits..."[2] The US Food and Drug Administration (FDA) subsequently conducted an extensive review of all recent paediatric antidepressant RCTs involving over 4000 children.[3][4] There were no fatalities in these trials. Most striking, however, only three of 15 RCTs for MDD showed efficacy on the primary outcome.[3] In fact, fluoxetine, which has a paediatric indication for depression, was the only antidepressant with more than one positive paediatric RCT supporting its use.[5][6] Although suicidality (ideation or attempts) was uncommon in these trials, the risk:benefit ratio was disturbing. The FDA concluded that, although suicidality was rare, the risk was significantly higher in children receiving antidepressants relative to placebo.[4] As a result, a black box warning regarding clinical worsening and suicide risk is now required on all antidepressants sold in the US,[7] and the FDA has issued proposed guidance about using antidepressants in children and teenagers.

This study is further evidence of the efficacy of fluoxetine for adolescents with depression, particularly when used in combination with CBT. It provides an important empirical basis for clinical decision making and is exemplary for the design of paediatric psychopharmacology RCTs.

Andrew C Leon, PhD
Professor of Biostatistics in Psychiatry and Professor of Public Health, Weill Medical College of Cornell University, NY, USA

Please visit http://www.ebmentalhealth.com/supplemental for reference list.

For correspondence: John S March MD MPH, Department of Psychiatry, Duke University Medical Center, 718 Rutherford Street, Box 3527, Durham, NC 27710, USA; jsmarch@acpub.duke.edu

Sources of funding: National Institute of Mental Health, USA.

(*From* Leon A. Fluoxetine plus cognitive therapy improves symptoms of major depressive disorder in adolescents. Evid Based Ment Health 2005;8(1):10; with permission.)

References

[1] Sackett DL, Rosenburg WMC, Gray JAM, et al. Evidence-based medicine: what it is and what it isn't. BMJ 1996;312:71–2.

[2] Greenhalgh T. Narrative based medicine: narrative based medicine in an evidence based world. BMJ 1999;318(7179):323–5.

[3] Guyatt G, Rennie D, editors. Users' guide to the medical literature. Essentials of evidence-based clinical practice. Chicago: AMA Press; 2002.

[4] March JS, Chrisman A, Breland-Noble A, et al. Using and teaching evidence-based medicine: the Duke University child and adolescent psychiatry model. Child Adolesc Psychiatr Clin N Am 2005;14(2):273–96.

[5] Sackett DL, Richardson WS, Rosenberg W, et al. Evidence-based medicine: how to practice and teach EBM. London: Churchill Livingstone; 2000.

[6] Gray GE. Concise guide to evidence-based psychiatry. Washington (DC): American Psychiatric Association; 2003.

[7] Guyatt G, Sackett D, Adachi J, et al. A clinician's guide for conducting randomized trials in individual patients. CMAJ 1988;139:497–503.

[8] Shaughnessy AF, Slawson DC, Bennett JH. Becoming an information master: a guidebook to the medical information jungle. J Fam Pract 1994;39:489–99.

[9] Leon AC. Fluoxetine plus cognitive behavioural therapy improves symptoms of major depressive disorder in adolescents. Evid Based Ment Health 2005;8(1):10.

[10] Guyatt G, Sackett DL, Cook DJ. How to use an article about therapy or prevention. A. Are the results of the study valid? Evidence-Based Medicine Working Group. JAMA 1993;270:2598–601.

[11] Guyatt G, Sackett DL, Cook DJ. How to use an article about therapy or prevention. B. What are the results and will they help me in caring for my patients? Evidence-Based Medicine Working Group. JAMA 1994;271:59–63.

[12] Greenhalgh T. How to read a paper: assessing the methodological quality of published papers. BMJ 1997;315:305–8.

[13] March J, Silva S, Petrycki S, et al. Fluoxetine, cognitive-behavioral therapy, and their combination for adolescents with depression: Treatment for Adolescents with Depression Study (TADS) randomized controlled trial. JAMA 2004;292:807–20.

[14] Szatmari P. The art of evidence-based child psychiatry. Evid Based Ment Health 2003;6(4):99–100.

[15] Hamilton JD. Evidence-based thinking and the alliance with parents. J Am Acad Child Adolesc Psychiatry 2004;43:105–8.

[16] Szatmari P. Evidence-based child psychiatry and the two solitudes. Evid Based Ment Health 1999;2(6):7.

[17] Steiner JF. Talking about treatment: the language of populations and the language of individuals. Ann Intern Med 1999;130:618–22.

[18] Straus SE, McAlister FA. Evidence-based medicine: a commentary on common criticisms. CMAJ 2000;163(7):837–41.

[19] Whittington CJ, Kendall T, Fonagy P, et al. Selective serotonin reuptake inhibitors in childhood depression: systematic review of published versus unpublished data. Lancet 2004;363(9418):1341–5.

[20] Geddes J, Szatmari P, Streiner D. The worm turns: publication bias and trial registers revisited. Evid Based Ment Health 2004;7(4):98–9.

[21] Plato. Phaedo. New York: Liberal Arts Press; 1951 [Church FJ, Trans.].

[22] Kleinmann A. The illness narratives: suffering, healing and the human condition. New York: Basic Books; 1988.

ELSEVIER
SAUNDERS

Child Adolesc Psychiatric Clin N Am
15 (2006) 289–302

CHILD AND
ADOLESCENT
PSYCHIATRIC CLINICS
OF NORTH AMERICA

Target-Symptom Psychopharmacology: Between the Forest and the Trees

Jeff Q. Bostic, MD, EdD[a],*, Yanni Rho, MD, MPH[b]

[a]*Harvard Medical School, Massachusetts General Hospital, Yawkey 6926,
55 Fruit Street, Boston, MA 02114-3139, USA*
[b]*Harvard Medical School, Cambridge Hospital, Cambridge, MA, USA*

In all branches of medicine, physicians start with presenting symptoms. In most cases, clinicians weave together pieces of the patient's history, physical examination, and laboratory findings to determine a diagnosis and then prescribe the appropriate treatments. Sometimes the diagnosis is relatively precise, and sometimes so too is the treatment. For example, if someone presents with a painful ear and fever, and otoscopic findings reveal fluid behind the tympanic membrane, an antibiotic may be prescribed for several weeks to treat otitis media. If, however, someone presents with fever, malaise, muscle aches, headache, and chills, culminating in the diagnosis of influenza, clinicians usually target the treatable symptoms, because there are no current satisfactory treatments for the influenza-causing viruses. The current absence of medications that adequately treat the myriad viruses causing influenza does not make the illness any less real, however.

In psychiatry, clinicians face these same diagnostic and treatment quagmires. Current psychopharmacologic approaches remain limited. For all current psychiatric disorders, psychopharmacology ameliorates symptoms but does not yet seem to cure or eliminate the biologic causes underlying any psychiatric disorder. In patients with ADHD, stimulants effectively reduce the magnitude of symptoms, but cessation of the medication usually leads to a return of the

Dr. Bostic has received research funding, honoraria, consulting fees, and speaker bureau funding from Abbott, Forest, GlaxoSmithKline, Lilly, and Pfizer Pharmaceuticals.

* Corresponding author.
E-mail address: roboz@adelphia.net (J.Q. Bostic).

symptoms. Few practicing clinicians would hold that neuroleptics or mood stabilizers eliminate schizophrenia or bipolar disorder, although most would contend these agents benefit patients substantially by reducing symptom severity and possibly the frequency of incapacitating episodes. For the pervasive developmental disorders, curative aspirations for secretin were high, but true successes in treatment using this information proved low [1]. Anxiety disorders may improve with psychopharmacologic treatments including benzodiazepines, buspirone, and, more recently, anticonvulsants, but too few patients are cured solely by following a course of any of these agents. Most recently, recognition of pediatric bipolar disorder has advanced, but it seems to be less responsive to any of the psychopharmacologic treatments deemed effective for adults [2].

This lack of a curative response to existing pharmacologic treatments does not make these psychiatric disorders any less real. Anyone who has observed a patient in the throes of mania readily appreciates the grossly aberrant rapid speech, grandiose delusions, high-risk behaviors, flight of ideas, and lack of sleep that characterize this disorder. This classic presentation of mania may be the exception rather than the rule [3], however, and may lead to underdiagnosis and undertreatment of patients experiencing significantly impairing psychopathology [4]. The current limitation, however, is the chasm existing between psychopharmacologic interventions and the underlying mechanisms these medications significantly affect.

Finding the forest but missing the trees: categorical diagnoses versus functionally impairing symptoms

Rather than obliterate an identified disorder, current pharmacotherapy for all psychopathologies is relegated to chopping away at certain amenable target symptoms, despite seeming advances in diagnostic precision and the identification of "new" disorders. Indeed, the number of disorders listed in the *Diagnostic and Statistical Manual* (*DSM*) has increased from 106 in *DSM-I* to 297 in *DSM-IV* [5], with additional diagnoses (eg, sex addiction, Internet addiction) ever looming on the horizon. The proliferation of diagnostic category nosology, however, remains limited as a vehicle to illuminate pathophysiology. Some have suggested that categorical descriptions have proven more useful for insurance coding and reimbursement [6] and perhaps for pharmaceutical companies to expand indications and patent, not patient, life.

The categorical diagnosis approach seems to be limited for multiple reasons. First, efforts to group the symptoms that truly describe a particular disorder and distinguish it from all others are far from perfect. Categorization schemes are ultimately heuristic efforts that it is hoped will correspond to relevant biologic processes, be it in brain regions or neurochemical anomalies. These categorizations help clinicians take one treatment road as opposed to another, because such categorizations suggest a patient suffers more from one general constellation of symptoms. For example, a patient may suffer more from depression than from mania, which would lead clinicians to choose very different classes of medications as a primary treatment (antidepressants versus mood stabilizers). Such categorizations, however, may not illuminate which symptoms within the disorder are the ones most likely to reveal the biologic underpinning for the etiological culprit to be targeted.

Second, the notion that one either has or does not have a disorder, based on having five of nine symptom criteria, although attractive to clinicians, is inadequate for the successful treatment of all patients. The *DSM-III* and subsequent versions have provided more attention to behaviors or observed signs than to inferred and nonobservable symptoms used in years past to yield psychiatric diagnoses. The *DSM* has helped psychiatry progress by focusing on symptoms that independent clinicians can observe.

Third, patients rarely present with distinct categorical entities. Patients rarely seem to have symptoms exclusively of one psychiatric disorder. More often than not, those with significant symptoms in one category have significant symptoms in other categories as well [7].

Fourth, developmental expression of certain disorders may further impede the application of current diagnostic categories in younger populations. Whereas otitis media and its treatment seem similar across the lifespan, psychiatric disorders seem to manifest differently at different life stages. Ultimately, psychiatric disorders may respond differently to psychopharmacologic treatments. Merinkangas and Avenevoli [8] suggested that anxiety and depression may in fact be part of a developmental sequence in which anxiety is expressed earlier in life than depression, diminishing the distance between these categories. Broader definitions have been proposed for eating disorders to take into account developmental changes that may mask criteria met for eating disorders in juvenile populations, and changes in defining alcohol abuse have similarly been proposed [9,10]. Therefore, across multiple disorders, symptom targets may change as the development of the individual, as well as of the disorder, changes over time. Sevin and colleagues [11] focused on diagnostic agreement in children dually diagnosed with developmental disabilities and other psychiatric diagnoses. In their study, patients had symptoms shifting diagnoses over a 10-year interval between conduct disorder, posttraumatic stress disorder, attention-deficit hyperactivity disorder (ADHD), mood disorder, psychotic disorders, and impulse-control disorders. The disagreements in diagnoses could result from clinician error but could also represent some change or evolution in symptom presentation with age.

At present, psychiatric illness is described mostly as disorders, or clusters of symptoms, rather than as diseases with a known cause. At issue is how much to embrace these categorical distinctions (for example, social phobia versus generalized anxiety disorder) in selecting psychopharmacologic treatment. Inadequate evidence exists to prove that the current psychopharmacologic treatment of social anxiety disorder is fundamentally or practically different from that of generalized anxiety. Indeed, current psychopharmacologic agents are widely used across these expanding categories of disorders, with selective serotonin reuptake inhibiting (SSRI) antidepressants prescribed as first-line treatment for patients with generalized anxiety disorder, obsessive-compulsive disorder, posttraumatic stress disorder, social anxiety disorder, separation anxiety disorder, and even selective mutism. Similarly, neuroleptics are used to treat juvenile psychosis. Seemingly dissimilar disease process states such as conduct disorder, pervasive developmental disorders (PDD), tic disorders, and bipolar disorder also use antipsychotic medications for treatment. Perhaps someday science will elucidate commonly shared genetic, neuroanatomic, and metabolic components among diverse disorders. At present, psychopharmacologic treatments are geared mostly toward treating a few symptoms of their respective disorders.

Most psychopharmacologic treatments have varied in their effectiveness across the lifespan. Most recently, antidepressants have been scrutinized. Admittedly, the collection of controlled trials of antidepressants for child and adolescent depression thus far has been unimpressive [12]. It remains unclear whether these trials failed because the diagnostic criteria (and rating scales) fail to capture juvenile depression adequately, raising questions whether categorization schemes describe younger populations adequately, or because the agents simply may not work as well in younger populations.

One alternative to the predicament of binary "have it or not" categorical diagnoses is to conceptualize symptoms as existing on a continuum. This conceptualization commonly occurs now with rating scales that measure symptoms as absent, mild, moderate, or severe. A dimensional, or spectrum, approach may help quantify symptom severity and therefore may capture some cases of psychopathology, particularly those that fall between the cracks of the existing categorical divisions [13]. Ghaemi [6] has described how personality disorders, for example, may be understood better on dimensional rather than categorical grounds. McHugh and Slavney [14] point out that, just as individuals differ in cognitive character, varying in smooth gradations from dull to bright, individuals also vary in their proneness to certain emotions, moods, and drives. One thus would expect most humans to have varying degrees of anxiety, depression, inattention, impulsivity, social fear, and other symptoms. Dimensional understanding encourages shifting the focus from the quantity of symptoms present to the quality or magnitude of the resultant impairment on that individual. Hyman [15] has recently suggested that depression should be considered on a continuum, much like cholesterol levels, and van Os [16] similarly has suggested that even psychotic symptoms exist on a continuum within the general population. Similarly, many psychiatric symptoms probably exist along a spectrum. The most severe presentations of these symptoms will ultimately impair some individuals, sometimes across all domains of functioning. More commonly, symptoms impair many persons only occasionally, for example, when situations stress a person's coping capabilities. The impacts of stress on brain architecture and functioning reveal biologic changes associated with these symptoms; an understanding of these changes may, ultimately, clarify targets for intervention

[17]. Patients probably vary as to where they fit on the anxiety spectrum, the depression spectrum, or even the reality-testing spectrum [18]. Increased attention given to where patients fall on multiple dimensions and the severity of symptoms on these spectra might allow treatment directed at the most impairing symptoms, across various diagnostic categories, for a particular individual.

The lack of understanding of specific biologic anomalies that sufficiently explain psychiatric disorders, the lack of clear biologic distinctions between disorders, the likely difference among illness manifestations across the lifespan, and the recognition that patients often have prominent symptoms differing in severity on several dimensions (such as anxiety, depression, attention, communication, and affect regulation) all suggest that prescribing medications based on diagnosing disorders will, for the short term, remain inadequate and ineffective. The stakes, however, are high. The current SSRI controversy illustrates how medication trials devised to measure psychopharmacologic treatments of a particular disorder, in which criteria are extrapolated from adults, can go awry and compromise treatment options that most clinicians believe can be useful for some symptoms but not for the entire symptom complex of the disorder. Attention to medication effects on component target symptoms may improve the choice of agents given an individual's constellation of symptoms. Coupling target-symptom response with particular agents might ultimately lead to a more specific understanding of pathophysiology as well.

Does it matter if a tree falls in the forest and no one hears it? Ignoring symptoms that are not consistent with a disorder

The limitations inherent in the prevailing categorization scheme probably influence current clinical decision making about selections of psychopharmacologic treatments. Two essential tasks are required by the clinician: (1) observing and further examining a wide variety of symptoms that may span many diagnostic categories, and (2) clarifying which of these symptoms have greatest impact on the particular patient. Attention to the patient's constellation of symptoms, even if they cut across disorders, and consideration of which symptoms existing medications affect may reveal better which medications would most benefit that patient. For example, instead of treating ADHD in a particular patient who seems to be most impaired by inattention but has accompanying anxiety when going to play after school and occasional temper outbursts, the treatment might focus on these specific symptoms. Focusing on the symptoms that most impact the patient and addressing those symptoms with medications and other types of therapies most likely to benefit them may provide more realistic expectations for medication treatment.

Ghaemi [6] has suggested a pluralistic approach in psychiatry, employing specific components of different treatment modalities matched with the patient's specific disorder states. Unlike the current eclectic approach, in which both psychotherapy and medication are summarily recommended for essentially all disorders, pluralism suggests a more sophisticated approach of identifying and implementing those particular treatment components (eg, specific psycho-therapeutic techniques such as empathy in depression but counterprojection for paranoia) as well as specific medications relevant to each disorder. Attention to which components of psychotherapy and psychopharmacology impact psycho-pathology ultimately should provide greater precision in treating the patient's unique symptom constellation.

Too many trees? Do disparate symptoms confuse treatment direction?

The identification and treatment of target symptoms has been proposed by a number of researchers in the treatment of a variety of disorders, including per-sonality disorders, conduct and oppositional defiant disorders, dementia and delirium, and PDD. For example, Ryden and Vinnars [19] and Dose [20] have proposed that target symptoms should be identified in personality disorders and treated accordingly. Dose [20] further suggested that underlying common neuro-chemical dysfunctions may exist in both axis I and axis II disorders. Therefore, the use of medications that typically have been specified for axis I disorders, such as anxiety, depression, mania, and schizophrenia, to treat the symptoms present in axis II disorders has been common practice that some patients and clinicians have found helpful.

Target-symptom approaches have been used perhaps most commonly among patients with PDD [21]. PDD often includes profound impairments warrant-ing aggressive clinical efforts. At times, parental or societal pressures may fuel desperate attempts by clinicians to try non–evidence-based "cures" or treat-ments that might alter the trajectory of an otherwise debilitating condition. Myhr [22] found a dimensional as opposed to categorical approach was useful when evaluating cases of PDD. Because thus far the *DSM-IV* distinctions have afforded little pharmacotherapy treatment precision, Myhr focused on treating irrita-bility, aggression, impulsivity, and sadness. Identifying symptoms and cou-pling them to medications likely to improve specific symptoms might provide pharmacologically responsive targets when pharmacotherapy is considered for these patients.

A wide variety of classes of medications have been used in the treatment of PDD to address the target symptoms of hyperactivity, temper tantrums, irritability, withdrawal, stereotypies, aggressiveness, self-injurious behavior, depression, and obsessive-compulsive behaviors [23]. Stimulants have been used for attentional difficulties, antidepressants and other serotonergic medications have been used for obsessional thoughts and repetitive behaviors, and a variety of medications including neuroleptics, anticonvulsants, and mood stabilizers have been used to address the aggression seen in autism [23,24]. The decisions to use these medications for PDD were based on accepted treatments for ADHD and obsessive and compulsive disorder; although often diagnostic criteria were not met, the potential benefits of these medications warrant their implementation. The recognition that many disorders share overlapping features further argues for consideration of symptoms across diagnostic categories and regardless of whether criteria for a disorder are satisfied.

Treatment of overlapping symptoms across disorders may simplify treatment when dealing with comorbid illnesses and when thinking about treatment in consumer-based terms. Arnold and colleagues [25] employed a "parent-defined target-symptom" to assess the efficacy of risperidone in the treatment of autism. Target symptoms were classified into seven categories: aggression to others, self-injurious behavior, property destruction, tantrums, yelling/screaming, stereotypy, and hyperactivity/impulsivity/agitation. What parents considered the most concerning symptoms became the target focus, and these target symptoms were detailed. For example, tantrums became described as "twice a day, lasting 10–25 minutes each, throwing self on floor, flailing arms, breaking furniture, hurting another child if in the way," and other. The Aberrant Behavior Checklist and the Clinical Global Impression of Improvement were administered to check collinearity of target-symptom ratings. Inter-rater reliability was high (0.9), even as these "parent-created" symptoms changed with treatment. Significant decreases in aggression, hyperactivity, tantrums, self-injury, stereotypy, and property destruction were detected after treatment, in this case, with risperidone.

Ultimately, two circumstances favor a target-symptom approach:

1. The more poorly a disorder is defined (that is, multiple phenotypes are present), and the more poorly the underlying etiology is understood, the more beneficial target-symptom approaches will be.
2. The more poorly a psychopharmacologic medication is understood, and the less its mechanism of action directly corresponds to the underlying disorder, the more beneficial a target-symptom approach will be.

Walking into the forest: components of a target-symptom psychopharmacology evaluation

What types of considerations should be included when using the target-symptom approach? First, diagnostic evaluations could be modified to include comprehensive evaluation of a wide variety of symptoms. Recruiting technological means such as questionnaires to assist in this effort will be helpful, given the ordinary clinician's time constraints in diagnostic situations. A paper or computer-administered instrument that covers multiple categories of symptoms will probably become an integral part of the electronic medical record as well as the basis for treatment planning. Appropriate instruments may be useful in clarifying and monitoring which symptoms are medication-responsive. Some measures focused on target symptoms are now available, such as the multi-informant, 13-item Target Symptom Rating Scale [26], which includes questions regarding family conflict, peer relationship problems, depression, anxiety, school difficulties, self-destructive behaviors, aggression, psychotic symptoms, substance problems, and impulsivity.

Currently, many instruments are available that amplify symptoms of ADHD, obsessive-compulsive disorder, depression, anxiety, mania, and other conditions, and most of these have been adapted for children. These instruments can probably provide a step along the way toward understanding certain significant symptoms (and similarly revealing some symptoms that may prove irrelevant or secondary). These instruments remain limited in determining recovery from a disorder (eg, Child Depression Rating Scale Score <10). With electronic access of these scales allowing immediate retrieval, these scales, or even specific items within them, may find their way into regular clinical practice. For example, approximately 90 different rating tools are described online at http://www.schoolpsychiatry.org.

Second, a target-symptom evaluation process need not restrict or exclude decisions about which diagnoses might be relevant. Clinical knowledge and supplementary tests can help focus on which disorders may be clinically relevant and further facilitate prioritizing which symptoms require most aggressive intervention. Thorough evaluation, wider than identifying a primary diagnosis, ascribes more attention to subthreshold or atypical symptoms [27] that may cause distress. In regular office practice, health economic factors have favored rapid identification of a disorder, with sometimes discouraging results for both patients and clinicians. Treatment can become relegated to prescription of a medication for the first diagnosis identified, particularly when more subtle, less conspicuous symptoms (such as obsessions) lurk beneath what is readily observable during a time-limited encounter.

Third, multiple sources of information may clarify prominent symptoms and, more importantly, indicate which symptoms most impact a child's functioning at school, with peers, and at home. Because many children and adolescents may have communication difficulties or simply may not have sufficient vocabulary or understanding to articulate their distress and symptoms accurately, inclusion of parent and teacher reports can help determine the full clinical picture for these children [28]. Psychopharmacologic evaluations may move toward tailoring treatment for the individual patient, rather than for the suspected identified disorder.

Taking down trees with current tools: symptom targets for common psychotropic agents

Certain symptoms are found across a variety of psychiatric disorders. Such symptoms include sadness, irritability, worthlessness, fatigue, anhedonia, insomnia, low energy, decreased concentration, and mood lability. Fortunately, research has been conducted to determine which psychotropic agents are effective in treating certain symptoms. For example, many of the SSRIs are effective in treating the symptom of sadness. As described elsewhere in this issue, emerging evidence now suggests that fluvoxamine may have greater benefit for pediatric anxiety symptoms than for pediatric depression symptoms. Mediating or promoting variables now being examined will probably increase precision in determining which symptoms are responsive to which medications, although pharmacogenetic approaches hold the highest promise.

What happens when the tree falls? Risk–benefit assessment of target-specific treatment

Medical decision making ordinarily involves the observation and collection of information (the art of medicine); coalescing this information to best determine syndromes, diseases, and treatments (the science of medicine); and, finally, making decisions with the patient, factoring in cultural, economic, interpersonal, religious, and ethical variables that influence patient participation or adherence (the ethics of medicine) [29]. This last component has become more notable recently, following the controversy surrounding the SSRIs, their use in the treatment of juvenile depression, and their putative link to suicidality. A small increased risk of suicidal comments and behaviors in juveniles was reported after review of the controlled trials. Many clinicians felt betrayed by pharmaceutical companies that had not provided access to all studies, including those that failed, in juvenile populations. Many patients felt betrayed by clinicians, who had not provided all the evidence for a treatment. This rift has accentuated the importance of clinicians partnering with patients in making decisions, further emphasizing the need to treat the individual rather than the disorder. In particular, psychopharmacology treatments often require months of treatment, requiring even greater consideration of how an agent will daily affect each patient's quality of life. As McHugh and Slavney [14] emphasize, all medications are toxic at some level and cannot be offered free of any injurious features. At a minimum, attention to and discussion of the wider effects of any medication on each patient's daily life, through more vigilant clinician monitoring of untoward effects, is vital. Although clinicians have always assessed for side effects, more formal efforts will probably emerge from clinicians as well as researchers to ensure that an individual's treatment includes specific consideration for the individual-specific side-effect profile.

Fig. 1 shows a sample side effect scale for patients or families to complete. This scale was modeled after the comprehensive Safety Monitoring Uniform Report Form (SMURF) now to be employed in publicly funded research settings. Administration of the SMURF requires approximately 25 minutes in research settings and therefore may not be feasible in regular clinical settings [30]. A simplified but comprehensive side-effect scale, which parents and teachers may

Patient Name:_____ **Date:**_____

EVALUATION OF MEDICATION SIDE EFFECTS

Please *CIRCLE* any side effects you have noticed in your child since the medication was started. The list is to help you think of side effects. These side effects may not be related to the medication, so please contact your clinician before changing or stopping the medication. Be prepared to discuss with your clinician when the side effect **started** (and stopped, if it has), if any **other illnesses** were occurring at that time, and **all other medications** your child was taking at this time.

VISUAL: Blurriness   Irritation or Redness   Watering   Dryness
Double Vision   Eye Pain   Eye Twitching   Light Bothering Eyes

HEARING: Ear Ache   Ear Infection   Poor Hearing   Ringing in the Ears

HEAD: Headache   Facial Pain   Face Muscle Weakness

NOSE: Nose bleeds   Nose Dryness   Sinus Congestion   Change in Smell

THROAT: Sore Throat   Hoarse Voice/Laryngitis   Difficulty Swallowing

MOUTH/LIPS: Mouth Ulcer/Sores   Gum Problems   Dental Problems   Sore/Swollen Tongue
Dry Mouth   Too Much Saliva   Drooling   Bad Taste in Mouth

CHEST: Pain   Tightness   Shortness of Breath   Wheezing   Coughing

BREAST: Swelling   Pain   Discharge

HEART: Rapid Heartbeat   Irregular Heartbeat   Slow Heartbeat

STOMACH: Pain/Discomfort   Heartburn/Reflux   Nausea   Vomiting

BOWELS: Diarrhea   Constipation   Blood in Stool   Bloated/Gassy
Stool Discoloration   Hemorrhoids

APPETITE: Increase   Decrease   Weight Gain (____lbs)   Weight Loss (____ lbs)
Taste Abnormality   Increased Thirst

URINATION: Painful   Difficulty   Increased   Change in Color/Smell
Bedtime Wetting   Daytime Wetting

MENSTRUAL: Irregular Periods   Cramping   Increased Bleeding   Breakthrough Bleeding
Midcycle Pain   Premenstrual Tension or Mood Changes

Fig. 1. Sample side-effect scale.

GENITAL: Genital Discomfort/Swelling   Discharge   Increased Urges/Interest in Sex
Decreased Urges/Interest in Sex   Sexual Dysfunction

MUSCLES, BONES, JOINTS: Pain   Swelling/Fluid Buildup   Cramps/Contractions
Numbness   Tingling   Restless Legs

MOVEMENT: Clumsiness/Poor Coordination Tics (twitches, blinking, making sounds)
Restlessness   Tremor, Trembling, or Shaking   Rigidity, Aches, Cramps

SKIN/HAIR: Rashes/Irritation   Pimples/Acne   Hives   Blisters   Dry Skin
Flaking Scalp   Sensitive to Sun   Oily skin/hair   Excessive Sweating
Change in Body Odor   Hair Problems (loss, brittle)   Easy Bruising

ENERGY: Tiredness/Fatigue   Sedation/Drugged Feeling   Withdrawn   Staring
Excessive Yawning   Overly Excited/Energetic   Too Keyed Up/Unable to Settle Down

SLEEP: Difficulty Falling Asleep   Interrupted Sleep   Early Morning Awakening
Sleeping Too Much   Awakening Not Feeling Rested   Drowsiness   Nightmares

STRANGE EXPERIENCES/THOUGHTS: Seeing Things That Are Not There
Hearing Things That Are Not There   Smelling/Tasing Things That Are Not There
Strange Physical Feelings   Strange Thoughts or Ideas

THINKING: Memory Problems   Concentration Difficulty   Confusion   Slowed Thinking
Speech Difficulty/Changes   Dizziness/Faintness   Loss of Consciousness

MOOD CHANGES: Depressed   Anxious/Nervous   Loss of Interest/Motivation
Irritable   "Manicky"

ACCIDENT/INJURY: Accidental Injury (describe):_____
Attempted Suicide   Self-Harmful Behavior (cutting on self, banging head, etc.)

ILLNESS: Upper Respiratory Infection   Lower Respiratory Infection   Gastrointestinal Virus
Bacterial Infection   Urinary Tract Infection   (Other) Fever   Allergies/Asthma
Swollen Glands   Feeling Flushed or Warm   Feeling Cold or Chills

Medical or Surgical Procedure (describe:)_____

Medicine(s) Added (names of): _____

ANY OTHER SIDE EFFECTS (Please Describe):_____

_____

Fig. 1 (*continued*).

complete, may provide a more expedient, comprehensive, clinic-friendly alternative. Like symptoms, side effects and their magnitude of impairment for an individual exist along a continuum. Treatment adherence will probably be facilitated by thorough attention to the various side effects and their impacts on the daily functioning of individual patients.

Forest preservation: problems and limitations with target-symptom treatment

Target-symptom treatment is a way station until underlying causes can be identified that afford more specific psychopharmacologic treatments. Until symptoms or disorders are comprehensively explained so that specific treatments can be matched to pathophysiologies, pharmacotherapy will remain ameliorative instead of curative. Moreover, target-symptom approaches remain reactive to symptoms once they have become problematic, rather than protective against the development or manifestation of psychopathology. Additionally, target-symptom approaches could foster irrational polypharmacy, particularly for conditions such as panic disorder. No one would suggest that the hyperventilation, palpitations, feelings of de-realization, nausea, and others should be treated separately with medications specific for each of these symptoms. In addition, a target-symptom approach may prove distressing to some patients. To have not a diagnosis but rather a set of target symptoms may overwhelm patients and their families searching for a parsimonious explanation for aberrant behaviors and functional impairment. Indeed, a disorder, even if only created by a *DSM* committee, may still exonerate and even unite patients and family members against a "chemical imbalance" enemy. The target-symptom approach is further hindered by a current tradition of psychotropic evaluation centering on treatment of disorders rather than specific symptoms. Patients may reject treatments that have not been "tested" for specific symptoms or simply may not invest in treatments if evidence cannot be provided that the particular target symptom does respond to a particular treatment.

Among the most concerning impacts of a target-symptom approach is that it might distract efforts to isolate the symptom constellation characteristic of a disease. Such an effort could obscure attention to identifying and correcting the organic pathophysiology or mechanism that underlies a disease. A target-symptom approach potentially could create the appearance of so many phenotypes that determination of appropriate interventions could become more difficult and once again slow progress toward elucidation of the underlying mechanism.

Balancing the clinical improvement of individual patients while working toward a better understanding of symptom presentations and their suggested underlying etiologic culprits remains vital. In addition, research efforts to determine which scales and measures best elicit target symptoms remains another crucial goal. Further research should also look specifically at target-symptom approaches in evaluating patient outcomes and clinical improvement as well as overall patient functioning as determined by patients, families, and school staff.

Protecting the forest and the trees within: summary

Diagnostic categories can go only so far in illuminating focused treatments for specific symptoms, particularly for patients experiencing symptoms crossing diagnostic categories. A psychopharmacologic treatment strategy focused on individuals and their specific symptom constellations, beyond disorders per se, may enhance medication selections for individual patients. Clinicians can examine specific symptoms impacting a particular patient and prioritize those symptoms that cause most impairment while considering which symptoms are most likely to respond to specific psychopharmacologic treatments. At the same time, risks of any treatment, particularly pharmacologic risks, can be more systematically determined and monitored to minimize negative impacts on each patient. A medical record that captures impairing symptoms, prioritizes them, configures in thorough assessment of side effects, and monitors response to these treatments will better match unique patients with optimal treatments.

References

[1] King BH, Bostic JQ. Psychopharmacology of autistic spectrum disorders: an update. Child Adolesc Psychiatr Clin N Am, in press.

[2] Kowatch RA, DelBello MP. Pharmacotherapy of children and adolescents with bipolar disorder. Psychiatr Clin North Am 2005;28(2):385–97.

[3] Akiskal HS. The prevalent clinical spectrum of bipolar disorders: beyond DSM-IV. J Clin Psychopharmacol 1996;16(2 Suppl 1):4S–14S.

[4] Cassano GB, Dell'Osso L, Frank E, et al. The bipolar spectrum: a clinical reality in search of diagnostic criteria and an assessment methodology. J Affect Disord 1999;54(3):319–28.

[5] Van Praag H. Reconquest of the subjective: against the waning of psychaitric diagnosing. Br J Psychiatry 1992;160:266–71.

[6] Ghaemi SN. The concepts of psychiatry: a pluralistic approach to the mind and mental illness. Baltimore (MD): Johns Hopkins University Press; 2003.

[7] Stefanis NC, Hanssen M, Smirnis NK, et al. Evidence that three dimensions of psychosis have a distribution in the general population. Psychol Med 2002;32(2):347–58.

[8] Merikangas KR, Avenevoli S. Epidemiology of mood and anxiety disorders in children and adolescents. In: Tsuang MT, Tohen M, editors. Textbook in psychiatric epidemiology. Hoboken (NJ): Wiley-Liss; 2002. p. 674–704.

[9] Lewinsohn PM, Striegel-Moore RH, Seeley JR. Epidemiology and natural course of eating disorders in young women from adolescence to young adulthood. J Am Acad Child Adolesc Psychiatry 2000;39(10):1284–92.

[10] Clark DB. The natural history of adolescent alcohol use disorders. Addiction 2004;99(Suppl 2): 5–22.

[11] Sevin JA, Bowers-Stephens C, Crafton CG. Psychiatric disorders in adolescents with developmental disabilities: longitudinal data on diagnostic disagreement in 150 clients. Child Psychiatry Hum Dev 2003;34(2):147–63.

[12] Bostic JQ, Rubin DH, Prince J, et al. Treatment of depression in children and adolescents. J Psychiatr Pract 2005;11(2):141–54.

[13] Kraemer HC, Noda A, O'Hara R. Categorical versus dimensional approaches to diagnosis: methodological challenges. J Psychiatr Res 2003;38:17–25.

[14] McHugh PR, Slavney PR. The perspectives of psychiatry. 2nd edition. Baltimore (MD): Johns Hopkins University Press; 1998.

[15] Garbarini N. Working better on drugs. Scientific American Mind 2005;14:8.

[16] van Os J, Hanssen M, Bijl RV, et al. Strauss (1969) revisited: a psychosis continuum in the general population? Schizophr Res 2000;45(1–2):11–20.

[17] Karten YJGOA, Cameron HA. Stress in early life inhibits neurogenesis in adulthood. Trends Neurosci 2005;28(4):171–2.

[18] Krabbendam L, Myin-Germeys I, De Graaf R, et al. Dimensions of depression, mania and psychosis in the general population. Psychol Med 2004;34(7):1177–86.

[19] Ryden G, Vinnars B. [Pharmacological treatment of borderline personality disorders. Several options for symptom reduction but nothing for the disorder per se]. Lakartidningen 2002; 99(50):5088–94 [in Swedish].

[20] Dose M. Psychopharmalogical treatment of personality disorders-risks and chances. Psychiatr Danub 1999;11(3–4):131–9.

[21] Hollander E, Phillips AT, Yeh CC. Targeted treatments for symptom domains in child and adolescent autism. Lancet 2003;362(9385):732–4.

[22] Myhr G. Autism and other pervasive developmental disorders: exploring the dimensional view. Can J Psychiatry 1998;43(6):589–95.

[23] Campbell M, Schopler E, Cueva JE, et al. Treatment of autistic disorder. J Am Acad Child Adolesc Psychiatry 1996;35(2):134–43.

[24] Posey DJ, McDougle CJ. The pharmacotherapy of target symptoms associated with autistic disorder and other pervasive developmental disorders. Harv Rev Psychiatry 2000;8(2):45–63.

[25] Arnold LE, Vitiello B, McDougle C, et al. Parent-defined target symptoms respond to risperidone in RUPP autism study: customer approach to clinical trials. J Am Acad Child Adolesc Psychiatry 2003;42(12):1443–50.

[26] Barber CC, Neese DT, Coyne L, et al. The Target Symptom Rating: a brief clinical measure of acute psychiatric symptoms in children and adolescents. J Clin Child Adolesc Psychol 2002;31(2):181–92.

[27] Rucci P, Maser JD. Instrument development in the Italy-USA Collaborative Spectrum Project. Epidemiol Psichiatr Soc 2000;9(4):249–56.

[28] Arnold LE, Aman MG, Martin A, et al. Assessment in multisite randomized clinical trials of patients with autistic disorder: the Autism RUPP Network. Research Units on Pediatric Psychopharmacology. J Autism Dev Disord 2000;30(2):99–111.

[29] Pellegrino ED, Thomasma DC. A philosophical basis of medical practice. New York: Oxford University Press; 1981.

[30] Greenhill LL, Vitiello B, Fisher P, et al. Comparison of increasingly detailed elicitation methods for the assessment of adverse events in pediatric psychopharmacology. J Am Acad Child Adolesc Psychiatry 2004;43(12):1488–96.

ELSEVIER
SAUNDERS

Child Adolesc Psychiatric Clin N Am
15 (2006) 303–310

CHILD AND
ADOLESCENT
PSYCHIATRIC CLINICS
OF NORTH AMERICA

Index

Note: Page numbers of article titles are in **boldface** type.

Changing Your Address?

Make sure your subscription changes too! When you notify us of your new address, you can help make our job easier by including an exact copy of your Clinics label number with your old address (see illustration below.) This number identifies you to our computer system and will speed the processing of your address change. Please be sure this label number accompanies your old address and your corrected address—you can send an old Clinics label with your number on it or just copy it exactly and send it to the address listed below.

We appreciate your help in our attempt to give you continuous coverage. Thank you.

W. B. Saunders Company	
SHIPPING AND RECEIVING DEPTS.	SECOND CLASS POSTAGE
151 BENIGNO BLVD.	PAID AT BELLMAWR, N.J.
BELLMAWR, N.J. 08031	

This is your copy of the
_____ **CLINICS OF NORTH AMERICA**

00503570 DOE—J32400   101   NH   8102

JOHN C DOE MD
324 SAMSON ST
BERLIN   NH   03570

XP-D11494

JAN ISSUE

Your Clinics Label Number

Copy it exactly or send your label along with your address to:
W.B. Saunders Company, Customer Service
Orlando, FL 32887-4800
Call Toll Free 1-800-654-2452

Please allow four to six weeks for delivery of new subscriptions and for processing address changes.